Enteroscopy

Guest Editor

DAVID R. CAVE, MD, PhD

GASTROINTESTINAL ENDOSCOPY CLINICS OF NORTH AMERICA

www.giendo.theclinics.com

Consulting Editor
CHARLES J. LIGHTDALE, MD

July 2009 • Volume 19 • Number 3

SAUNDERS an imprint of ELSEVIER, Inc.

W.B. SAUNDERS COMPANY
A Division of Elsevier Inc.

1600 John F. Kennedy Blvd. • Suite 1800 • Philadelphia, Pennsylvania 19103-2899

http://www.giendo.theclinics.com

GASTROINTESTINAL ENDOSCOPY CLINICS OF NORTH AMERICA Volume 19, Number 3
July 2009 ISSN 1052-5157, ISBN-13: 978-1-4377-1221-6, ISBN-10: 1-4377-1221-5

Editor: Kerry Holland

© **2009 Elsevier ■ All rights reserved.**

This journal and the individual contributions contained in it are protected under copyright by Elsevier, and the following terms and conditions apply to their use:

Photocopying
Single photocopies of single articles may be made for personal use as allowed by national copyright laws. Permission of the Publisher and payment of a fee is required for all other photocopying, including multiple or systematic copying, copying for advertising or promotional purposes, resale, and all forms of document delivery. Special rates are available for educational institutions that wish to make photocopies for non-profit educational classroom use. For information on how to seek permission visit www.elsevier.com/permissions or call: (+44) 1865 843830 (UK)/(+1) 215 239 3804 (USA).

Derivative Works
Subscribers may reproduce tables of contents or prepare lists of articles including abstracts for internal circulation within their institutions. Permission of the Publisher is required for resale or distribution outside the institution. Permission of the Publisher is required for all other derivative works, including compilations and translations (please consult www.elsevier.com/permissions).

Electronic Storage or Usage
Permission of the Publisher is required to store or use electronically any material contained in this journal, including any article or part of an article (please consult www.elsevier.com/permissions). Except as outlined above, no part of this publication may be reproduced, stored in a retrieval system or transmitted in any form or by any means, electronic, mechanical, photocopying, recording or otherwise, without prior written permission of the Publisher.

Notice
No responsibility is assumed by the Publisher for any injury and/or damage to persons or property as a matter of products liability, negligence or otherwise, or from any use or operation of any methods, products, instructions or ideas contained in the material herein. Because of rapid advances in the medical sciences, in particular, independent verification of diagnoses and drug dosages should be made.

Although all advertising material is expected to conform to ethical (medical) standards, inclusion in this publication does not constitute a guarantee or endorsement of the quality or value of such product or of the claims made of it by its manufacturer.

Gastrointestinal Endoscopy Clinics of North America (ISSN 1052-5157) is published quarterly by Elsevier Inc., 360 Park Avenue South, New York, NY 10010-1710. Months of issue are January, April, July, and October. Business and Editorial Offices: 1600 John F. Kennedy Blvd., Suite 1800, Philadelphia, PA, 19103-2899. Customer Service Office: 6277 Sea Harbor Drive, Orlando, FL 32887-4800. Periodicals postage paid at New York, NY and additional mailing offices. Subscription prices are $259.00 per year of US individuals $386.00 per year for US institutions, $133.00 per year for US students and residents, $286.00 per year for Canadian individuals, $471.00 per year for Canadian institutions, $362.00 per year for international individuals, $471.00 per year for international institutions, and $185.00 per year for Canadian and foreign students/residents. To receive student/resident rate, orders must be accompanied by name of affiliated institution, date of term, and the *signature* of program/residency coordinator on institution letterhead. Orders will be billed at individual rate until proof of status is received. Foreign air speed delivery is included in all *Clinics* subscription prices. All prices are subject to change without notice. **POSTMASTER:** Send address change to *Gastrointestinal Endoscopy Clinics of North America*, Elsevier Periodicals Customer Service, 11830 Westline Industrial Drive, St. Louis, MO 63146. **Customer Service: 1-800-654-2452 (US). From outside the United States, call 1-314-453-7041. Fax: 1-314-453-5170. E-mail: JournalsCustomerService-usa@elsevier.com (for print support) or JournalsOnlineSupport-usa@elsevier.com (for online support).**

Reprints. For copies of 100 or more, of articles in this publication, please contact the Commercial Reprints Department, Elsevier Inc., 360 Park Avenue South, New York, NY 10010-1710. Tel. (212) 633-3812; Fax: (212) 482-1935; E-mail: reprints@elsevier.com.

Gastrointestinal Endoscopy Clinics of North America is covered in *Excerpta Medica, MEDLINE/PubMed (Index Medicus), and MEDLINE/MEDLARS.*

Printed and bound by CPI Group (UK) Ltd, Croydon, CR0 4YY

Transferred to Digital Print 2011

Contributors

CONSULTING EDITOR

CHARLES J. LIGHTDALE, MD
Professor, Department of Medicine, Columbia University Medical Center, New York

GUEST EDITOR

DAVID R. CAVE, MD, PhD
Professor, Department of Medicine, University of Massachusetts Medical School, Worcester, Massachusetts

AUTHORS

PAUL A. AKERMAN, MD
Clinical Assistant Professor, Brown University; and University Gastroenterology, Providence, Rhode Island

DANIEL CANTERO, MD
Chief, Endoscopy, National Hospital of Paraguay, Asuncion, Paraguay

MICHEL DELVAUX, MD, PhD
Department of Internal Medicine and Digestive Pathology, Hôpitaux de Brabois, Vandoeuvre les Nancy, France

ROBERTO DE FRANCHIS, MD
Department of Medical Sciences, Head, Gastroenterology 3 Unit, University of Milan, IRCCS Policlinico, Mangiagalli, Regina Elena Foundation, Milan, Italy

CHRISTIAN ELL, MD, PhD
Department of Internal Medicine II, Dr. Horst Schmidt Klinik Medical School of the University of Mainz, Wiesbaden, Germany

GÉRARD GAY, MD
Department of Internal Medicine and Digestive Pathology, Hôpitaux de Brabois, Vandoeuvre les Nancy, France

LAUREN B. GERSON, MD, MSc
Associate Professor of Medicine, Division of Gastroenterology & Hepatology, Stanford University School of Medicine, Stanford, California

JONATHAN A. LEIGHTON, MD
Professor of Medicine, Division of Gastroenterology and Hepatology, Department of Internal Medicine, Mayo Clinic, Scottsdale, Arizona

BLAIR S. LEWIS, MD
Clinical Professor of Medicine, Department of Gastroenterology, Columbia University School of Medicine, New York, New York

SIMON K. LO, MD
Director of Endoscopy, Division of Digestive Diseases, Clinical Professor, Department of Medicine, Cedars-Sinai Medical Center, David Geffen School of Medicine at UCLA, Los Angeles, California

ANDREA MAY, MD, PhD
Department of Internal Medicine II, HSK Wiesbaden, Teaching Hospital-Johannes Gutenberg University, Wiesbaden, Germany

SHABANA F. PASHA, MD
Assistant Professor of Medicine, Division of Gastroenterology and Hepatology, Department of Internal Medicine, Mayo Clinic, Scottsdale, Arizona

SHIRLEY C. PASKI, MSc, MD
Section of Gastroenterology, Department of Internal Medicine, University of Chicago Medical Center, Chicago, Illinois

MARCO PENNAZIO, MD
Head, Small Bowel Disease Section, 2nd Division of Gastroenterology, Department of Medicine, San Giovanni Battista University Teaching Hospital, Turin, Italy

JÜRGEN POHL, MD, PhD
Department of Internal Medicine II, Dr. Horst Schmidt Klinik Medical School of the University of Mainz, Wiesbaden, Germany

EMANUELE RONDONOTTI, MD, PhD
Department of Medical Sciences, Gastroenterology 3 Unit, University of Milan, IRCCS Policlinico, Mangiagalli, Regina Elena Foundation, Milan, Italy

ANDREW S. ROSS, MD
Digestive Disease Institute, Virginia Mason Medical Center, Seattle, Washington

VALERIA SALADINO, MD
Department of Medical Sciences, Gastroenterology 3 Unit, IRCCS Policlinico, Mangiagalli, Regina Elena Foundation, Milan, Italy

HARALD SCHMIDT, MD
Oskar-Ziethen-Hospital, Sana Clinic Lichtenberg, Medical Clinic I, Berlin University-Teaching Hospital (Charité), Berlin, Germany

HANS-JOACHIM SCHULZ, MD
Professor of Internal Medicine, Oskar-Ziethen-Hospital, Sana Clinic Lichtenberg, Medical Clinic I, Berlin University-Teaching Hospital (Charité), Berlin, Germany

CAROL E. SEMRAD, MD
Department of Internal Medicine, Section of Gastroenterology, University of Chicago Medical Center, Chicago, Illinois

KEIJIRO SUNADA, MD
Assistant Professor of Medicine, Departments of Endoscopic Research and International Education, Jichi Medical University, Shimotsuke, Tochigi, Japan

CHRISTINA A. TENNYSON, MD
Assistant Professor of Clinical Medicine, Department of Gastroenterology, Columbia University School of Medicine, New York, New York

BENNIE R. UPCHURCH, MD
Visiting Assistant Professor of Medicine, Cleveland Clinic Lerner College of Medicine, Cleveland, Ohio

JAN HEIN T.M. VAN WAESBERGHE, MD, PhD
Department of Radiology, VU University Medical Center, Amsterdam, The Netherlands

STIJN J.B. VAN WEYENBERG, MD
Department of Gastroenterology and Hepatology, VU University Medical Center Amsterdam, The Netherlands

JOHN J. VARGO, MD, MPH
Head, Section of Therapeutic Endoscopy, Digestive Disease Institute, Cleveland Clinic; and Associate Professor of Medicine, Cleveland Clinic Lerner College of Medicine, Cleveland, Ohio

FEDERICA VILLA, MD
Department of Medical Sciences, Gastroenterology 3 Unit, IRCCS Policlinico, Mangiagalli, Regina Elena Foundation, Milan, Italy

HIRONORI YAMAMOTO, MD, PhD
Professor of Medicine, Departments of Endoscopic Research and International Education, Jichi Medical University, Shimotsuke; and Director, Endoscopy Center, Jichi Medical University Hospital, Tochigi, Japan

Contents

Foreword xiii

Charles J. Lightdale

Preface xv

David R. Cave

Enteroscopy: An Overview 315

Christina A. Tennyson and Blair S. Lewis

Although the small intestine has long been considered the final frontier of endoscopy, a vast amount of progress has led to increased diagnostic and therapeutic capabilities. With the increasing prevalence of capsule endoscopy, the need for enteroscopy also continues to increase. The endoscopic options currently available include double and single balloon–assisted enteroscopy, spiral enteroscopy, and lastly, intraoperative enteroscopy. The majority of published literature has focused on double balloon enteroscopy, but further studies have to provide information on the safety and yield of the newer techniques. Although intraoperative enteroscopy may be practiced less frequently, it has a role in the management of lesions that may not be approachable by other endoscopic means and a role in the guidance of surgical management.

Technology and Indications 325

Keijiro Sunada and Hironori Yamamoto

Double-balloon endoscopy (DBE) was developed based on the principle of preventing stretching of the intestinal tract by anchoring the convoluted intestinal tract with an endoscope and overtube fitted with inflatable balloons. The DBE system includes the main body of the endoscope with a built-in air channel, a balloon attached to the tip of the endoscope, an overtube with a hydrophilic coating equipped with an inflatable balloon, and a balloon controller that safely inflates/deflates the two balloons. At present, there are three different types of endoscopes for DBE. The indications for DBE include the diagnosis or treatment of various small intestinal conditions such as obscure gastrointestinal bleeding, Crohn's disease, and benign and malignant tumors. In addition, DBE can be used to approach the surgically modified intestinal tract; conventional endoscopes have difficulty in that situation. DBE can be used for colonoscopy in cases in which it is difficult to insert a conventional colonoscope. In the future, DBE will have the potential for wider use in routine colonoscopy because the insertion technique is easy and reliable.

Single-balloon Enteroscopy 335

Bennie R. Upchurch and John J. Vargo

Single-balloon enteroscopy has emerged as a viable alternative to double-balloon enteroscopy in the management of small bowel disease.

Technically, it is easier to perform, may be more efficient, and in the limited literature available, seems to provide similar diagnostic and therapeutic yield when compared with double-balloon enteroscopy. This review provides up-to-date views on this emerging technology and its application.

Balloon Enteroscopy: Single- and Double-Balloon Enteroscopy **349**

Andrea May

Balloon enteroscopy is a method that allows endoscopic inspection of the entire small bowel, or large parts of it, while simultaneously making it possible to obtain histologic samples and carry out treatment measures. Studies of double-balloon enteroscopy (DBE) have confirmed the high diagnostic yield of the procedure, with an acceptably low complication rate (approximately 1% for diagnostic DBE and 3% to 4% for therapeutic DBE). The principal indication for the procedure is midgastrointestinal bleeding, that is, when the bleeding source is located in the small bowel. With good patient selection, the diagnostic yield here is 70% to 80%, and this has a substantial influence on subsequent treatment measures. Single-balloon enteroscopy appears to be a simplification of the technique that is easier to handle, but few original studies have been published on the topic to date, and the results of prospective and controlled studies with larger numbers of patients must therefore be awaited. At present, DBE must still be regarded as the standard method for diagnostic and therapeutic endoscopy in the small bowel, avoiding the need for intraoperative enteroscopy or therapeutic laparotomy.

Spiral Enteroscopy and Push Enteroscopy **357**

Paul A. Akerman and Daniel Cantero

Spiral enteroscopy is a new technique for endoscopic evaluation of the small bowel. Currently, more than 3000 cases have been performed worldwide. The Discovery SB device has been approved by the Food and Drug Administration and has been granted a CE mark. The technique is safe and effective for management and detection of small bowel pathology. Recent studies of spiral enteroscopy have demonstrated diagnostic yield, total time of procedure, and depth of insertion that compare favorably with double and single balloon enteroscopy. The strengths of spiral enteroscopy are rapid advancement in the small bowel and controlled, stable withdrawal that facilitates therapy. Future studies will be needed to compare competing technologies. Push enteroscopy is a readily available, safe and effective technique for detecting and treating proximal gut pathology. If performed without an overtube, complications are rare. Use of a dedicated push enteroscope with an overtube is generally reserved for specific indications in which a moderate increase in depth of insertion into the small bowel is required. When capsule endoscopy and deep small bowel enteroscopy are not available, push enteroscopy is a reasonable option with low risk and moderate yield. Push enteroscopy will remain an important part of the armamentarium of the modern endoscopist.

Intraoperative Enteroscopy **371**

Hans-Joachim Schulz and Harald Schmidt

Current options for the diagnosis and management of small bowel lesions include push enteroscopy (PE), video capsule endoscopy (VCE), single-balloon enteroscopy (SBE), double-balloon enteroscopy (DBE), and intraoperative enteroscopy (IOE). IOE, the ultimate diagnostic and therapeutic modality for small bowel disorders, is a major surgical and endoscopic procedure. It should be reserved for cases that cannot be managed with others modalities because of the difficulties of the procedure and significant morbidity. The indication for IOE have diminished in recent years because of the development of VCE and DBE. IOE is reserved for patients with massive mid-gut bleeding, lesions not accessible by balloon enteroscopy, and lesions difficult or impossible to treat by balloon enteroscopy. There are special indications in Crohn disease and in Peutz-Jeghers syndrome. Our own results and a review of the literature are presented.

Techniques, Tricks, and Complications of Enteroscopy 381

Simon K. Lo

Small bowel endoscopy has made tremendous advances over the last 8 years. The introduction of capsule endoscopy, double-balloon enteroscopy, single-balloon enteroscopy and spiral overtube-assisted enteroscopy have completely removed the mystery in investigating the small intestine. These new procedures are challenging and timeconsuming to perform. A brief overview on the technical issues and complications related to these small bowel endoscopy procedures is presented.

Enteroscopy and its Relationship to Radiological Small Bowel Imaging 389

Stijn J.B. Van Weyenberg, Jan Hein T.M. Van Waesberghe, Christian Ell, and Jürgen Pohl

The field of radiological small bowel imaging is changing rapidly, as is small bowel enteroscopy. New techniques allow the depiction of intraluminal, mural, and extraintestinal features of various small bowel disorders, such as Crohn disease, small bowel polyposis syndromes, small intestinal malignancies, and celiac disease. For patients requiring repeated small bowel imaging, modalities that do not use ionizing radiation, such as ultrasound or magnetic resonance imaging, should be considered.

Enteroscopy in the Diagnosis and Management of Obscure Gastrointestinal Bleeding 409

Marco Pennazio

Capsule endoscopy and balloon-assisted enteroscopy, have revolutionized our approach to the diagnosis and management of patients with obscure gastrointestinal bleeding, largely replacing intraoperative enteroscopy and conventional barium studies. Despite its limitations, capsule endoscopy may well be the most reasonable initial diagnostic strategy to evaluate most patients with obscure gastrointestinal bleeding, leaving balloon-assisted enteroscopy in reserve as a complementary tool. This article reviews the data on enteroscopy, with particular emphasis on the use of capsule endoscopy and balloon-assisted enteroscopy for the diagnosis and management of patients with obscure gastrointestinal bleeding.

Enteroscopy in the Diagnosis and Management of Crohn Disease 427

Shabana F. Pasha and Jonathan A. Leighton

Crohn disease is a chronic disorder that can affect any part of the gastrointestinal tract, and is characterized by mucosal and transmural inflammation of the bowel wall. The disease most commonly involves the small bowel. Evaluation of patients with suspected Crohn disease has traditionally involved the use of ileocolonoscopy, push enteroscopy, and barium small bowel radiography. A large proportion of patients with mild small bowel disease or involvement of the mid small bowel can potentially be missed if only these tests are utilized. Enteroscopy is defined as direct visualization of the small bowel using a fiber optic or wireless endoscope. Following recent advances in technology, enteroscopy currently plays a pivotal role not only in the diagnosis of small bowel Crohn disease but also in the management of its complications, such as bleeding and strictures. Enteroscopy may have additional roles in the future, including the objective assessment of mucosal response to therapy, and surveillance for small bowel malignancy. This article focuses on the utility of enteroscopy, and its advantages and limitations in the evaluation and longterm management of Crohn disease.

Enteroscopy in the Diagnosis and Management of Celiac Disease **445**

Emanuele Rondonotti, Federica Villa, Valeria Saladino, and Roberto de Franchis

Esophagogastroduodenoscopy (EGD) with 3 to 6 biopsies in the descending duodenum is the gold standard for the diagnosis of celiac disease. At the time of the first diagnosis of celiac disease, an extensive evaluation of the small bowel is not recommended. However, video capsule endoscopy, because of its good sensitivity and specificity in recognizing the Endoscopic features of celiac disease, can be considered a valid alternative to EGD in patients unable or unwilling to undergo EGD with biopsies. Capsule endoscopy is also a possible option in selected cases with strong suspicion of celiac disease but negative first-line tests. In evaluating patients with refractory or complicated celiac disease, in whom a complete evaluation of the small bowel is mandatory (at least in refractory celiac disease type II patients) because of the possible presence of complications beyond the reach of conventional endoscopes, both capsule endoscopy and balloon-assisted enteroscopy have been found to be helpful. In these patients, capsule endoscopy offers several advantages: it is well tolerated, it allows inspection of the entire small bowel, and it is able to recognize subtle mucosal changes. However, in this setting, capsule endoscopy should ideally be coupled with imaging techniques that provide important information about the thickness of the wall of the intestine and about extraluminal abnormalities. Although deep enteroscopy (such as balloon enteroscopy) is expensive, time-consuming, and potentially risky in these frail patients, they may have a key role, because they make it possible to take tissue samples from deep in the small intestine.

Small Bowel Tumors **461**

Shirley C. Paski and Carol E. Semrad

Although rare, small bowel tumors may cause significant morbidity and mortality if left undetected. New endoscopic modalities allow full examination of the small bowel with improved diagnosis. However, isolated mass lesions may be missed by capsule endoscopy or incomplete balloon-assisted enteroscopy. Therefore the use of radiologic imaging and intraoperative enteroscopy for diagnosis should not be forgotten. Endoscopic resection of small bowel polyps and certain vascular tumors is possible but requires proper training. Advances in endoscopic tools are likely to broaden the endoscopic management of small bowel tumors. This article describes the general features of small bowel tumors, clinical presentation, and diagnostic tests followed by a description of the more common tumor types and their management.

Outcomes Associated with Deep Enteroscopy **481**

Lauren B. Gerson

The purpose of this article is to describe the available data regarding the short- and long-term outcomes associated with deep enteroscopy. Deep enteroscopy can be defined as the use of an enteroscope to examine small bowel distal to the ligament of Treitz or proximal to the distal ileum. The term deep enteroscopy includes double-balloon, single-balloon, and spiral enteroscopy. Comparisons are made with push enteroscopy and intraoperative enteroscopy, the major therapeutic endoscopic options available to the gastroenterologist before the introduction of deep enteroscopy. The article concludes with a discussion regarding complications associated with deep enteroscopy and cost-effectiveness of management strategies for obscure bleeding. Proposed changes to the current algorithm for management of obscure bleeding are suggested.

Endoscopic Retrograde Cholangiopancreatography in the Surgically Modified Gastrointestinal Tract **497**

Andrew S. Ross

Endoscopic retrograde cholangiopancreatography (ERCP) in the patient with altered intestinal anatomy secondary to surgery presents significant challenges to the endoscopist. Navigating anastamoses, cannulation using a forward viewing endoscope in a retrograde position and use of specialized instruments encompass just a few of the unique issues which arise when attempting ERCP in patients with surgically altered anatomy. This article focuses on instruments, technique and a review of the published literature to date on performing ERCP in this group of patients.

Novel Applications of Balloon Endoscopy **509**

Michel Delvaux and Gérard Gay

Double-balloon endoscopy has been available for investigation of the small bowel since 2001, concomitantly with capsule endoscopy. Beyond established indications, endoscopic examination of the small bowel is currently performed in many clinical conditions involving the small bowel, which were under investigated in the past. Biopsies of lesions observed by capsule endoscopy or balloon enteroscopy can be taken and the lesions can sometimes be treated during a balloon Endoscopic procedure. Double-balloon endoscopy can be used in patients when conventional endoscopy was incomplete. The main applications of double-balloon endoscopy are the examination of patients with a surgically modified gastrointestinal tract and colonoscopy after a previously failed attempt to reach the cecum. In the latter indication, using a dedicated double-balloon colonoscope, the success rate of cecal intubation may be nearly 100%.

Index **519**

FORTHCOMING ISSUES

October 2009

Advances in Biliary and Pancreatic Endoscopy

Peter Stevens, MD, *Guest Editor*

Jaunary 2010

Endoluminal Therapy of Esophageal Diseases

Herbert Wolfson, MD, *Guest Editor*

April 2010

CT Colonography

Jacques Van Dam, MD, PhD, and
Subhas Bannerjee, MD, *Guest Editors*

RECENT ISSUES

April 2009

Enhanced Endoscopic Imaging

Grace H. Elta, MD, and
Kenneth K. Wang, MD, *Guest Editors*

January 2009

Gastrointestinal Motility and Neurogastroenterology

Richard W. McCallum, MD, FACP, FACG, *Guest Editor*

October 2008

Endoscopic Sedation: Preparing for the Future

Lawrence B. Cohen, MD,
and James Aisenberg, MD, *Guest Editors*

THE CLINICS ARE NOW AVAILABLE ONLINE!

Access your subscription at:
www.theclinics.com

Foreword

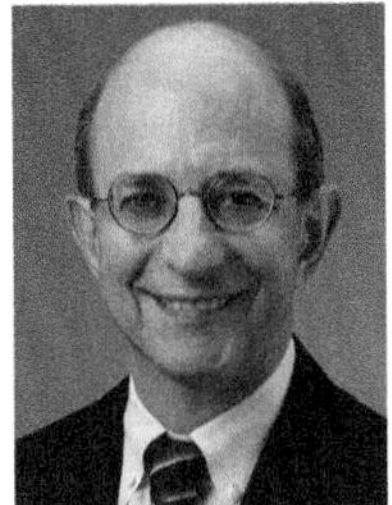

Charles J. Lightdale, MD
Consulting Editor

Enteroscopy is a thriving infant in the field of gastrointestinal endoscopy. With a huge impetus from the invention of the video capsule, enteroscopy was reborn at the right time. The double-balloon enteroscope appeared almost simultaneously, and now there are competitive capsules and enteroscopes, which almost guarantee further improvements and developments. Perfect timing really, as the understanding of small-intestinal disease has expanded exponentially in recent years. Indeed, the new capacity to visually explore the small intestine has in turn furthered the understanding of the pathogenesis and extent of diseases affecting this long, complex organ. The window has been opened for tissue acquisition and for therapy throughout the entire length of the small intestine.

Of course, there are difficulties and limitations at this stage, but this has not stopped a growing band of gastroenterologists who have embraced this new opportunity to diagnose and treat small-intestinal disease. There is much to be learned, but the potential for patient benefits are huge. The usual cynics and naysayers, who wondered whether enteroscopy could really be of value, are backing off. It is gratifying to see a developing field that truly has "legs." The video capsule and double-balloon enteroscope are huge booster rockets, but there is plenty more to come.

David Cave was quick to grasp the importance of the emergence of enteroscopy as a major new focus in gastrointestinal endoscopy. As a leader in academic gastroenterology, he has steadily promoted the critical role of clinical research in enteroscopy as a fundamental aspect of its orderly development. I am very appreciative that he agreed to be the guest editor of this issue of the *Gastrointestinal Endoscopy Clinics of North America* on the subject of enteroscopy. He has had the cooperation of the foremost experts as authors, and he has absolutely nailed it. If you are a gastrointestinal endoscopist ready to explore the previously unseen and untouchable, or if

Gastrointest Endoscopy Clin N Am 19 (2009) xiii–xiv
doi:10.1016/j.giec.2009.04.017
1052-5157/09/$ – see front matter © 2009 Elsevier Inc. All rights reserved.
giendo.theclinics.com

you are already on board, but want to be completely updated, you must have this issue of the *Clinics*.

Charles J. Lightdale, MD
Department of Medicine
Columbia University Medical Center
161 Fort Washington Avenue, Room 812
New York, NY 10032, USA

E-mail address:
CJL18@columbia.edu (C.J. Lightdale)

Preface

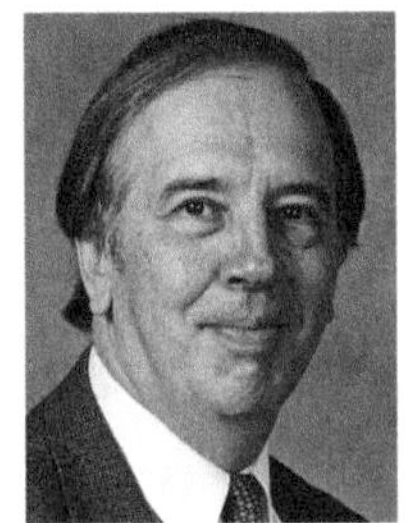

David R. Cave, MD, PhD
Guest Editor

At the turn of the 21st century, interest in the small bowel was at a low ebb, in large part due to its inaccessibility. In 2001, this started to change with the Food and Drug Administration approval of the M2A video capsule (Given Imaging,Yoqneam, Israel). This imaginative device, which reminded many of us of the science fiction movie "Fantastic Voyage," for the first time provided a noninvasive view of most of the mucosa of the entire length of the small intestine. This stimulus has resulted in the publication of thousands of abstracts and hundreds of peer-reviewed articles. In 8 short years, the device and its successors and competitors have gone from curiosities to mainstream clinical and investigative tools. Somewhere around a million of these devices have been deployed, and most have been excreted! The indications, contraindications, and complications of this technology are now quite well understood. There are, however, areas of clinical application and investigation where it is still underused. New capsules are being developed with additional and therapeutic possibilities.

In 2001, the double balloon enteroscope, developed by Dr Yamamoto and Fujinon Corp, became available in Japan. This novel device was rapidly deployed around the world and has spawned a plethora of innovations, collectively referred to as deep enteroscopes. These, for the first time, have allowed both diagnostic and therapeutic approaches to the entire length of the small intestine and facilitated examination of the surgically modified gastrointestinal tract.

Thanks to the outstanding contributions of an international panel of experts who have contributed to this issue, we now have in one place a compendium of not only the latest views of the technologies mentioned above, but also an up-to-the-minute appreciation of how they might be used in the optimal care of patients, which is the universal objective. The issue is divided into two sections. First, new technologies are presented, and they include video capsule endoscopy, balloon and spiral enteroscopy, the newest radiological imaging techniques, and the long-standing gold standard of intraoperative enteroscopy, along with reviews of techniques, tricks, complications, and outcomes. The second section covers disease management and how these technologies contribute to its improvement. Articles on obscure gastrointestinal bleeding, Crohn disease, celiac disease, and small-bowel tumors are included.

Gastrointest Endoscopy Clin N Am 19 (2009) xv–xvi
doi:10.1016/j.giec.2009.04.016 giendo.theclinics.com
1052-5157/09/$ – see front matter © 2009 Elsevier Inc. All rights reserved.

In addition, an article on the use of the new enteroscopes in the colon is included as an entrée into a novel application of the technology.

I would like to thank all the contributors who have made the time to write their articles, particularly because these techniques they have written about take a lot of time and have further eroded the time available for writing.

I would also like to thank Charlie Lightdale, MD, for providing me with the opportunity to assemble this contribution to endoscopic research and clinical application. It should provide a major resource for anyone interested in small-bowel endoscopy, for both trainees and experts, for years to come.

Last but not least, I would like to thank Kerry Holland and her staff at Elsevier for their support and very professional management of this project.

David R. Cave, MD, PhD
Department of Medicine
University of Massachusetts Medical School
55 Lake Avenue North Worcester
MA 01655, USA

E-mail address:
caved@ummhc.edu

Enteroscopy: An Overview

Christina A. Tennyson, MD, Blair S. Lewis, MD*

KEYWORDS

- Enteroscopy • Double balloon • Overtubes
- Capsule endoscopy • Sprial endoscopy

The small bowel has long been considered the final frontier of the gastrointestinal tract because it was unable to be routinely examined by way of endoscopic techniques. It was believed to be an organ where little happened. Using a colonoscope or longer enteroscope only allowed for visualization of a relatively short section of the small bowel. Other options for enteroscopy were limited and available at few centers. After the advent of capsule endoscopy and the development of new endoscopic techniques for investigating the small bowel, enteroscopy has undergone tremendous development within the past several years. The increasing widespread use of capsule endoscopy after its introduction in 2001 has led to an increased interest and need to examine the small bowel.

Enteroscopy is a companion to capsule endoscopy. Capsule endoscopy provides a thorough examination of the small bowel, but does have limitations. Capsule endoscopy examinations may be hindered by incomplete examinations, poor preparations, or limited mucosal visualization, rapid transit through particular segments, and a unidirectional field of view. In addition, capsule endoscopy does not allow for therapeutic interventions. When an area appears abnormal on capsule endoscopy, enteroscopy can reexamine the area and obtain biopsies. Enteroscopy can be performed for therapeutic intervention, such as cauterization, polypectomy, stricture dilation, or removal of foreign bodies, including retained capsules. Lesions can be tattooed to target subsequent surgical interventions. Enteroscopy can assist in performing biliary procedures and/or examining the stomach and duodenum in patients with a Roux-en-Y after bariatric surgery. In addition, enteroscopy may have a role in patients with continued bleeding after negative capsule endoscopy. Enteroscopy may also be indicated in patients with unexplained malabsorption, diarrhea, refractory celiac disease, or radiographic abnormalities of the small bowel.[1–3]

TECHNIQUES

Until recent years, the options for endoscopic evaluation of the small bowel had been fairly limited. Pediatric colonoscopes, measuring approximately 135 cm, were initially

Division of Gastroenterology, Mount Sinai School of Medicine, 1067 Fifth Avenue, New York, NY 10128, USA
* Corresponding author.
E-mail address: blairslewismdpc@Covad.net (B.S. Lewis).

Gastrointest Endoscopy Clin N Am 19 (2009) 315–324
doi:10.1016/j.giec.2009.04.005 giendo.theclinics.com
1052-5157/09/$ – see front matter © 2009 Elsevier Inc. All rights reserved.

used to examine to the depth of the proximal jejunum. Longer enteroscopes, measuring up to approximately 2.5 m, were later constructed that could be advanced slightly further into the proximal to midjejunum. Although these instruments were longer, it was difficult to push distally because of the multiple bends of the small bowel. Overtubes also have been used in an attempt to attain deeper small bowel intubation, although they achieved only limited success. With the use of longer instruments or overtubes, navigation into the small bowel was limited, secondary to formation of loops or stretching of the intestine.[4]

In addition to longer instruments or the use of overtubes, other types of enteroscopy were developed. These techniques were not widely adopted because of their time-consuming nature and inefficiencies. Rope-way enteroscopy and sonde enteroscopy were two of these techniques. In rope-way enteroscopy, a patient swallowed a guide string, which traveled the entire gastrointestinal tract, emerged from the anus, and was then exchanged with a stiffer Teflon tube.[5] An endoscope was then passed through the oral or anal route. The procedure allowed intubation of the small bowel, but it was invasive and time consuming and never gained widespread acceptance. Sonde enteroscopy involved swallowing a thin endoscope with balloon tip that was dragged through the small intestine by peristalsis and allowed examination of the small bowel upon withdrawal.[6] The procedure was also time consuming and did not provide an opportunity for therapeutic interventions.

The forms of enteroscopy available include balloon-assisted enteroscopy (using a double or single balloon method), intraoperative enteroscopy, and spiral enteroscopy. Intraoperative enteroscopy, long considered the gold standard of enteroscopy, has largely been replaced. The newer techniques provide a stable, less invasive platform to view the bowel and can be repeated at a later time if indicated. Most of the published literature has involved double balloon enteroscopy because it has been available for a longer period of time.

BALLOON-ASSISTED ENTEROSCOPY

Double Balloon Enteroscopy

Double balloon enteroscopy, enabling total intubation of the small bowel, was developed by Dr. Hinori Yamamoto and first described in 2001.[7] It is also known as "push and pull" enteroscopy. Two types of endoscopes, EN-450P5 and EN-450T5, are available for diagnostic and therapeutic use respectively (Fujinon Inc, Saitama, Japan). Both devices consist of a 200-cm enteroscope coupled with a 140-cm soft flexible polyurethane overtube. The diagnostic EN-450P5 is slightly thinner, with an external diameter of 8.5 mm, forceps channel diameter of 2.2 mm, and total resulting external diameter of 12.2 mm. The therapeutic EN-450T5 is slightly larger, with an external diameter of 9.4 mm, forceps channel diameter of 2.8 mm, and total resulting external diameter of 13.2 mm. A hydrophilic coating is present on the inner and outer surfaces of the overtube, resulting in minimal friction. Water is injected through a catheter to activate the hydrophilic surface of the overtube. Latex balloons, located at the tip of the overtube and tip of the enteroscope, are inflated and deflated using a hand switched, but automatic pressure-regulated pump. The balloons are inflated to 45 mm Hg because this amount allows sufficient force to hold the balloon in place, allow insertion of the endoscope, and does not result in patient discomfort.[8] The device allows for the small bowel to be pleated onto the overtube. It allows for significantly deeper intubation than push enteroscopy. Although it has been speculated that bowel insufflation with carbon dioxide, instead of air, may improve patient comfort during the procedure, there are no data to support its use.[9,10]

Double balloon enteroscopy can be performed through the peroral and peranal route. These are also known as the antegrade and retrograde approaches. The examination is labor intensive and involves a series of repetitive maneuvers that have been described by Yamamoto.[7] The balloons, attached to the scope and overtube tips, hold the wall of the small bowel in place at various times during the examination. Withdrawal of the 2 inflated balloons pleats the bowel over the overtube. The enteroscope is first advanced as far as possible distal to the ligament of Treitz without causing significant looping, and the enteroscope balloon is then inflated. Next, the overtube is advanced to the enteroscope's tip, and the overtube balloon is inflated. This holds the scope in place and prevents looping during further advancement of the scope. The enteroscope balloon is next deflated, and the scope is advanced to the point of maximal insertion. When the scope is fully advanced, the enteroscope tip balloon is again inflated to hold position. The overtube balloon is next deflated, the overtube advanced to the enteroscope's tip, and the overtube balloon is inflated. With both balloons inflated at the distal end, the entire assembly is pulled backward to pleat the scope onto the overtube. For a retrograde approach, the ileocecal valve must be intubated by both balloons, and the assembly is advanced. During an examination, the series of maneuvers may be performed more than 12 times. The length of the procedure varies, but it often lasts 1 to 2 hours.

Localization of a lesion identified at capsule endoscopy is challenging. An endoscopist must determine if the lesion is within the reach of a push enteroscope or if deeper intubation of the small bowel is needed. If a double balloon enteroscopy is performed, one must decide whether to pursue the lesion from an oral or transrectal approach. There has been little published data to guide clinicians. Because capsule transit times vary amongst individuals, it is not possible to use the total capsule passage time to guide the approach of double balloon enteroscopy. Mark Appleyard has suggested that the percentage of small bowel total transit time to a lesion be used to determine approach (personal communication, 2005). The time of capsule passage from the pylorus to a specific lesion is divided by the total small bowel transit time. He has suggested that lesions seen within 10% of passage time may be reached with push enteroscopy. Lesions from 10% to 70% passage time may be reached through the oral approach, whereas those found over 70% of the passage time may be reached through the retrograde approach. This technique has been applied in a small study involving 47 double balloon enteroscopy procedures in 42 patients.[11] Gay and colleagues[11] found that capsule endoscopy reliably indicated the need for a transrectal double balloon enteroscopy approach if the transit time to a lesion was greater than or equal to 75% of the total transit time. The study is limited by the small number of patients and small number of procedures performed through the transrectal approach. It has also been suggested that retrograde double balloon enteroscopy be performed first when looking for neuroendocrine tumors because these occur much more commonly in the ileum.[12]

The depth of the examination of small bowel enteroscopy is difficult to assess. The reporting of depths of insertion for enteroscopy has not been extensively studied, is subjective, and may be exaggerated.[13] For double balloon enteroscopy, a method of assessing depth of insertion, described using an ex vivo porcine endoscopy training device, appears to accurately estimate insertion depth. In this method developed by May and colleagues,[14] the endoscopist measures the depth of insertion with each cycle of scope insertion and subtracts any backward slippage of the apparatus.

Using double balloon enteroscopy, it has been possible to view the entire small bowel, although this is rarely achieved with one examination. Combined approaches using antegrade with retrograde routes are frequently performed. Yamamoto and colleagues[15] reported total enteroscopy using both approaches in 86% of patients. A subsequent European study reported total enteroscopy in 45% of patients using both approaches.[16] Initial American experience with the procedure achieved total enteroscopy of the small bowel in only 5% of cases.[17] It appears that total intubation of the small bowel cannot be achieved in every patient. Every small bowel lesion may not be amenable to endoscopic, or nonsurgical, therapy. Difficulty in pleating the small bowel in double balloon enteroscopy may be caused by surgical adhesions or by fat in the mesentery in obese patients. Endoscopists may encounter more difficulty in intubating the small bowel through the retrograde approach in particular. In a small retrospective study, procedure failure occurred in 21% of retrograde cases and was associated with earlier abdominal or pelvic surgery.[12]

The complications of double balloon enteroscopy may be caused by the procedure itself or may be secondary to anesthesia. The most commonly reported complications include pancreatitis, bleeding, and perforation.[18–20] Parotitis has also been reported after double balloon enteroscopy.[21] Complications are more frequent in therapeutic procedures as compared with diagnostic procedures. In an international multicenter study, the rates of complications were 0.8% and 4.3% for diagnostic and therapeutic procedures, respectively.[19] Polypectomy of large polyps in the small bowel, measuring more than 3 cm, appears to be associated with the highest risk and has a reported complication rate of 10%.[18] Complications secondary to anesthesia occur less than 1% of the time and include aspiration, respiratory depression, and pneumonia.[9]

The contraindications for double balloon enteroscopy are not well defined. Relative contraindications to balloon-assisted endoscopy include altered surgical anatomy, coagulopathy, present/recurrent pancreatitis, and high-grade bowel obstruction.[10] Since the Fujinon double balloons are constructed of latex, a latex allergy is a relative contraindication, and the procedure should be performed only if the benefits outweigh the risks. Large esophageal or gastric varices should also be considered a contraindication for balloon-assisted enteroscopy because of potential overtube trauma and bleeding. In addition, an endoscopist should proceed with caution in patients with severe mucosal inflammation, such as severe Crohn or celiac disease.

Double balloon enteroscopy can provide a targeted examination and endoscopic therapy for bleeding lesions within the small bowel. Although angioectasias are a major cause of obscure gastrointestinal bleeding and can be controlled with endoscopic cautery, the depth of intubation with push enteroscopy alone was limited.[22] In a prospective study of patients with suspected small bowel bleeding, double balloon enteroscopy had a diagnostic yield of 73% compared with a yield of 44% for push enteroscopy.[23] In the same study by May and colleagues[23], double balloon enteroscopy identified additional small lesions deeper in the small bowel in 78% of patients with findings on push enteroscopy. The overall diagnostic yield from double balloon enteroscopy has ranged from 43% to 80%, with the most common indication being obscure gastrointestinal bleeding.[15–17,24] In a study by Fry and colleagues,[25] approximately 24% of patients referred for double balloon enteroscopy had sources explaining the cause of bleeding within reach of a conventional endoscope. Double balloon enteroscopy can replace intraoperative enteroscopy in patients with bleeding in the mid to distal small bowel and offers several advantages. Double balloon enteroscopy provides shorter procedure times, a less invasive approach, and the ability to repeat examination if indicated.

Procedure guidelines recommend capsule endoscopy in patients with obscure gastrointestinal bleeding after a normal upper endoscopy and colonoscopy are done.[26,27] A pooled data analysis of capsule endoscopy demonstrated that there is a 20% overall miss rate and that 10% of cases have a bleeding source outside of the small bowel.[28] Previous studies had demonstrated that capsule endoscopy has demonstrated a slightly increased yield of small bowel lesions when compared with double balloon enteroscopy.[29,30] In a larger study and a meta-analysis, capsule endoscopy and double balloon enteroscopy were found to be comparable when the entire small bowel is examined.[31,32] Although capsule endoscopy and double balloon enteroscopy are complementary procedures, there still may be lesions missed on capsule examinations. If a capsule endoscopy study is negative, it is estimated that only 5% to 11% of patients experience further bleeding when followed for more than 1 year.[33,34] A minority of patients may continue to bleed, and the management of these cases is difficult. One approach is to perform a repeat capsule endoscopy, and another approach is to perform double balloon enteroscopy. In a study, repeat capsule endoscopy was performed in 24 patients; the procedure revealed additional findings in 75% of cases and lead to a change in management in 62%.[35] There are limited data for the role of double balloon enteroscopy after negative capsule studies. In the proximal small bowel, the capsule may travel rapidly and fail to detect significant pathology.[36] In a small series by Chong and colleagues[37] using double balloon enteroscopy, four patients had findings consisting of two gastrointestinal stromal tumors, one adenocarcinoma, and one lymphoma after negative capsule studies. Another small case series described five lesions, consisting of tumors, varices, and polyps, missed on capsule endoscopy, but found using alternative techniques, including double balloon enteroscopy.[36] It also may be difficult to identify small bowel diverticula on capsule endoscopy.[38]

Another role for double balloon enteroscopy is to retrieve a retained capsule and thus prevent surgical intervention. Capsule retention is defined as having a capsule endoscope remain in the gastrointestinal tract for a minimum of 2 weeks as defined by the International Conference on Capsule Endoscopy consensus statement.[39] Capsules retention can also be defined as capsules that remain in the gastrointestinal tract permanently unless removed by endoscopic, surgical, or medical therapy. The choice to proceed with endoscopic or surgical management depends on the cause of the retention, indication for the examination, and condition of the patient. In a patient with severe bleeding or severe Crohn strictures, surgical intervention may be the optimal strategy to remove the capsule and correct the initial problem. In a patient with less severe symptoms or a patient who may respond to medical treatment alone, double balloon enteroscopy is an option to retrieve the retained capsule. The antegrade approach can be used if the capsule is a retained nonsteroidal antiinflammatory drug or Crohn stricture is sufficiently proximal. Alternatively, it is possible to use the retrograde approach, dilate the stricture(s), and remove the capsule. Great care needs to be taken with complex or acutely inflamed strictures because of the risk for perforation.[40]

Single Balloon Enteroscopy

Single balloon enteroscopy is another new type of balloon-assisted enteroscopy with a single balloon on the tip of the overtube (Olympus Optical, Tokyo, Japan). There is no balloon on the tip of the enteroscope. The SIF-Q180 scope has a working length of 200 cm, 9.2 mm outer diameter, and a 2.8 mm working channel.[41] The flexible overtube measures 140 cm in length, has a diameter of 13.2 mm, and also contains a hydrophilic coating to minimize friction. The overtube and balloon are constructed from silicon. Because there is no balloon to attach to the tip of the enteroscope, the assembly of the apparatus is quicker than that of the double balloon device. The balloon is inflated by a hand-operated pressure-controlled pump similar to that of the double balloon system. The single balloon technology was introduced in 2008, and there are few published studies available. There has been no direct comparison of single versus double balloon enteroscopy; however, both methods may allow total small bowel intubation in certain patients.

The technique of single balloon enteroscopy is similar to double balloon enteroscopy. The scope is advanced to its maximal position without looping and the enteroscope tip is deflected into a U-turn to hook onto the small bowel. The overtube is then advanced to the distal portion of the scope, the overtube balloon is inflated, the enteroscope tip is returned to a luminal view, and the assembly is withdrawn. The series of maneuvers are repeated. The procedure can be used for the antegrade and retrograde routes. Tsujikawa and colleagues[41] first reported their experiences in 78 procedures in 41 patients referred for suspected midgastrointestinal bleeding, Crohn disease, abdominal pain, and abdominal tumor. The mean procedure times were 62.8 minutes and 70.4 minutes for the oral and anal routes, respectively. Total enteroscopy was achieved in 25% (6/24) of the patients attempted. In a single center study by Kawamura and colleagues,[42] single balloon enteroscopy was used in 37 examinations in 27 patients. Procedure times averaged 83 minutes and 90 minutes for the oral and anal routes respectively; however, total enteroscopy was only achieved in 12.5% (1/8) cases where it was attempted.

The 2 balloon-assisted techniques have been used to perform endoscopic retrograde cholangiopancreatography (ERCP) in patients with altered anatomy after Roux-en-Y.[43,44] Patients requiring this technique may have had gastric bypass or a hepaticojejunostomy after liver transplant. These examinations are particularly labor intensive and use forward-viewing instruments that may result in lower cannulation rates. The cannulation rates using balloon-assisted techniques are less than those in standard ERCPs and have been reported to be between 60% and80%.[45] The endoscopist must reach the Roux-en-Y located approximately 1 m past the ligament of Trietz, appropriately identify the afferent limb, and then proceed to the second portion of the duodenum.

Spiral Enteroscopy

In addition to balloon-assisted enteroscopy, enteroscopy using a novel spiral overtube has been developed.[46,47] The Endo-Ease Discovery SB (Spirus Medical, Stoughton, Massachusetts) allows endoluminal advancement using a spiral overtube. The device is used for antegrade enteroscopy procedures and allows the small bowel to be pleated onto the overtube and scope. The overtube is polyvinyl chloride, measures 118 cm with a 21-cm spiral element at the tip, and has two handles for rotation. There are two available models consisting of a standard 5.5-mm spiral element and a lower 4.5-mm spiral element. Although earlier prototypes were placed over a pediatric colonoscope, the newer devices are used with 200-cm long enteroscopes.[46,47] The outer diameter of the device and endoscope assembly measures approximately 16 mm.

The technique was originally described in 75 patients by Akerman and colleagues[46] in 2008 using the Fujinon EN-450T5 and Olympus SIF-Q180. As described by Akerman, the inside of the overtube is coated with a proprietary lubricant, the overtube placed over the enteroscope, and secured. Additional lubricant is placed on the outside of the device and it is passed orally using push and rotation until past the ligament of Trietz. After this, advancement is made by clockwise rotation until the point of maximum depth of insertion. The enteroscope is then unlocked from the overtube and advanced through the overtube as far as possible. The enteroscope is then withdrawn using a "hook and suction" technique, comparable to single balloon enteroscopy, while rotating the overtube. This process is usually repeated three times. Withdrawal is performed by counterclockwise rotation of the overtube device, and the bowel is slowly unpleated from the overtube/enteroscope assembly.

In the initial description by Akerman and colleagues, the estimated average depth of insertion was 243 cm and 256 cm (range 50–380 cm) using the two types of enteroscopes. The average time to reach maximum depth was less than 20 minutes, and there were no reported complications. Since the mean total procedure time was less than thirty minutes, this technique is markedly faster than double balloon–assisted enteroscopy. In addition to increased speed, the technique also allows the enteroscope to be removed and reintroduced if needed, while holding the position deep in the small bowel. The spiral overtube may be helpful when procedures such as polypectomies are performed. There have been no comparisons of balloon and spiral enteroscopy to date. It is unclear whether diagnostic yields and depth of insertion are equivalent to those in balloon-assisted enteroscopy.

Intraoperative Enteroscopy

Intraoperative enteroscopy has long been considered the gold standard of enteroscopy, and it allows for total small bowel endoscopic examination. Although colonoscopes are routinely used for the examination, enteroscopes may also be used. There are several techniques of intraoperative enteroscopy. The instrument does not need to be sterile. The scope may be introduced through the oral route or through a surgically created enterotomy, using a sterile plastic sheath placed over the instrument.

In the oral technique of intraoperative enteroscopy, the scope is passed orally into the proximal jejunum before the laparotomy. When a patient is intubated and the instrument is passed orally, it may be necessary to deflate the endotracheal cuff to avoid trauma. Placing before laparotomy facilitates passage of the scope because it may be difficult to advance the instrument around the ligament of Trietz once the laparotomy is performed. In an open abdomen, the endoscope may excessively bow along the greater curvature of the stomach. To prevent colonic distention, which can lead to difficulties with subsequent abdominal closure, a noncrushing clamp is placed across the ileocecal valve. The surgeon grasps the endoscope tip and holds a short segment of bowel to allow endoscopic inspection during intubation. Dim overhead lights allow internal and external examination of the transilluminated bowel by the endoscopist and surgeon. After an area is examined, the small bowel is pleated onto the shaft of the endoscope, and the next section of bowel is examined. Mucosal trauma often occurs with pleating of the small bowel, and thus, it is best to examine the bowel with intubation. Trauma may cause artifact and have a similar appearance to angioectasias. Any identified lesions are marked by the surgeon with a suture placed on the serosal surface of the small intestine. The endoscope is later withdrawn, and sites of resection are identified by the sutures.

An alternative technique used in intraoperative enteroscopy is to create an enterotomy. The examination may be performed in a laparoscopically assisted manner with a small incision.[48] The endoscope, covered by a sterile plastic sheath, is placed through the enterotomy and advanced. The site of the enterotomy may be determined by findings at capsule endoscopy or be performed in the mid-small bowel to allow for proximal and distal intubation.

Intraoperative endoscopy has been used for several reasons. With the development of new techniques for enteroscopy, intraoperative endoscopy may be performed less frequently; however, not all lesions may be amenable to endoscopic therapy. It is useful for small intestinal bleeding sites identified on capsule endoscopy that are not approachable by endoscopic means. It also may be useful when surgical guidance is needed to limit small bowel resection. An example may be in a patient with hereditary hemorrhagic telangiectasia syndrome with diffuse small bowel lesions limited to the jejunum requiring resection. Intraoperative enteroscopy has also been used to perform multiple polypectomies in those with small bowel polyposis, such as Peutz-Jeghers syndrome. The specimens can be removed by the enterotomy-limiting resection. In patients with suspected multicentric carcinoid, intraoperative enteroscopy may identify small nonpalpable lesions and tumor resection. Intraoperative enteroscopy may also be helpful in identifying diaphragm disease of the small bowel to facilitate resection. These lesions are not palpable, and endoscopic guidance is often necessary intraoperatively.

SUMMARY

Although the small intestine has long been considered the final frontier of endoscopy, a vast amount of progress has led to increased diagnostic and therapeutic capabilities. With the increasing prevalence of capsule endoscopy, the need for enteroscopy also continues to increase. The endoscopic options currently available include double- and single balloon–assisted enteroscopy, spiral enteroscopy, and lastly, intraoperative enteroscopy. The majority of published literature has focused on double balloon enteroscopy, but further studies have to provide information on the safety and yield of the newer techniques. Although intraoperative enteroscopy may be practiced less frequently, it has a role in the management of lesions that may not be approachable by other endoscopic means and a role in the guidance of surgical management.

REFERENCES

1. Upchurch B, Vargo J. Small bowel enteroscopy. Rev Gastroenterol Disord 2008;8:169–77.
2. Hadithi M, Al-toma A, Oudejans J, et al. The value of double balloon enteroscopy in patients with refractory celiac disease. Am J Gastroenterol 2007;102:987–96.
3. Fry L, Bellutti M, Neumann H, et al. Utility of double balloon enteroscopy for the evaluation of malabsorption. Dig Dis 2008;26:134–9.
4. Yamamoto H, Kita H. Double balloon endoscopy: from concept to reality. Gastrointest Endosc Clin N Am 2006;16:347–61.
5. Classen M, Fruhmorgen P, Koch H. Peroral enteroscopy of the large and small intestine. Endoscopy 1972;4:157–9.
6. Seensalu R. The sonde examination. Gastrointest Endosc Clin N Am 1999;9:37–59.
7. Yamamoto H, Sekine Y, Sato Y, et al. Total enteroscopy with a nonsurgical steerable double-balloon method. Gastrointest Endosc 2001;53:216–20.
8. Yamamoto H, Yano T, Kita H, et al. New system of double balloon enteroscopy for diagnosis and treatment of small intestinal disorders. Gastroenterology 2003;125:1556 [author reply].
9. Pohl J, Blancas JM, Cave D, et al. Consensus report of the 2nd International Conference on double balloon enteroscopy. Endoscopy 2008;40:156–60.
10. Gerson L, Flodin J, Miyabayashi K. Balloon-assisted enteroscopy: technology and troubleshooting. Gastrointest Endosc 2008;68:1158–67.
11. Gay G, Delvaux M, Fassler I. Outcome of capsule endoscopy in determining indication and route for push and pull enteroscopy. Endoscopy 2006;38:49–58.
12. Mehdizadeh S, Han N, Cheng D, et al. Success rate of retrograde double balloon enteroscopy. Gastrointest Endosc 2007;65:633–9.

13. Schembre D, Ross A. Spiral enteroscopy: a new twist on overtube-assisted endoscopy. Gastrointest Endosc 2009;69:333–5.
14. May A, Nachbar L, Schneider M, et al. Push and pull enteroscopy using the double-balloon technique: methods of assessing depth of insertion and training of the enteroscopy technique using the Erlanger endo-trainer. Endoscopy 2005;37(1):66–70.
15. Yamamoto H, Kita H, Sunada K, et al. Clinical outcomes of double-balloon endoscopy for the diagnosis and treatment of small intestinal diseases. Clin Gastroenterol Hepatol 2004;2:1010–6.
16. May A, Nachbar L, Ell C. Double-balloon enteroscopy (push-and-pull enteroscopy) of the small bowel: feasibility and diagnostic and therapeutic yield in patients with suspected small bowel disease. Gastrointest Endosc 2005;62:62–70.
17. Mehdizadeh S, Ross A, Gerson L, et al. What is the learning curve associated with double balloon enteroscopy? Technical details and early experience in 6 U.S. Tertiary Care Centers. Gastrointest Endosc 2006;64:740–50.
18. May A, Nachbar L, Pohl J, et al. Endoscopic interventions in the small bowel using double balloon enteroscopy:feasibility and limitations. Am J Gastroenterol 2007;102:527–35.
19. Mensink P, Haringsma J, Kucharzik TF, et al. Complications of double balloon enteroscopy (DBE): a multicenter study. Endoscopy 2007;39:613–5.
20. Groenen MJM, Moreels TGG, orlent H, et al. Acute pancreatitis after double balloon enteroscopy: an old pathogenic theory revisited as a result of a new endoscopic tool. Endoscopy 2006;38:82–5.
21. Kekilli M, Onal I, Kurt M, et al. Parotitis during oral double-balloon enteroscopy: an unexpected but benign finding. Am J Gastroenterol 2009;104:533–4.
22. Askin M, Lewis B. Push enteroscopic cauterization: long-term follow-up of 83 patients with bleeding small intestinal angiodysplasia. Gastrointest Endosc 1996;43:580–3.
23. May A, Nachbar L, Schneider M, et al. Prospective comparison of push enteroscopy and push-and-pull enteroscopy in patients with suspected small-bowel bleeding. Am J Gastroenterol 2006;101:2016–24.
24. Di Caro S, May A, Heine DG, et al. The European experience with double-balloon enteroscopy: indications, methodology, safety, and clinical impact. Gastrointest Endosc 2005;62:545–50.
25. Fry L, Bellutti M, Neumann H, et al. Incidence of bleeding lesions within reach of conventional upper and lower endoscopes in patients undergoing double-balloon enteroscopy for obscure gastrointestinal bleeding. Aliment Pharmacol Ther 2009;29:342–9.
26. Raju GS, Gerson L, Das A, et al. American Gastroenterological Association. American Gastroenterological Association (AGA) Institute medical position statement on obscure gastrointestinal bleeding. Gastroenterology 2007;133:1694–6.
27. ASGE technology committee, Disario JA, Petersen BT, et al. Enteroscopes. Gastrointest Endosc 2007;66:872–80.
28. Lewis B, Eisen G, Friedman S. A pooled analysis to evaluate results of capsule endoscopy trials. Endoscopy 2005;37:960–5.
29. Kameda N, Higuchi K, Shiba M, et al. A prospective, single-blind trial comparing wireless capsule endoscopy and double-balloon enteroscopy in patients with obscure gastrointestinal bleeding. J Gastroenterol 2008;43:434–40.
30. Hadithi M, Heine D, Jacobs A, et al. A prospective study comparing video capsule endoscopy with double balloon enteroscopy in patients with obscure gastrointestinal bleeding. Am J Gastroenterol 2006;101:52–7.

31. Fukumoto A, Tanaka S, Shishido T, et al. Comparison of detectability of small bowel lesions between capsule endoscopy and double balloon endoscopy for patients with suspected small bowel disease. Gastrointest Endosc 2009;69(4):857–65.
32. Pasha SF, Leighton JA, Das A, et al. Double-balloon enteroscopy and capsule endoscopy have comparable diagnostic yield in small-bowel disease: a meta-analysis. Clin Gastroenterol Hepatol 2008;6(6):671–6.
33. Lai LH, Wong GL, Chow DK, et al. Long-term follow-up of patients with obscure gastrointestinal bleeding after negative capsule endoscopy. Am J Gastroenterol 2006;101:1224–8.
34. Macdonald J, Porter V, McNamara D. Negative capsule endoscopy in patients with obscure GI bleeding predicts low rebleeding rates. Gastrointest Endosc 2008;68:1122–7.
35. Jones BH, Fleischer DE, Sharma VK, et al. Yield of repeat wireless video capsule endoscopy in patients with obscure gastrointestinal bleeding. Am J Gastroenterol 2005;100:1058–64.
36. Postgate A, Depott E, Burling D, et al. Significant small-bowel lesions detected by alternative diagnostic modalities after negative capsule endoscopy. Gastrointest Endosc 2008;68:1209–14.
37. Chong AK, Chin BW, Meredith CG. Clinically significant small-bowel pathology identified by double-balloon enteroscopy but missed by capsule endoscopy. Gastrointest Endosc 2006;64:445–9.
38. Hussain S, Esposito S, Rubin M. Identification of small bowel diverticula with double-balloon enteroscopy following non-diagnostic capsule endoscopy. Dig Dis Sci 2008 [epub ahead of print December 3, 2008].
39. Cave D, Legnani P, deFranchis R, et al. ICCE consensus for capsule retention. Endoscopy 2005;37:1065–7.
40. Tanaka S, Mitsui K, Shirakawa K, et al. Successful retrieval of video capsule endoscopy retained at ileal stenosis of Crohn's disease using double-balloon endoscopy. J Gastroenterol Hepatol 2006;21:922–3.
41. Tsujikawa T, Saitoh Y, Andoh A, et al. Novel single-balloon enteroscopy for diagnosis and treatment of the small intestine: preliminary experience. Endoscopy 2008;40:11–5.
42. Kawamura T, Yasuda K, Tanaka K, et al. Clinical evaluation of a newly developed single-balloon enteroscope. Gastrointest Endosc 2008;68:1112–6.
43. Dellon E, Kohn G, Morgan D, et al. Endoscopic retrograde cholangiopancreatography with single-ballon enteroscopy is feasible in patients with prior Roux-en-Y anastomosis. Dig Dis Sci 2009;54:1798–803.
44. Koornstra J. Double balloon enteroscopy for endoscopic retrograde cholangio-pancreaticography after Roux-en-Y reconstruction: case series and review of the literature. Neth J Med 2008;66:275–9.
45. Chu Y, Yang C, Yeh Y, et al. Double balloon enteroscopy application in biliary tract disease, therapeutic and diagnostic functions. Gastrointest Endosc 2008;68:585–91.
46. Akerman PA, Agrawal D, Cantero D, et al. Spiral enteroscopy with the new DSB overtube: a novel technique for deep peroral small-bowel intubation. Endoscopy 2008;40:974–8.
47. Akerman PA, Agrawal D, Chen W, et al. Spiral enteroscopy: a novel method of enteroscopy by using the Endo-Ease Discovery SB overtube and a pediatric colonoscope. Gastrointest Endosc 2009;69:327–32.
48. Hotokezaka M, Jimi S, Hidaka H, et al. Intraoperative enteroscopy in minimially invasive surgery. Surg Laparosc Endosc Percutan Tech 2007;17:492–4.

Technology and Indications

Keijiro Sunada, MD[a], Hironori Yamamoto, MD, PhD[a,b,*]

KEYWORDS

- Enteroscopy • Small intestine • Double-balloon endoscopy
- Obscure gastrointestinal bleeding (OGIB)

The double-balloon endoscope (**Fig. 1**) has been commercially available since 2003, after Yamamoto et al[1] reported the clinical application of double-balloon enteroscopy (DBE) in 2001. DBE is now available worldwide, and its usefulness for the diagnosis and treatment of various diseases has been demonstrated.[2] The practical application of capsule endoscopy was achieved at about the same time, and strategies for diagnosing and treating small intestinal diseases using these methods are now being investigated. Unlike capsule endoscopy, DBE allows the operator to control function at will in real time, and the technology can be applied not only to diagnosis but also to various treatments such as hemostasis, polypectomy, and dilation. In addition, DBE can access the surgically bypassed intestinal tract, which is inaccessible to the current generation of video capsules. It can also be applied to the treatment and diagnosis of biliary tract diseases through the bypassed tract such as a Roux-en-Y afferent limb. Application of DBE to colonoscopy has been reported recently, and it is being used not only for cases of difficult insertion[3] but also for routine colonoscopy.[4] The technology and indications for DBE are described in this paper.

PRINCIPLE OF DBE

Normally it is difficult to advance an endoscope through the convoluted intestinal tract. Insertion would be easier if the intestinal tract could be straightened. However, without straightening, the endoscope cannot be inserted very far unless loop formation is prevented by manual pressure on the abdominal wall (**Fig. 2**A). In DBE, the flexible overtube holding the intestinal tract from inside with a balloon substitutes for manual pressure. The intestinal tract anchored from inside with the overtube balloon is not stretched further as the endoscope is advanced. Thus, the force of insertion is

[a] Department of Endoscopic Research and International Education, Jichi Medical University, 3311-1 Yakushiji, Shimotsuke, Tochigi 329-0498, Japan
[b] Endoscopy Center, University Hospital 3311-1 Yakushiji, Shimotsuke, Tochigi, Japan 329-0498
* Corresponding author. Department of Endoscopic Research and International Education, Jichi Medical University, 3311-1 Yakushiji, Shimotsuke, Tochigi, Japan 329-0498.
E-mail address: yamamoto@jichi.ac.jp (H. Yamamoto).

Gastrointest Endoscopy Clin N Am 19 (2009) 325–333
doi:10.1016/j.giec.2009.04.015 giendo.theclinics.com
1052-5157/09/$ – see front matter © 2009 Elsevier Inc. All rights reserved.

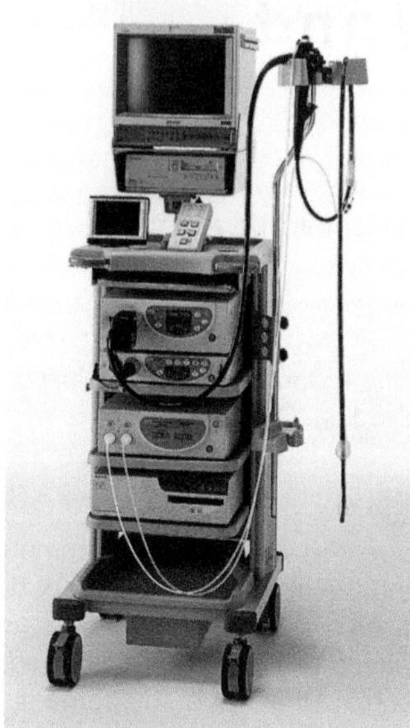

Fig. 1. DBE system.

transmitted effectively to the tip of the endoscope, and the endoscope can be advanced to the deeper portion of the intestine (**Fig. 2**B).

For deep insertion, a balloon is also attached to the tip of the endoscope. At the deepest site reached by the endoscope in the first insertion, the balloon at the tip of

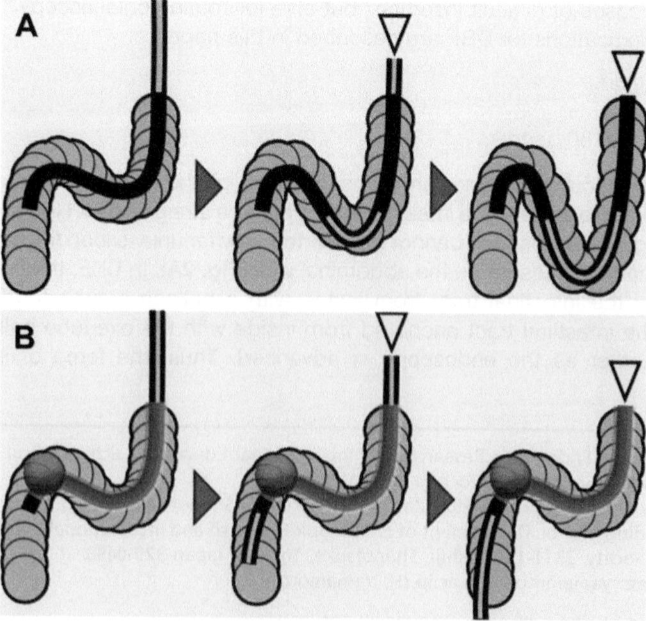

Fig. 2. (*A*) Stretching of a curved intestine during insertion of an endoscope. (*B*) Prevention of stretching of the intestine by the overtube balloon.

the endoscope is inflated to anchor the scope within the intestinal tract. The endoscope then cannot slip back on insertion of the overtube. In this fashion, the length of insertion through the small intestine is pleated back over the overtube. By repeating this procedure, deep insertion becomes possible.

TECHNOLOGY

System Composition

The system includes an endoscope capable of attachment of a balloon at the tip, a flexible overtube with a balloon attached to the tip, and a balloon controller (automatic pressure control) that controls the inflation/deflation of both balloons. A light source and a monitor are also required.

Endoscopy

In the DBE endoscope, an air channel (**Fig. 3**) is arranged so that the balloon attached to the tip can be inflated or deflated. In addition, apart from scale lines marking each 5 cm, as in a conventional endoscope, a wider white line is added as a mark to avoid over insertion when the overtube is inserted (**Fig. 4**). Over insertion may result in the balloon at the tip of the scope being stripped off.

At present, 3 types of endoscopes for DBE are on the market. The EN-450P5 (effective length 2000 mm, outer diameter 8.5 mm, forceps caliber 2.2 mm) has a thin diameter, features good flexibility with adequate rigidity, and is mainly used for diagnosis. The EN-450T5 (effective length 2000 mm, outer diameter 9.4 mm, forceps caliber 2.8 mm) can be used for various treatments because of the larger accessory channel. The EC-450BI5 (effective length 1520 mm, outer diameter 9.4 mm, forceps caliber 2.8 mm) has a shorter working length and is mainly used for the large intestine and postoperative intestinal tract. With this endoscope, most of the endoscopic retrograde cholangiopancreatography (ERCP) devices, which are too short for a 2-m scope, can be used for treatment in the bile duct system of postoperative patients with Roux-en-Y anastomosis.

The viewing angle of the EN-450P5 is 120 degrees, whereas the EN-450T5 and EC-450BI5 have a wider viewing angle of 140 degrees. The operational angle for each instrument tip is 180 degrees up–down and 160 degrees right–left, and each exhibits good operability.

Overtube

At present, 3 types of overtubes corresponding to the individual endoscopes are available. A flexible material is used for the main body to enable holding the intestinal tract while it is curved. A hydrophilic coating is applied to the outer and inner surface of the overtube to reduce friction between the endoscope and overtube lubricated by the injection of water.

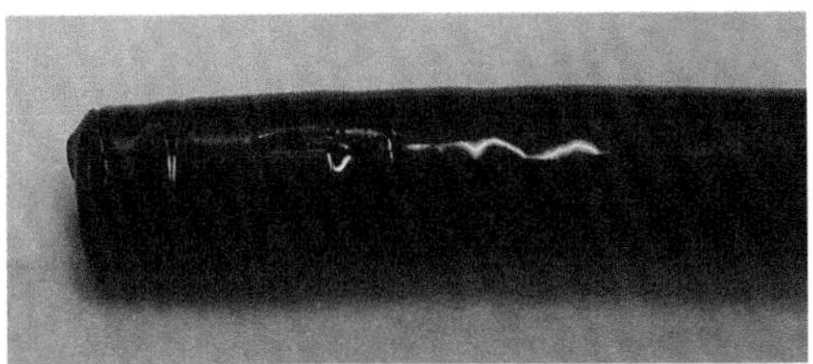

Fig. 3. Outlet of the air channel at the DBE scope tip.

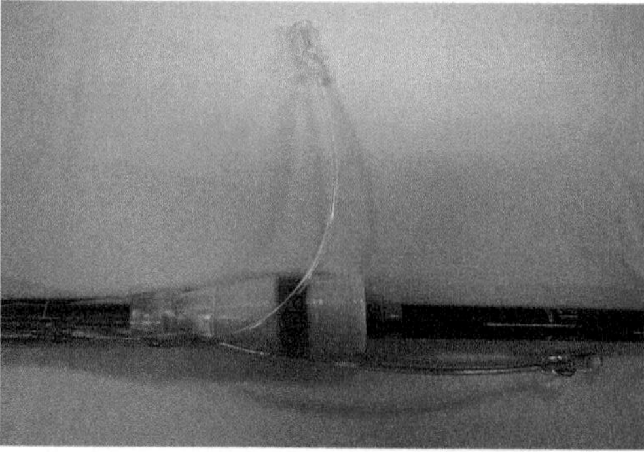

Fig. 4. The white line as the distance marker at 155 cm on the endoscope shaft.

In addition, a valve is attached to the proximal end of the overtube in a skirtlike shape (**Fig. 5**) to prevent back flow of intestinal fluid from the inside of the tube. If the surface of the main body of the endoscope is dry, friction may be generated, and in this situation a lubricating gel may be applied.

Balloon controller

The present balloon controller (PB-20) is more compact than those used previously. A simple push maneuver of the buttons on the controller can control insufflation/deflation of the air to and from the 2 balloons. A monitor is available for visual confirmation of the condition of the 2 balloons and to prevent mishandling (**Fig. 6**). The air supply to the balloons is controlled by pressure, with dilating pressure set at 45 mmHg, which is safe and effective for anchoring the intestinal tract without rupture of the small intestine, as confirmed by animal experiments. (The setting specified for the actual instrument is 5.6 kPa or lower for the air supply, to be maintained at about 6 kPa.)

Insertion Techniques

The DBE scope can be inserted anterograde or retrograde. Here, only anterograde insertion is described. The ideal shape of the small intestine for endoscope insertion is the creation of a large concentric circle. The small intestine without adhesions can move freely in the peritoneal cavity to achieve this configuration. Therefore, the endoscope should be inserted in such a way that the intestinal tract is moved toward the endoscope, and not with the endoscope chasing the intestinal tract. In particular,

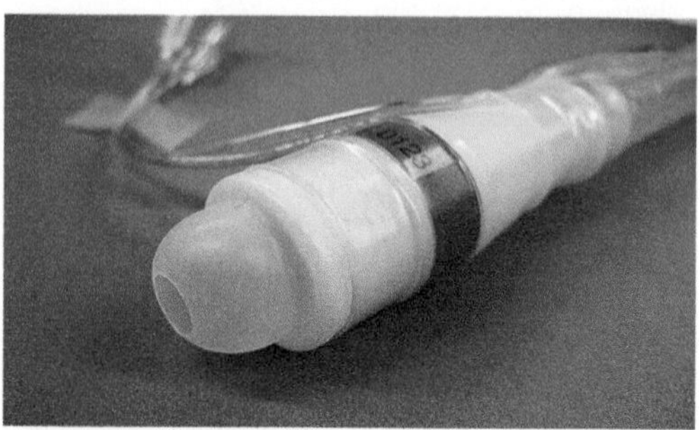

Fig. 5. Skirtlike shape back flow prevention valve.

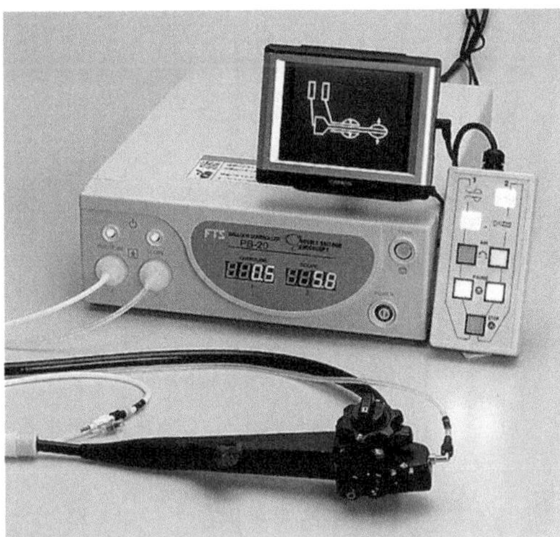

Fig. 6. Balloon controller with balloon monitor.

efficient insertion can be achieved by gently pushing while performing small back-and-forth movements (jiggling) without too much angle at the tip of the endoscope.

Excess air in the intestinal tract can be an obstacle to effective shortening of the intestinal tract. Thus, for DBE insertion, air insufflation should be kept to the minimum. The use of a plastic hood on the tip of the endoscope (**Fig. 7**) helps to minimize air insufflations. SubstitutingCO_2 for air aids efficient DBE insertion, because CO_2 is rapidly absorbed, thereby facilitating shortening of the intestinal tract.

Anterograde insertion

For insertion of the DBE into the stomach, a single operator initiates insertion of the endoscope (**Fig. 8**A). When the endoscope is passed from the incisura to the antrum, the assistant moves the overtube to the white line marked on the endoscope (**Fig. 8**B). Next, the operator inserts the endoscope from the descending limb of the duodenum to the third portion of the duodenum and inflates the balloon at the tip of the endoscope (**Fig. 8**C, D). Then the assistant moves the overtube along the endoscope to the region of the white line and inflates the overtube balloon (**Fig. 8**E, F). In the first insertion after entering the duodenum, shortening of the small intestine is not performed before proceeding to the second stroke. The endoscope is further inserted after deflating the balloon at the tip of the endoscope and then the balloon is inflated at the deepest point (**Fig. 8**G–I). In many cases, the endoscope crosses over the ligament of Treitz (duodeno-jejunal junction) at the second stroke. After deflation of the

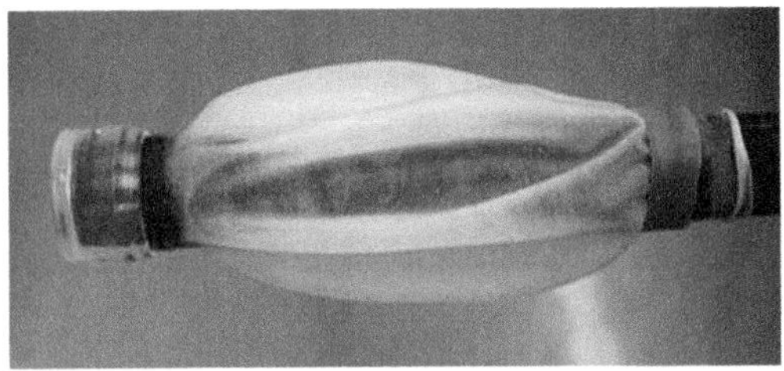

Fig. 7. Short transparent hood attached to the DBE scope.

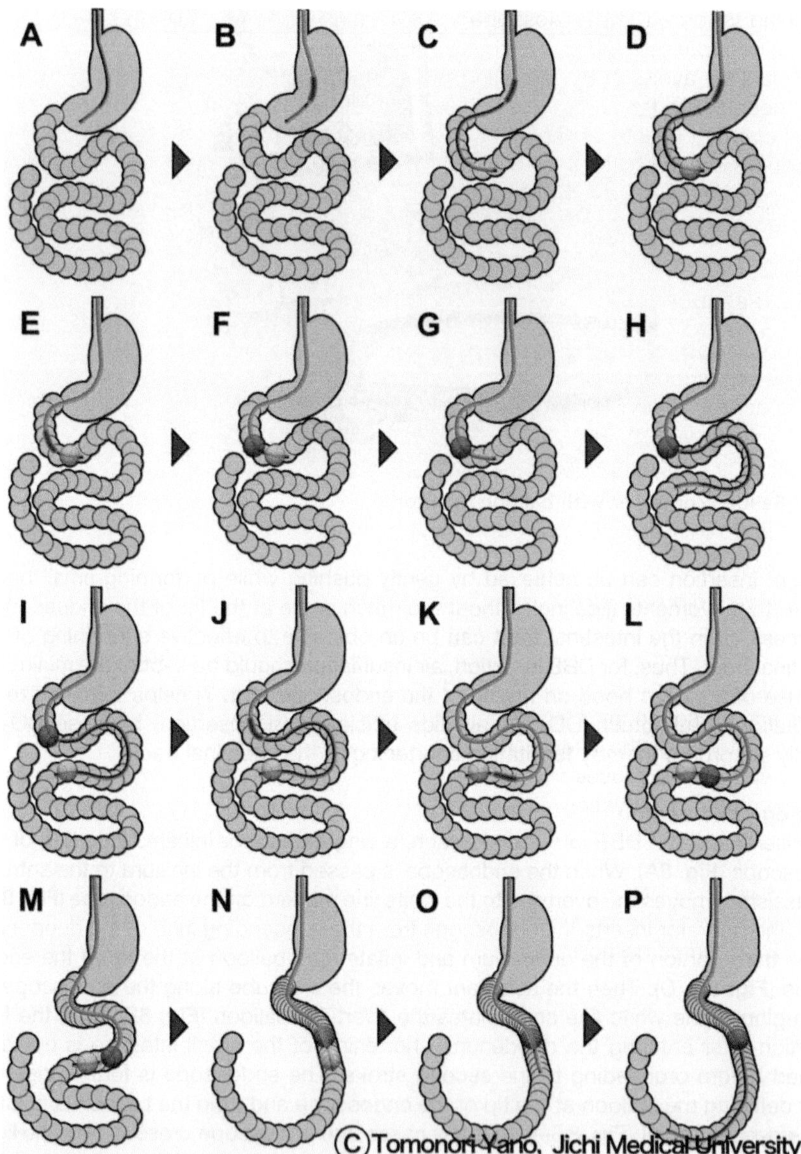

Fig. 8. (*A–P*) Insertion images through the mouth. (*Courtesy of* Tomonori Yano, Tochigi, Japan.)

overtube balloon, the overtube is moved again to the white line, and then the balloon is inflated (**Fig. 8**J–L). At this point both balloons are inflated at the end of the scope, anchoring the intestinal tract from the inside. When the endoscope and the overtube are pulled proximally, the portion of the small intestine that the endoscope has passed is pleated back over the overtube (**Fig. 8**M, N). At the same time, the intestinal tract beyond the scope is straightened. The intubated intestinal tract is further straightened by jiggling the endoscope and overtube on shortening. If the operator notes pain in the patient or resistance to the endoscope, no more shortening should be performed. If shortening is forced, the endoscope will slip back when the holding power of the balloons is surpassed. Excessive shortening may contribute to the risk of pancreatitis and should be avoided. By repeating these procedures the endoscope can be inserted deep inside the small intestine (**Fig. 8**O, P).[5]

If the operator is not familiar with this technique, it is helpful to perform maneuvers under fluoroscopic control, which allows for confirmation of the correct configuration of the scope and overtube. However, when the technique is mastered, fluoroscopy is rarely necessary.

ROLE OF THE ENDOSCOPE BALLOON

The main purpose of the endoscope balloon is to anchor the intestinal tract so that the tip of the endoscope does not slip back when the overtube is inserted. In DBE, either the endoscope balloon or the overtube balloon or both are kept inflated at all times to maintain anchorage in the intestinal tract, making steady insertion of the endoscope possible. The endoscope balloon is particularly useful for inserting the endoscope deep inside the small intestine and in cases in which insertion is difficult.

The endoscope balloon is useful not only for assisting insertion but also in the following situations.

1. Selective radiographic imaging tests: by obstructing the intestinal tract by inflation of the endoscope balloon, back flow of the contrast medium can be prevented and radiological contrast imaging in the distal intestinal tract can be performed. This technique is particularly useful for the evaluation of stenotic lesions.
2. Immersion endoscopy: the endoscope balloon can be used to facilitate observation of the interior of the intestinal tract under water by inflation and creation of an obstruction that causes water to accumulate. In some cases of small intestinal hemorrhage, observation under water allows a clear view of the bleeding point. The endoscope balloon can also be useful for observation under water during an ultrasonic examination using a miniprobe.
3. Stabilization of the endoscope in endoscopic treatment: stabilization of the endoscope tip with the endoscope balloon is useful in some cases of endoscopic therapy such as balloon dilation of intestinal stenoses.

INDICATIONS

Although DBE was developed for observation and treatment of the deep portions of the small intestine, target organs are not limited to the small intestine. DBE can be performed when it is advantageous compared with conventional endoscopy. In the small intestine, such cases include:

1. Diagnosis/treatment of obscure GI bleeding[6]
2. Diagnosis/treatment of benign and malignant lesions[7,8]
3. Diagnosis of inflammatory bowel diseases[9,10]
4. Diagnosis/treatment of stenotic lesions[11,12]

In the large intestine they include:

1. Application in cases of difficulty with insertion.[3]
2. Application to colonoscopy without sedation.[4]
3. Application to endoscopic treatment such as endoscopic submucosal dissection (ESD).

In addition, DBE is used for diagnosis/treatment of bile duct/pancreatic disease in the reconstructed intestinal tract after various surgeries.[13–16] The endoscope alone may be used as a small-caliber endoscope for colonoscopy in children and for use in a stenotic intestinal tract. Recovery of a foreign body using the overtube can be applied to any part of the intestinal tract, from the esophagus to the large intestine.

CONTRAINDICATIONS

Similar to standard endoscopy, patients with poor cardiopulmonary function, multiple comorbidities, or possible perforation are contraindications for DBE. Although there has been debate whether intestinal obstruction should be a contraindication to conventional endoscopy, DBE can be used in cases of intestinal obstruction without ischemia. In cases in which it is difficult to determine whether DBE should be performed, DBE should be performed only if the advantages of diagnosis and treatment outweigh the risks.

In children or patients who are uncooperative with testing, performance of DBE under general anesthesia should be considered.

SUMMARY

The indications, contraindications, and techniques of DBE have been described. The uniquely shaped DBE endoscope with 2 balloons, one at the tip of the endoscope and other at the tip of the overtube, make endoscopic observation and treatment possible along the entire small intestine for the first time without operative intervention. Indications for DBE include not only diseases of the small intestine but also diseases located anywhere in the digestive tract, from the esophagus to the large intestine, for which use of a small-caliber endoscope and a flexible overtube is advantageous. In the future, DBE can be expected to be useful for patients with various digestive tract diseases with the further development of DBE endoscopes, ancillary devices, and new technology.

REFERENCES

1. Yamamoto H, Sekine Y, Sato Y, et al. Total enteroscopy with a nonsurgical steerable double-balloon method. Gastrointest Endosc 2001;53:216–20.
2. Yamamoto H, Kita H, Sunada K, et al. Clinical outcomes of double-balloon endoscopy for the diagnosis and treatment of small-intestinal diseases. Clin Gastroenterol Hepatol 2004;2:1010–6.
3. Pasha SF, Harrison ME, Das A, et al. Utility of double-balloon colonoscopy for completion of colon examination after incomplete colonoscopy with conventional colonoscope. Gastrointest Endosc 2007;65:848–53.
4. Das A. Future perspective of double balloon endoscopy: newer indications. Gastrointest Endosc 2007;66:S51–3.
5. Yamamoto H, Sugano K. A new method of enteroscopy – the double-balloon method. Can J Gastroenterol 2003;17:273–4.
6. Ohmiya N, Yano T, Yamamoto H, et al. Diagnosis and treatment of obscure GI bleeding at double balloon endoscopy. Gastrointest Endosc 2007;66:S72–7.
7. Iwamoto M, Yamamoto H, Kita H, et al. Double-balloon endoscopy for ileal GI stromal tumor. Gastrointest Endosc 2005;62:440–1 [discussion: 441].
8. Kuno A, Yamamoto H, Kita H, et al. Double-balloon enteroscopy through a Roux-en-Y anastomosis for EMR of an early carcinoma in the afferent duodenal limb. Gastrointest Endosc 2004;60:1032–4.

9. Sunada K, Yamamoto H, Hayashi Y, et al. Clinical importance of the location of lesions with regard to mesenteric or antimesenteric side of the small intestine. Gastrointest Endosc 2007;66:S34–8.
10. Oshitani N, Yukawa T, Yamagami H, et al. Evaluation of deep small bowel involvement by double-balloon enteroscopy in Crohn's disease. Am J Gastroenterol 2006;101:1484–9.
11. Sunada K, Yamamoto H, Kita H, et al. Clinical outcomes of enteroscopy using the double-balloon method for strictures of the small intestine. World J Gastroenterol 2005;11:1087–9.
12. Fukumoto A, Tanaka S, Yamamoto H, et al. Diagnosis and treatment of small-bowel stricture by double balloon endoscopy. Gastrointest Endosc 2007;66: S108–12.
13. Sunada K, Yamamoto H. Double-balloon endoscopy: past, present, and future. J Gastroenterol 2009;44:1–12.
14. Kuga R, Furuya CK Jr, Hondo FY, et al. ERCP using double-balloon enteroscopy in patients with Roux-en-Y anatomy. Dig Dis 2008;26:330–5.
15. Monkemuller K, Fry LC, Bellutti M, et al. ERCP with the double balloon enteroscope in patients with Roux-en-Y anastomosis. Surg Endosc 2008; in press.
16. Chu YC, Yang CC, Yeh YH, et al. Double-balloon enteroscopy application in biliary tract disease – its therapeutic and diagnostic functions. Gastrointest Endosc 2008;68:585–91.

Single-balloon Enteroscopy

Bennie R. Upchurch, MD[a,*], John J. Vargo, MD, MPH[a,b]

KEYWORDS

- Enteroscopy • Single-balloon enteroscopy
- Gastrointestinal hemorrhage
- Double-balloon enteroscopy • Small intestine

Some of the most exciting developments in gastrointestinal (GI) endoscopy in the last decade have been capsule endoscopy and double-balloon endoscopy. These technologies have had an impact on small bowel endoscopy. Although only a small portion of the pathology affecting the small bowel is located between the ligament of Treitz and the ileocecal valve, there has been increased recognition and understanding of the diseases affecting the small intestine as technology has enhanced our ability to visualize this area of the GI tract. The term "mid gut" has been used to describe the deeper portions of the small bowel, and this area has long been considered poorly accessible to the endoscopist.[1] Standard endoscopy using traditional upper endoscopes can reach up to the second or third first portion of the duodenum. Push enteroscopy with or without the use of an overtube can reach distances of 75 to 80 cm past the ligament of Treitz. Colonoscopy in expert hands may frequently reach 10 to 20 cm beyond the ileocecal valve. Thus, most of the small bowel is inaccessible by traditional endoscopic means. In addition, radiographic studies and surgery have significant limitations with regard to diagnostic yield and invasiveness, respectively. With the development of capsule endoscopy and approval by the US Food and Drug Administration in 2001, the small bowel can now be completely visualized, abolishing the notion that the small bowel remained as a final frontier.[2] Numerous studies throughout the world have demonstrated the abilities of capsule endoscopy as a sensitive diagnostic modality.[3,4] The advent of double-balloon enteroscopy in 2001 has provided further diagnostic capabilities to investigate the diseases of the small bowel, but has also provided a necessary tool to allow therapeutic interventions, in many cases using the same techniques and tools that have been used with traditional endoscopes. In recent years, single-balloon enteroscopy has emerged as an additional enteroscopy system with a technique both familiar and unique, and

[a] Cleveland Clinic Lerner College of Medicine, 9500 Euclid Avenue, NA 21, Cleveland, OH 44195, USA
[b] Section of Therapeutic Endoscopy, Digestive Disease Institute, 9500 Euclid Avenue, A30, Cleveland Clinic, Cleveland, OH 44195, USA
* Corresponding author.
E-mail address: upchurb@ccf.org (B.R. Upchurch).

Gastrointest Endoscopy Clin N Am 19 (2009) 335–347
doi:10.1016/j.giec.2009.04.010 giendo.theclinics.com
1052-5157/09/$ – see front matter © 2009 Elsevier Inc. All rights reserved.

the ability to provide similar diagnostic and therapeutic potential to that of the double-balloon enteroscopy system. This review provides up-to-date views on this emerging technology and its application.

BACKGROUND

Conceptually, the length, tortuosity, and the tendency for the small intestine to stretch and form redundant loops are the challenges for the endoscopist to overcome with the insertion of a traditional endoscope, regardless of the length of the endoscope or the technique. Yamamoto successfully addressed the stretching of the intestine by the use of a balloon affixed to an overtube that held the bowel in place while advancing the endoscope. A second balloon affixed to the endoscope tip anchored the scope in a deeper portion of the bowel, and the balloon overtube was then advanced to meet the endoscope balloon. Both balloons were then inflated and gently pulled back to pleat the small bowel onto the overtube and the process repeated until the objective was reached.[5] This early proof of concept witnessed by Dr. Yamamoto and colleagues before the turn of the century has ushered in a new era in the performance of endoscopy, particularly in the management of small bowel disease. In fact, the use of overtubes in endoscopy has had a resurgence in recent years with the increasing acceptance of balloon-assisted enteroscopy and the Spirus overtube (Spirus Medical Inc, Stoughton, Massachusetts), which uses a novel "rotate to advance" insertion method.[6,7]

INDICATIONS

Although the list of indications for small bowel enteroscopy is continually expanding, the most common indication remains obscure GI bleeding.[1–4,6,8–14] Several current indications for small bowel enteroscopy are listed in **Table 1**. The AGA Institute Technical Review on obscure gastrointestinal bleeding defines this as bleeding from the GI tract that persists or recurs without an obvious cause after esophagogastroduodenoscopy (EGD), colonoscopy, and radiographic evaluation of the small bowel.[3] Although only 5% to 7% of obscure GI bleeding is ultimately deemed to be from the small bowel, these patients tend to have more investigations, longer periods of anemia, higher transfusion requirements, decreased quality of life, increased physician visits, and increased health care expenditure.[15] Correspondingly, the widespread use of capsule endoscopy and increasing availability of deep enteroscopy has improved our care of these patients.[3,8–10,12–15]

Guidelines published on deep enteroscopy are limited, but push enteroscopy guidelines and proposed algorithms governing the use of double-balloon enteroscopy are available.[3,7,16] Enteroscopy receives a grade B recommendation, and is seen as a complementary examination to capsule endoscopy, particularly as a therapeutic option if pathology is suspected beyond the reach of push enteroscopy.[16] Based on limited data suggesting that single-balloon enteroscopy is as useful as double-balloon enteroscopy, presumably single-balloon enteroscopy can be substituted for double-balloon enteroscopy in these algorithms (**Fig. 1**).[2,17]

SINGLE-BALLOON ENTEROSCOPY SYSTEM

The single-balloon enteroscopy system (Olympus, Tokyo, Japan) consists of the early prototype XFIF Q160Y enteroscope or the commercially available SIF Q260 enteroscope, an overtube balloon control unit (MAJ1440) and a silicone splinting tube with balloon (ST-SB-1). The enteroscope is a high-resolution video endoscope that works

Table 1
Indications for deep enteroscopy

Common (not reachable by other means)
Obscure GI bleeding
Chronic diarrhea
Iron deficiency anemia
Abnormal SBFT/CTE
Abnormal capsule endoscopy findings
Peutz-Jegher polyps
Refractory celiac sprue
Retained foreign bodies
Intestinal strictures
Crohn disease
Large small bowel mass needing resection
Unusual
Mid gut carcinoids
ERCP in Roux-en-Y situations
Abdominal symptoms in gastric bypass patients
Protein-wasting enteropathy
Jejunal stenting
PEG placement in gastric bypass anatomy
Previously failed colonoscopy
No/not yet established
When push enteroscopy is probably adequate
When ileoscopy is sufficient for Crohn evaluation
Abdominal pain alone
Small bowel obstruction

Abbreviations: CTE, computed tomographic enterography; ERCP, endoscopic retrograde cholangiopancreatography; GI, gastrointestinal; PEG, percutaneous endoscopic gastrostomy; SBFT, small bowel follow-through.

Data from Lo S. Technical matters in double balloon enteroscopy. Gastrointest Endosc 2007;66:S15–8.

with current Olympus EVIS processors (240, 260, and SL). Narrowband imaging is available with the EVIS EXERA II system. It has an outer diameter of 9.2 mm, a working length of 2000 mm, and channel size of 2.8 mm. The field of view is 140°, and the depth of view is 3 to 100 mm. The splinting tube is a silicone overtube with an inflatable balloon affixed at its distal tip, and a small raised circumferential tab on its proximal end. Some investigators suggest the tab at the end of the proximal splinting tube enhances the user's control when sliding the overtube along the enteroscope.[18] The distal end of the tube is radiopaque, which can be beneficial for confirming overtube position with fluoroscopic guidance. The inner diameter of the tube is 11 mm, the outer diameter is 13.2 mm, the working length of the splinting tube is 1320 mm, and the total length is 1400 mm. With the addition of a small amount of water through a small port on the proximal end of the splinting tube, a hydrophilic coating enhances the sliding of the enteroscope through the overtube. Additional water can be flushed throughout the procedure, as needed to lessen friction or wash away debris that collects between the enteroscope and the splinting tube. The balloon is inflated and deflated by a balloon control unit with a pressure range of −6 kPa to +6 kPa. This pressure allows for atraumatic traction on the small bowel mucosa. There is an alarm and pause safety feature that alerts the user to elevated pressures. Once activated, this alarm feature must be reset to continue, and the balloon pressure is maintained at a prescribed level to avoid injury. The overtube balloon control unit has one button for inflation, one button for

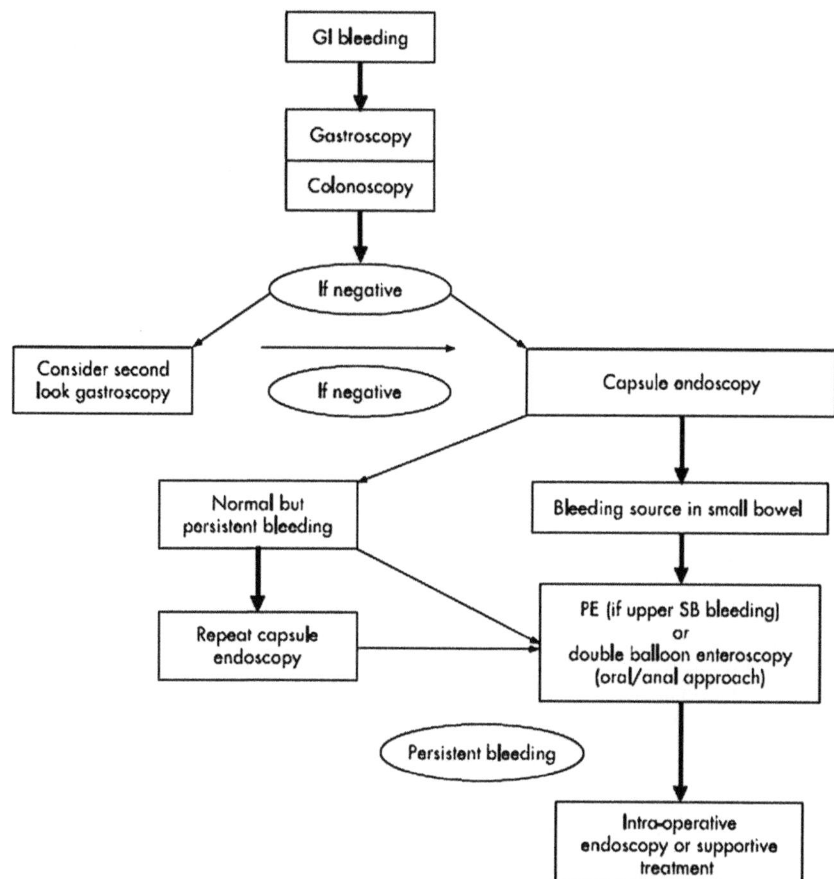

Fig. 1. Proposed role of capsule endoscopy and enteroscopy in obscure gastrointestinal bleeding. (*Reproduced from* Sidhu S, Sanders DS, Morris AJ. Guidelines on small bowel enteroscopy and capsule endoscopy in adults. Gut 2008;57:125–36; with permission from BMJ Publishing Group Ltd.)

deflation, and a third control for the pause/cancel feature. All features are available on the unit or the wired remote control module (*courtesy of* olympusamerica.com).

INSERTION TECHNIQUE

The insertion method is similar to that of double-balloon enteroscopy and has been described by others.[5,8,13,18,19] The method used by Tsujikawa and colleagues, outlined in brief, involves the grasping of the intestine by first angulating the tip of the scope after the initial deep insertion to the duodenum. Then with the balloon deflated, the splinting tube is advanced over the scope until it reaches the bending section of the scope. The balloon is then inflated and the scope and splinting tube are pulled back to shorten the bowel. The angulation of the tip of the scope and hooking behind a fold if possible serve to achieve the same stabilizing effect of the scope tip balloon of the double-balloon system. The endoscope can then be further advanced beyond its position near the end of the splinting tube while the inflated balloon holds the small bowel in place, thereby allowing the pushing force of the operator applied to the endoscope to be transmitted to the distal end of the endoscope without further stretching of the intestine.[20] Then in a similar fashion to the double-balloon technique, the overtube balloon is used to pleat the small bowel onto the overtube. With serial inflations and deflations of the overtube balloon, and hooking and grasping with the endoscope tip, the endoscope is advanced deep into the small bowel with the "push and pull" technique. The depth of insertion can be estimated by counting folds in 10-cm increments during withdrawal or counting the 40-cm push and pull reduction cycles, as described by May and colleagues.[13] When the entire small bowel needs to be visualized, endoclips or tattoo ink are used to mark the limit of the initial study; total enteroscopy is achieved by reaching the mark from the opposite approach on a subsequent examination. Ideally, as in double-balloon endoscopy, the balloon is not inflated in the area of the proximal duodenum to avoid trauma to the papilla and lessen the risk of pancreatitis.

There have been modifications of the single-balloon enteroscopy insertion technique by others. Hartmann and colleagues described an alternative method of single-balloon enteroscopy insertion. At the point of reinflation of the splinting tube balloon near the end of the endoscope, rather than doing the "pull back maneuver" with the splinting tube and angulated scope tip, the angulation is released and the endoscope steered to find the lumen. The overtube with the balloon still inflated is pulled back while simultaneously pushing the endoscope forward. These investigators believed this method works best with two examiners and is more efficient without sacrificing the depth of insertion or safety.[21] Although arriving at this alternative method independently, Manno and colleagues performed four procedures using the conventional technique described by Tsujikawa, and four procedures using the alternative method described by Hartmann to prospectively evaluate the two techniques. In this study, the alternative method described by Hartmann allowed a lower mean procedure time (58.3 versus 65.9 minutes for the oral approach and 66.4 versus 74.1 minutes for the anal approach, using the alternative technique and the conventional technique, respectively). The depth of insertion did not differ significantly between the conventional and alternative techniques (240 versus 250 cm for the oral approach and 180 versus 160 cm for the anal approach, using the alternative technique and the conventional techniques, respectively). The results were not felt to correlate with the experience of the operators, as both endoscopists were experienced with the performance of double-balloon enteroscopy.[22]

PREPARATION AND SEDATION

No preparation is needed in most cases for single-balloon enteroscopy by the oral route. However, in the author's institution, 2 L of a polyethylene glycol (PEG) bowel preparation is used for all inpatients and the standard 4 L bowel preparation for inpatient and outpatient retrograde examinations. The use of the limited bowel preparation for oral examinations in the typically nonambulatory inpatients has improved visibility deep in the small bowel, where dark bile and debris can sometimes compromise deep enteroscopy and capsule examinations. Patient tolerance is variable, however, as many have difficulty with the sheer volume of a PEG preparation, and find it particularly arduous and unconventional before an oral endoscopic examination. Reports in the literature seem to demonstrate similar heterogeneity to double-balloon enteroscopy, with the use of general anesthesia, propofol monitored anesthesia care (MAC), and conscious sedation in the performance of single-balloon enteroscopy.[17–23]

DISCUSSION

Just as double-balloon enteroscopy has literally extended our therapeutic interventions deep into the small bowel, single-balloon enteroscopy has similarly shown an ability to offer nearly every treatment option available through standard endoscopes. With an identical working length, and similar platform to the double-balloon enteroscopy system, devices developed for these enteroscopy systems are compatible. Understandably, double-balloon enteroscopy is the de facto standard in deep enteroscopy that must be used to evaluate single-balloon enteroscopy. Early reports on the use of single-balloon enteroscopy since its appearance in 2006 involving the prototype XSIF Q160 and its commercially available successor, the SIF Q180, have suggested a high diagnostic yield and similar therapeutic potential to that of the double-balloon endoscope. Several series examining the usefulness of single-balloon enteroscopy are summarized in **Table 2**.[18,20,24–31] Ohtsuka and colleagues helped to develop the single-balloon enteroscope in cooperation with Olympus Medical Systems and are credited with the first comparison of single-balloon with double-balloon enteroscopy. They performed 102 procedures in 65 patients with suspected small intestinal disease. Seventy-nine of the procedures were done with the single-balloon enteroscopy system and 11 with double-balloon enteroscopy. Antegrade and retrograde procedures were performed. Thirty-six of the patients were referred for suspected GI bleeding. Single-balloon enteroscopy was performed by the single person insertion method in most cases, whereas double-balloon enteroscopy required two operators. In 21 cases the cause of bleeding was identified, but in nine cases no explanation for bleeding was found. Examination time for antegrade insertion was 65.3 minutes for single-balloon enteroscopy and 74 minutes for antegrade double-balloon endoscopy. Single-balloon enteroscopy retrograde insertion averaged 57.5 minutes and 56.3 minutes for retrograde double-balloon enteroscopy. There were no complications. Depth of insertion was not recorded, as is the case with many reported series. The investigators concluded it was easy to set up the single-balloon enteroscopy system and perform the procedure with a single operator. Although not specifically reported, they felt they were able to achieve a high diagnostic yield and obtain high-quality images with the single-balloon enteroscope, using their experience with the double-balloon enteroscopy system as a point of reference.[17]

Ramchandani and colleagues studied 60 patients with suspected small bowel disease using the prototype single-balloon enteroscopy system. All patients underwent antegrade examinations; 10 underwent antegrade and retrograde procedures. Depth of insertion was determined by carefully recording the length of the scope inserted during each push and pull maneuver. Fluoroscopy was used intermittently. Enteroscopy was performed under MAC. Mean procedure time was 63 minutes. The mean depth of insertion was 260 cm beyond the ligament of Treitz. Total enteroscopy was possible in 5 out of 10 cases (50%). Indications for single-balloon enteroscopy included obscure GI bleeding,[18] or chronic abdominal pain with abnormal imaging studies,[21] malabsorption syndrome,[11] polyposis syndromes,[9] and foreign body.[1] Enteroscopic findings were arteriovenous malformations (AVMs),[7] ulcers,[15] polyps,[6] diffuse enteritis,[2] mass lesions,[3] and effacement of jejunual folds.[3] Diagnostic yield in cases of obscure GI bleeding, chronic abdominal pain, and malabsorption syndrome were 77%, 61%, and 63%, respectively.[29]

Reports of ERCP in altered anatomy patients using the single-balloon enteroscope seem to be frequent in the recent literature.[28,32,33] Dellon and colleagues successfully performed ERCP in three of four patients with Roux-en-Y anastomosis for various indications using the single-balloon enteroscope to traverse the biliary limb. The ERCP

Table 2
Single-balloon enteroscopy series

Series	Number of Patients/ Cases	Number of Cases with GI Bleeding	Mean Procedure Time (min)			Depth of Insertion (cm)		Rate of Total Enteroscopy (%)	Overall Yield (%)	Yield in GI Bleeding (%)	Complications
			Antegrade	Retrograde	Overall	Antegrade	Retrograde				
K. Ohtsuka	30/48	14	68.3	54.7	—	N/A	N/A	71	—	46	0
T. Tsujikawa	41/78	12	62.8	70.4	—	270 (from pylorus)	199	25 (43 if no prior surgery)	54	33	Aspiration pneumonia, mucosal tear, peritonitis
T. Kawamura	27/37	11	83	90	—	N/A	N/A	12.5	40.7	—	1 perforation
M. Ramchanani	60	18	—	—	63	260	N/A	50	—	77	0
P. Okolo	17	4	—	—	33	193	N/A	0	—	75	0
M. Lapalus	10	5	—	—	120	N/A	N/A	N/A	—	60 treatment rendered	0
K. Kobayashi	14/17	6	—	—	—	N/A	N/A	"I near total enteroscopy"	65	—	0
L. Helmstaeder	28/32	32	57	62	—	239	165	N/A	62.5	50 treatment rendered	0
J. Forman	26/28	28	—	—	54.9	N/A	N/A	N/A	—	69.2	Fever despite prophylactic antibiotics in patient with prosthetic valve

that was unsuccessful was due to inability to see the enteroenteroscopy site. Conscious sedation was used successfully for all patients. Procedure times were somewhat longer than for standard ERCP.[33] The breadth of clinical applications seems to be as comprehensive for single-balloon enteroscopy as that of double-balloon enteroscopy and likely will increase over time.[2,34–36] The use of single-balloon enteroscopy in the management of small bowel Crohn strictures, the placement of jejunal feeding tubes, and gastrostomy tube placement in altered surgical anatomy will be likely areas to target, as they have been successful for double-balloon enteroscopy.[11]

Single-balloon enteroscopy has established itself as an effective tool in the management of patients with small bowel disease. In the series included in **Table 2**, the yield of single-balloon enteroscopy was 58.5% in GI bleeding and 50 to 60% of the cases were therapeutic. This diagnostic yield and therapeutic impact seems to be comparable to many reported series on double-balloon enteroscopy, particularly for studies focusing on obscure GI bleeding. In a study by May and colleagues,[12] the average insertion depth for double-balloon enteroscopy was 230 cm. The overall diagnostic yield was 73%. In a retrospective review of 237 cases at six tertiary centers in the United States by Mehdizadeh and colleagues, average double-balloon enteroscopy peroral insertion depth was 360 cm from the pylorus. Retrograde procedures with a successful small bowel intubation examined an average of 181 cm.[37] A systematic review of the literature to determine the diagnostic and therapeutic yield of double-balloon enteroscopy in patients with obscure GI bleeding by Pasha and colleagues,[10] analyzed 13 studies (n = 906). In this analysis a potential bleeding source was detected in 66% of patients.

In patients in whom a target has been identified, either by traditional imaging or capsule endoscopy, the location and anticipated depth of the lesion may guide the choice of the enteroscopy platform, if more than one is available. In addition, the route of insertion is directed by the initial localization. In some cases, clinical parameters may guide the enteroscopy without the need for an initial diagnostic study. One common scenario would be overt bleeding with frank hematochezia and no colonic source seen on recent colonoscopy. In this setting, without signs or symptoms to suggest a torrential upper GI bleed, proceeding with a retrograde enteroscopy may be the most appropriate next step clinically.

From available data, there may be some minor limitations on depth of insertion with single-balloon enteroscopy compared with the average maximal depth reached with double-balloon enteroscopy. In examinations directed by capsule or other imaging, with lesions localized to the proximal or mid small bowel, or perhaps the more distal ileum, a successful deep insertion with either enteroscopy system would likely suffice to reach and address pathology. Conversely, when the pathology is localized to the distal jejunum or proximal ileum, or when total enteroscopy is needed in a patient with AVMs throughout the small bowel, it would be desirable to have an enteroscopy platform that could more commonly accomplish total enteroscopy, thereby offering the opportunity to potentially effect therapeutics throughout the small bowel. Double-balloon enteroscopy might have an advantage in this setting if it consistently has deeper insertion depth. Nonetheless, there have been numerous studies in Occidental populations that suggest a low rate of complete enteroscopy with double-balloon enteroscopy compared with studies from the Orient. This brings into question whether it is a realistic expectation for the endoscopist with either of the enteroscopy systems to consistently accomplish total enteroscopy in Occidental patients.[6,8–14,37]

COMPLICATIONS

Complications of single-balloon enteroscopy reported in the literature include the usual risks related to sedation and conventional endoscopy, but to date have not included reports of pancreatitis as seen with double-balloon enteroscopy (see **Table 2**). This may be related in part to the recognition of this risk early in the performance of double-balloon enteroscopy, and the subsequent caution that has been exercised to avoid inflating any enteroscope balloon in the area of the ampulla. Over time, however, as the volume of these procedures increase, it would be expected that similar complications will arise with single-balloon enteroscopy as those seen with double-balloon enteroscopy. In discussions of informed consent, it would be advisable to include the potential for pancreatitis with any deep enteroscopy procedure, particularly with the use of a balloon overtube. The risk of postprocedure abdominal pain and ileus might also be incorporated into these discussions, if they prove to be reported occasionally as they have been with double-balloon enteroscopy. Using carbon dioxide (CO_2) for insufflation rather than air has been reported by some to cause less postprocedure pain, and possibly to enhance the depth of insertion in double-balloon enteroscopy.[11] This concept clearly could be applied to each deep enteroscopy platform, and deserves further prospective studies. Patients who are allergic to latex should avoid double-balloon enteroscopy due to the latex balloons, but can be successfully evaluated with single-balloon enteroscopy, as the splinting tube and balloon are made from silicone.

ADDITIONAL CONCERNS

There have been several concerns raised on the use of deep enteroscopy platforms. These include the use of resources, particularly the time to perform the procedure, the number of endoscopic personnel, setup time, cost of equipment, and reimbursement. In reported series, the time to perform double-balloon enteroscopy and single-balloon enteroscopy varies depending on the series, and perhaps the experience of the operator.[10,37] The learning curve may not be as steep for single-balloon enteroscopy as that described with double-balloon enteroscopy.[11,17–20,22,24–27,29,30] Single-balloon and double-balloon enteroscopy systems can be used by a single user with minor adaptation of the technique. An assistant to control the splinting tube while the endoscopist controls the enteroscope is more typical, however, and this second operator can vary at different centers from a nurse or fellow to the use of two physician operators. Setup time is shorter with the single-balloon enteroscopy system, without the need to install the scope tip balloon used with the double-balloon enteroscope. Some investigators have suggested that single-balloon enteroscopy is more intuitive to learn and more efficient.[17–20,26] If the depth of insertion with single-balloon enteroscopy is a significant limitation, these advantages would be nullified, except in cases when the anticipated pathology is deemed within reach. With double-balloon enteroscopy, the additional setup time and the additional time for two balloon cycles rather than one, the somewhat more cumbersome balloon control panel, and at times overly flexible scope, may all be forgivable when the location of the lesion is deemed to be more likely reachable only with the double-balloon enteroscope. Comparison studies between these two systems are needed to confirm whether the double-balloon system offers improved overall clinical usefulness. If so, then a slightly longer setup time and longer procedure time may be an acceptable compromise.

One reason the single-balloon enteroscope is believed to have less pleating ability, and therefore less potential depth of insertion, is that the hooking of the bowel with the endoscope tip on the single-balloon enteroscope is not as effective a grasping maneuver as with the scope tip balloon on the double-balloon enteroscope. Fortunately, there do not seem to be an increased number of mucosal tears or perforation related to the "pullback maneuver" with single-balloon enteroscopy using the hooked scope tip rather than the scope tip balloon on the double-balloon enteroscope. In the author's experience, the stiffer nature of the Olympus single-balloon enteroscope compared with the double-balloon enteroscope is an attribute when traversing the colon for retrograde studies, without the need for a stiffening wire. Clearly, there are unique attributes to each of these platforms that must be taken into consideration with their application in clinical practice.

COST

Capital expenditures for both enteroscopy systems can be substantial. The enteroscope alone can cost many thousands of dollars ($37,500 for the Olympus enteroscope and $47,400 for the Fujinon therapeutic enteroscope).[7] Ideally, the equipment would be compatible with the endoscopist's current endoscopy system to avoid the need to purchase an entirely new endoscopic platform. With a working length of more than 2 m, many of the standard devices such as biopsy forceps, snares, and catheters are too short. Equipment manufacturers have been gradually improving the range of devices available for these long enteroscopes. Even with the appropriate length, however, equipment that has moving parts or thin flexible shafts is not always reliable when used deep in the small bowel. Even in expert hands, interventional procedures can become lengthy and tedious when the objective is reached but none of the available tools will extrude from the scope or deploy once in the lumen. Lubricants such as vegetable oil, silicone, or simple water-soluble lubricants injected down the accessory channel may facilitate passage of therapeutic devices through the enteroscope.

REIMBURSEMENT

Reimbursement for deep enteroscopy is a major challenge for the endoscopist, as there are currently no specific billing codes for single-balloon or double-balloon enteroscopy procedures. A recent American Society for Gastrointestinal Endoscopy (ASGE) Technology Status Report included a summary of available billing codes for enteroscopy. Current Procedural Terminology (CPT) codes 44360 to 44373 encompass "small intestinal endoscopy, enteroscopy beyond the second portion of the duodenum, not including the ileum ..." and codes 44376 to 44397 refer to "small intestinal endoscopy, enteroscopy, beyond the second portion of the duodenum, including the ileum." For antegrade single-balloon or double-balloon enteroscopy, the jejunal codes (44360 to 44373) or the ileal codes (44376 to 44397) can be used. These can be used in conjunction with the standard codes for EGD (43235 to 43259) if the EGD is necessary for more than transit to the deep small bowel, such as for biopsy, ablation, or polypectomy within reach of a standard upper endoscope. For the retrograde procedures with deep ileal intubation, ileal codes (44376 to 44397) can be combined with colonoscopy codes (45378 to 45385) if the colonoscopy entails more than transit to the ileum, with therapeutic intervention provided in the colon. When using the push enteroscopy codes, there is a substantial discrepancy between the level of reimbursement and the amount of time and technical difficulty in the performance of the deep enteroscopy procedures in comparison with push enteroscopy. The 22 modifier can be used with the primary CPT code for the unusual procedural services. Documentation should reflect the increased degree of difficulty, increased duration, along with the usual comparisons. The code for fluoroscopy (76003) with a 26 modifier should also be documented when used.[7] In some cases, these efforts may result in improved reimbursement.

SUMMARY

Single-balloon enteroscopy has emerged as a viable alternative to double-balloon enteroscopy in the management of small bowel disease. Technically, it is easier to perform, may be more efficient, and in the limited literature available, seems to provide similar diagnostic and therapeutic yield when compared with double-balloon enteroscopy. The incremental increased depth of insertion of double-balloon enteroscopy over that of single-balloon enteroscopy may not fully explain the higher yield reported in some studies. Studies that fully compare these two platforms are needed.

MAJOR POINTS

1. The most common indication for deep enteroscopy is obscure GI bleeding.
2. Enteroscopy has an important role in the evaluation of suspected small bowel disease.
3. Single-balloon enteroscopy may be more intuitive, easier to set up, and more efficient than double-balloon enteroscopy, but has a slightly less maximal depth of insertion.
4. Single-balloon enteroscopy has similar diagnostic and therapeutic yield to that of double-balloon enteroscopy, particularly in obscure GI bleeding.
5. Prospective comparative studies are needed to determine if one deep enteroscopy system is superior to the other.

REFERENCES

1. Ell C, May A. Mid-gastrointestinal bleeding: capsule endoscopy and push-and-pull enteroscopy give rise to a new medical term. Endoscopy 2006;38:73–5.
2. Upchurch B, Vargo J. Small bowel enteroscopy. Rev Gastroenterol Disord 2008;8(3):169–77.
3. Raju G, Gerson L, Das A, et al. American Gastroenterological Association (AGA) Institute technical review on obscure gastrointestinal bleeding. Gastroenterology 2007;133:1697–717.
4. Pennazio M, Eisen G, Goldfarb N. ICCE consensus for obscure gastrointestinal bleeding. Endoscopy 2005;37:1046–50.
5. Yamamoto H, Sekine Y, Sato Y, et al. Total enteroscopy with a nonsurgical steerable double-balloon method. Gastrointest Endosc 2001;53:216–20.
6. Akerman P, Cantero D, Avila J, et al. The spiral enteroscopy experience in 101 consecutive patients: safety and efficacy using the discovery SB. Gastrointest Endosc 2008;67(5):AB92–3.
7. DiSario J, Petersen B, Tierney W, et al. Enteroscopes. Gastrointest Endosc 2007;66:872–80.
8. May A, Nachbar L, Wardak A, et al. Double-balloon enteroscopy: preliminary experience in patients with obscure gastrointestinal bleeding or chronic abdominal pain. Endoscopy 2003;35:985–91.
9. Heine GDN, Hadithi M, Groenen MJM, et al. Double-balloon enteroscopy: indications, diagnostic yield, and complications in a series of 275 patients with suspected small-bowel disease. Endoscopy 2006;38:42–8.

10. Pasha SF, Leighton JA, Das A, et al. Diagnostic yield and therapeutic utility of double-balloon enteroscopy (DBE) in patients with obscure gastrointestinal bleeding (OGIB): a systematic review. Gastrointest Endosc 2007;65:AB366 [abstract].
11. Lo S. Technical matters in double balloon enteroscopy. Gastrointest Endosc 2007;66:S15–8.
12. May A, Nachbar L, Schneider M, et al. Prospective comparison of push enteroscopy and push-and-pull enteroscopy in patients with suspected small-bowel bleeding. Am J Gastroenterol 2006;101:2016–24.
13. May A, Ell C. Push-and-pull enteroscopy using the double-balloon technique/double-balloon enteroscopy. Dig Liver Dis 2006;38:932–8.
14. May A. Current status of double balloon enteroscopy with focus on the Wiesbaden results. Gastrointest Endosc 2007;66:S12–4.
15. Lin S, Rockey D. Obscure gastrointestinal bleeding. In: Rockey DC, editor. Gastroenterol Clin N Am. Philadelphia: W B Saunders Company; 2005. p. 679–98.
16. Sidhu S, Sanders DS, Morris AJ, et al. Guidelines on small bowel enteroscopy and capsule endoscopy in adults. Gut 2008;57:125–36.
17. Ohtsuka K, Kashida H, Kodama K, et al. Observation and treatment of small bowel diseases using single balloon endoscope. Gastrointest Endosc 2008;67:AB271 [abstract].
18. Ohtsuka K, Kashida H, Kodama K. Diagnosis and treatment of small bowel diseases with a newly developed single balloon endoscope (new instrument and technique). Dig Liver Dis 2008;20:134–7.
19. Tsujikawa T, Saito Y, Fujiyma Y. Single balloon enteroscopy: is it feasible? Tech Gastrointest Endosc 2008;10:62–5.
20. Tsujikawa T, Saitoh Y, Andoh A, et al. Novel single-balloon enteroscopy for diagnosis and treatment of the small intestine: preliminary experiences. Endoscopy 2008;40:11–5.
21. Hartmann D, Eickhoff A, Tamm R, et al. Balloon-assisted enteroscopy using a single-balloon technique. Endoscopy 2007;39:E276 [comment].
22. Manno M, Mussetto A, Conigliaro R. Preliminary results of alternative simultaneous technique for single-balloon enteroscopy. Endoscopy 2008;40:538 [letter].
23. Vargo JJ, Upchurch B, Dumot JA, et al. Clinical utility of the Olympus single-balloon enteroscope: the initial U.S. experience. Gastrointest Endosc 2007;65:AB90 [abstract].
24. Forman J, Karp B, Uradomo L, et al. Single balloon enteroscopy of the small bowel: diagnostic and therapeutic yield in patients with obscure gastrointestinal bleeding. Gastrointest Endosc 2007;65:AB172 [abstract].
25. Helmstaedter L, Hartmann D, Eickhoff A, et al. First experiences with the Olympus single balloon enteroscopy system. Gastrointest Endosc 2008;67:AB298 [abstract].
26. Kobayashi K, Haruki S, Yokoyama K, et al. Clinical experience with a new model single-balloon enteroscope (XSIF-Q260Y) for the diagnosis and treatment of small-intestinal diseases. Gastrointest Endosc 2007;65:AB162 [abstract].
27. Lapalus M, Ponchon T, Chemali M, et al. Single-balloon enteroscopy: a preliminary experience. Gastrointest Endosc 2006;65:AB184 [abstract].
28. Okolo PI, Lauder N. Single balloon augmented enteroscopy (SBAE): initial experience at a single institution. Gastrointest Endosc 2007;65:AB341 [abstract].
29. Ramchandani M, Reddy D, Rao G, et al. Diagnostic yield and therapeutic impact of single balloon enteroscopy; a series of 60 patients with suspected small bowel disease. Gastrointest Endosc 2008;67:AB269 [abstract].

30. Kawamura T, Yasuda K, Cho E, et al. Clinical evaluation of newly developed single balloon enteroscopy. Gastrointest Endosc 2007;65:1112–6.
31. Nista E, Riccioni M, Spada C, et al. A new method of enteroscopy: the single-balloon enteroscope. Gastrointest Endosc 2007;65:AB174 [abstract].
32. Monkemuller K, Fry L, Belluti M, et al. ERCP using single-balloon instead of double-balloon enteroscopy in patients with Roux-en-Y anastomosis. Endoscopy 2008;40:E19–20.
33. Dellon ES, Kohn GP, Morgan DR, et al. Endoscopic retrograde cholangiopancreatography with single-balloon enteroscopy is feasible in patients with a prior Roux-en-Y anastomosis. Dig Dis Sci 2008;. Available at: ncbi.nlm.nih.gov. Accessed September, 2008.
34. Tominaga K, Lida T, Nakamura Y, et al. Small intestinal perforation of endoscopically unrecognized lesions during peroral single-balloon enteroscopy. Endoscopy 2008;40:E213–4.
35. Yumori A, Okubo H, Takahashi H, et al. Gastrointestinal: mantle cell lymphoma diagnosed by balloon enteroscopy. J Gastroenterol Hepatol 2008;23:1623 [comment].
36. de Melo S. Single-balloon enteroscopy-guided hemostasis of an anastomotic ulcer in a patient with simultaneous enteric-drained pancreas-kidney transplant. Endoscopy 2008;40:E164 [comment].
37. Mehdizadeh S, Han N, Cheng D, et al. Success rate of retrograde double-balloon enteroscopy. Gastrointest Endosc 2007;65:633–9.

Balloon Enteroscopy: Single- and Double-Balloon Enteroscopy

Andrea May, MD, PhD

KEYWORDS

- Double-balloon enteroscopy • Single-balloon enteroscopy
- Balloon-guided enteroscopy • Small-bowel endoscopy
- Push-and-pull enteroscopy

Until only a few years ago, it was not possible to access most of the small bowel using endoscopic techniques that avoided the need for surgery. Video capsule endoscopy and balloon enteroscopy thus represent decisive breakthroughs in this field. Capsule endoscopy is a safe method, which, in most cases, allows endoscopic visualization of the entire small bowel. A substantial disadvantage of the method is the inability to obtain histologic samples and carry out endoscopic treatments. In addition, the interpretation of nonspecific findings is not easy in some cases and requires confirmation and checking using a second procedure.

Flexible enteroscopy using push enteroscopy and balloon enteroscopy is a more invasive procedure in comparison with capsule endoscopy. However, it provides all the advantages of conventional endoscopy. Push enteroscopy became established in the 1980s, but it is associated with only a limited depth of penetration into the small bowel. This limitation was overcome through the development of balloon enteroscopy.[1,2] In optimal cases, the entire small bowel, or at least considerable proportions of it, can be visualized using balloon enteroscopy (usually by combining the oral and anal examinations). Depending on the endoscopist's level of experience, the rate of complete enteroscopy using the double-balloon method is around 40% to 80% (maximum 86%).[3,4] With single-balloon enteroscopy, the rates are currently up to a maximum of 25%.[5] In 2001, the DBE system developed by Dr. Yamamoto was presented for the first time in Japan, and in 2003 by the author's own research group in Germany.[6,7] In the meantime, the system has become established throughout the world for diagnostic and therapeutic small-bowel examinations, and it is now being used widely in routine clinical work. In addition to the classic indication for small-bowel endoscopy, the DBE technique has a variety of other potential uses as well, for

Department of Internal Medicine II, HSK Wiesbaden, Teaching Hospital-Johannes Gutenberg University, Ludwig-Erhard-Strasse 100, 65199 Wiesbaden, Germany
E-mail address: andrea.may@hsk-wiesbaden.de

Gastrointest Endoscopy Clin N Am 19 (2009) 349–356
doi:10.1016/j.giec.2009.04.003 giendo.theclinics.com
1052-5157/09/$ – see front matter © 2009 Elsevier Inc. All rights reserved.

example, in difficult colonoscopies, or for access to the pancreatic and biliary tract in patients with a surgically modified gastrointestinal tract, or for access to the stomach in patients who have undergone obesity surgery. Another balloon enteroscopy system was recently introduced that is equipped with only one balloon at the tip of the overtube and is, therefore, known as single-balloon enteroscopy (SBE).[5] The two systems and their potential clinical applications are briefly presented in the following sections.

DOUBLE-BALLOON ENTEROSCOPY

The double-balloon enteroscopy (DBE) system (Fujinon, Inc, Saitama, Japan) consists of a high-resolution video endoscope, with a working length of 200 cm and a flexible overtube made of polyurethane. Latex balloons are attached at the tip of the enteroscopy and also on the overtube, and can be filled with air or emptied using a pressure-controlled pump. The principle of the DBE technique is based on alternating pushing and pulling maneuvers, allowing the small bowel to be threaded onto the overtube step by step.[5,6] Two different types of devices are currently available with the double-balloon system: the EN450-P5 model, with a working channel of 2.2 mm and an outer diameter of 8.5 mm, and the EN450-T5 model, with a working channel of 2.8 mm and an outer diameter of 9.4 mm. The corresponding overtubes have diameters of 12.2 and 13.2 mm respectively, with an overall length of 145 cm.

SINGLE-BALLOON ENTEROSCOPY

The SBE system was recently introduced (Olympus, Inc, Tokyo, Japan). The enteroscope (XSIF Q260Y) is also a high-resolution video endoscope, with a working length of 200 cm. The enteroscope is equipped with a working channel that is 2.8 mm in diameter, and its outer diameter is 9.2 mm. The overtube has an overall length of 140 cm, consists of silicone, and has a latex-free balloon made of silicone at its distal end. In contrast to the DBE system, a balloon is not attached to the tip of the enteroscope, and stable positioning in the small bowel is achieved during withdrawal of the scope by angling the tip of the endoscope. Insufflation of the overtube balloon is performed using a pressure-controlled pump.

In principle, the double-balloon system can, of course, also be used as a single-balloon enteroscope, by dispensing with the balloon attached to the enteroscope tip.[8,9]

EXAMINATION PROCEDURE OF DBE AND SBE

For both DBE and SBE, the examination procedures are described in detail elsewhere.[2,5,6] The patient only needs to fast before the oral examination (approximately 12 hours for food, approximately 4 hours for clear liquids). For a retrograde procedure, standard colonoscopy preparation is necessary. Preparation before antegrade procedures is not generally necessary but may be useful in patients with suspected stenoses or diabetic neuropathy with delayed transit.

The examination itself is usually performed either with conventional conscious sedation or with propofol. There is, however, a wide range of sedation options, and selection is related to local conditions and policies. In most cases of antegrade or retrograde balloon enteroscopy, conscious sedation (ie, with midazolam, pethidine, and/or fentanyl) is sufficient. For antegrade balloon enteroscopy that may last more than an hour, deep monitored sedation, for example, with propofol, is widely accepted. General anesthesia with intubation is not customary in Germany and is restricted to individual cases, for example, in children, but it is used more often in other countries. For retrograde DBE, as for colonoscopy, conscious sedation is sufficient in most cases. However, deep monitored anesthesia with propofol can be used, as well as no sedation in selected cases.

Depending on experience, radiologic fluoroscopy can be used as an aid in balloon enteroscopy, especially early on the learning curve. Fluoroscopy can be very useful, particularly when adhesions are expected following prior abdominal surgery. When stenoses are expected, for example, in patients with Crohn disease, radiology is certainly useful, as the intraluminal injection of radiographic contrast material allows for assessment of the complexity of impassable stenoses. Radiographic imaging is essential when endoscopic retrograde cholangiopancreatography (ERCP) is being performed with balloon enteroscopy.[3]

Following positive reports on the use of carbon dioxide insufflation in colonoscopy and ERCP, a prospective two-center study has now been published that has demonstrated substantial advantages of carbon dioxide insufflation for DBE as well.[10] Patient comfort is markedly improved, as reflected in reduced perception of pain. In addition, the depth of penetration seems to be markedly improved. Despite these positive data, the use of carbon dioxide is not yet generally established. This could change if the experience is confirmed by further studies. These results could probably also be applied to SBE.

INDICATION FOR DBE AND SBE

On the basis of the extensive published data on DBE, suspected or known mid-gastrointestinal bleeding (MGI) represents the principal indication for the procedure.[11–16] The same certainly also applies to SBE,[5,17] as there is no difference in the indications for the two enteroscopy methods. Lesions that have been discovered using other imaging procedures, such as magnetic resonance enteroclysis, can be diagnostically checked using balloon enteroscopy and histologically confirmed if necessary. If there is a suspicion of small-bowel obstruction, balloon endoscopy is preferable to capsule endoscopy as a diagnostic step, in view of the risk of capsule retention.[17]

In addition to hemostatic procedures, balloon endoscopy can also be used in the small bowel to carry out resection of mucosal lesions—flat or polypoid—as well as for balloon dilation of stenoses, preoperative marking of pathologic findings, foreign-body removal (eg, retained capsules, parts of dentures, plastic prostheses, and gastrostomy bumpers), and also, in a few cases, for implantation of self-expanding metal stents.[4,11,12,15,18,19]

DBE is also suitable for obtaining access to a surgically modified gastrointestinal tract, for example, in ERCP after Billroth II operations or gastric resection with Roux-en-Y reconstruction,[20,21] as well as for access to the biliary system or residual stomach after obesity surgery.[22] Another area of application seems to be difficult ileocolonoscopy.[23–26] For colonoscopy and ERCP, there have also been reports of experience in the form of case series and a case report using the single-balloon technique.[7,8]

Mid-Gastrointestinal Bleeding

MGI is defined as small-bowel bleeding, located between the papilla and the ileocecal valve.[27] The first comparative studies of capsule endoscopy and double-balloon endoscopy showed that the two methods had a similar diagnostic yield.[28–30] In comparison with push enteroscopy, a much higher diagnostic yield can be achieved with DBE, as expected, because much more of the small bowel can be visualized.[1,31] No studies comparing DBE with SBE have so far been published. The high diagnostic yield of DBE, at around 60% to 80%, is also associated with a high percentage of direct therapeutic implications for the patient.[3,11–13,16] Most publications on DBE have reported a high rate of endoscopic interventions, at between 35% and 65%. The first original studies in Asia on SBE show a slightly lower diagnostic yield of around 40% to 50%,[4,17] whereas the rate of endoscopic interventions was only 5% to 20%. However, the data are still too limited in comparison with DBE for a valid assessment to be possible. In addition, it is well known that angiodysplasias, which can generally be well treated endoscopically, are much more frequent in the Western hemisphere than in Asia.

Crohn Disease

Balloon enteroscopy is certainly not one of the standard procedures in the initial diagnosis of Crohn disease, or for follow-up examinations in patients with known Crohn disease. DBE and SBE only have a place in patients with obstructive Crohn disease, as it allows dilation to be performed. In rare cases, direct visual observation and histologic sampling may be required to confirm Crohn carcinoma. In addition, the inflammatory components in a stenotically altered segment of the small bowel can be more reliably assessed with direct visualization, and this is important for the patient's subsequent drug treatment. The need for endoscopic dilation treatment or surgical treatment can also be assessed effectively.[3]

Polyposis Syndrome

Patients with polyposis syndromes—familial adenomatous polyposis (FAP), Peutz-Jeghers syndrome—in the colon and/or small bowel usually undergo surgery, and therefore often have considerable numbers of adhesions. Balloon enteroscopy is therefore difficult in these patients, and complete enteroscopy will not be possible in most of the cases. Based on the experience of the author, insertion depth with SBE is lower than when using DBE in this special group of patients, because the balloon at the tip of the scope facilitates to hold a stable position while pushing forward the overtube. However, there are no published data on this topic. Balloon enteroscopy, therefore, has a place here for therapeutic endoscopy with polypectomy after screening with, for example, capsule endoscopy. In the case of Peutz-Jeghers syndrome, the management can be changed as small-bowel involvement can be expected in more than 90% of the Peutz-Jeghers patients. Particularly in symptomatic Peutz-Jeghers patients (with anemia and/or obstruction), balloon enteroscopy can be used as the first diagnostic procedure, with an expectation that treatment will be needed.[32]

Small-Bowel Tumors

The frequency of small-bowel tumors in patients with MGI is between 5% and 10%. Up to 60% of the tumors are malignant.[33] Balloon enteroscopy represents the procedure of choice for patients with suspected small-bowel tumors, because it allows for histologic sampling. Additionally, singular small bowel mass lesions might be missed by capsule endoscopy in a substantial percentage.[34] In treatment of refractory celiac disease, balloon enteroscopy is similarly the procedure of choice, because tissue can be obtained for identifying T-cell lymphomas.[35] The same applies to the staging of gastrointestinal lymphomas beyond the stomach—although there are, as yet, insufficient data here for balloon enteroscopy to be used as the standard examination.

COMPLICATIONS

On the basis of published data, including the German double-balloon registry (less than 4000 DBE procedures), relevant complications in diagnostic DBE can be expected in approximately 1% of cases. The most severe complication here is certainly pancreatitis, with a risk of approximately 0.3% in oral DBE. As in conventional endoscopy, the risk is higher in therapeutic enteroscopy, at around 3% to 4%.[36,37] In findings similar to those of the prospective Munich colon polypectomy study, it has been found that the complication risk (bleeding and perforation) may reach as much as 10%, particularly with large, broad-based polyps.[19] Experience is indispensable here to minimize complications.

With regard to the mortality rate associated with DBE, the only data available are from the German double-balloon registry, where the mortality rate is 0.05% (death after pancreatitis and complicated postoperative course after perforation during polypectomy for a small-bowel polyp).

Insufficient data are currently available with regard to the expected complication rates in diagnostic and therapeutic SBE. Perforation as a severe complication of a diagnostic examination has only been reported in one of the two original studies that have been published to date (1 of 37 examinations in 27 patients).[17] In the other study,[4] a deep mucosal tear was described, which was treated with clips (1 of 78 examinations in 41 patients). This was caused by the flexed endoscope tip during advancement of the overtube. It is conceivable that this inverted endoscope tip technique might, in fact, lead to a higher rate of relevant mucosal injuries, but the question cannot as yet be answered due to the limited number of cases. A recommendable alternative to the angulation of the tip of the enteroscope is the power suction technique.[38]

CONTRAINDICATIONS FOR DBE AND SBE

The contraindications for balloon endoscopy correspond to those for conventional endoscopy in the upper and lower gastrointestinal tract. Adhesions are not contraindications for the examination, but represent limitations of it, as the depth of penetration into the small bowel can be restricted by fixed small-bowel loops. Probably, these adhesions play a more important role for the SBE technique than for the DBE technique, because of the missing balloon at the tip of the scope, but actually, there are no published data to prove this. In addition, adhesions can lead to considerable discomfort for the patients during and after the examination. In patients with a latex allergy, "allergy prophylaxis," comparable with the prophylaxis administered in patients with contrast allergies in ERCP, is advisable when the double-balloon system is used. There are no evidence-based data on the necessity for this measure, however.

SUMMARY

Balloon enteroscopy has become established throughout the world for diagnostic and therapeutic examinations of the small bowel, and it is now used universally in clinical routine work. The main advantages of the method in comparison with other imaging procedures (eg, capsule endoscopy and MRI) are that it allows histologic sampling and endoscopic therapy. With appropriate patient selection, relevant pathologic findings can be detected in a high percentage of cases (70%–80%) with DBE, leading in turn to direct therapeutic implications for the patient. Endoscopic therapy can be performed in more than 50% of patients with MGI. The complication rates with diagnostic and therapeutic double-balloon endoscopy are acceptably low. The recently introduced technique of SBE represents a simplification of the method, and the initial preliminary data for it have been positive, although the rate of complete enteroscopies seems to be markedly lower. It remains to be seen whether a significant reduction in the detection rate for relevant findings is associated with the method. On the basis of currently available data, DBE must continue to be regarded as the standard procedure at present. Larger prospective studies on SBE, and, above all, prospective studies comparing the two systems, will have to be awaited before conclusive assessments can be made.

REFERENCES

1. May A, Nachbar L, Schneider M, et al. Prospective comparison of push enteroscopy and push-and-pull enteroscopy in patients with suspected small-bowel bleeding. Am J Gastroenterol 2006;101:2016–24.
2. Gerson LB, Flodin JT, Miyabayashi K. Balloon-assisted enteroscopy: technology and troubleshooting. Gastrointest Endosc 2008;68:1158–67.
3. Pohl J, Blancas JM, Cave D, et al. Consensus report of the 2nd international conference on double balloon endoscopy. Endoscopy 2008;40:156–60.
4. Yamamoto H, Kita H, Sunada K, et al. Clinical outcomes of double-balloon endoscopy for the diagnosis and treatment of small-intestinal diseases. Clin Gastroenterol Hepatol 2004;2:1010–6.
5. Tsujikawa T, Saitoh Y, Andoh A, et al. Novel single-balloon enteroscopy for diagnosis and treatment of the small intestine: preliminary experiences. Endoscopy 2008;40:11–5.
6. Yamamoto H, Sekine Y, Sato Y, et al. Total enteroscopy with a nonsurgical steerable double-balloon method. Gastrointest Endosc 2001;53:216–20.
7. May A, Nachbar L, Wardak A, et al. Double-balloon enteroscopy: preliminary experience in patients with obscure gastrointestinal bleeding or chronic abdominal pain. Endoscopy 2003;35:985–91.
8. May A, Nachbar L, Ell C. Push-and-pull enteroscopy using a single-balloon technique for difficult colonoscopy. Endoscopy 2006;38:395–8.
9. Mönkemüller K, Fry LC, Bellutti M, et al. ERCP using single-balloon instead of double-balloon enteroscopy in patients with Roux-en-Y anastomosis. Endoscopy 2008;40(Suppl 2):E19–20.
10. Domagk D, Bretthauer M, Lenz P, et al. Carbon dioxide insufflation improves intubation depth in double-balloon enteroscopy: a randomized, controlled, double-blind trial. Endoscopy 2007;39:1064–7.
11. Ell C, May A, Nachbar L, et al. Push-and-pull enteroscopy in the small bowel using the double-balloon technique: results of a prospective European multicenter study. Endoscopy 2005;37:613–6.
12. May A, Nachbar L, Ell C. Double-balloon enteroscopy (push-and-pull enteroscopy) of the small bowel: feasibility and diagnostic and therapeutic yield in patients with suspected small bowel disease. Gastrointest Endosc 2005;62:62–70.
13. Heine GD, Hadithi M, Groenen MJ, et al. Double balloon enteroscopy: indications, diagnostic yield, and complications in a series of 275 patients with suspected small-bowel-diseases. Endoscopy 2006;38:42–8.
14. Mehdizadeh S, Ross A, Gerson L, et al. What is the learning curve associated with double-balloon enteroscopy? Technical details and early experience in 6 U.S. tertiary care centers. Gastrointest Endosc 2006;64:740–50.
15. Sun B, Rajan E, Cheng S, et al. Diagnostic yield and therapeutic impact of double-balloon enteroscopy in a large cohort of patients with obscure gastrointestinal bleeding. Am J Gastroenterol 2006;101:2011–5.
16. Zhong J, Ma T, Zhang C, et al. A retrospective study of the application on double-balloon enteroscopy in 378 patients with suspected small-bowel diseases. Endoscopy 2007;39:208–15.

17. Kawamura T, Yasuda K, Tanaka K, et al. Clinical evaluation of a newly developed single-balloon enteroscope. Gastrointest Endosc 2008;68:1112–6.
18. Sunada K, Yamamoto H, Kita H, et al. Clinical outcomes of enteroscopy using the double-balloon method for strictures of the small intestine. World J Gastroenterol 2005;11:1087–9.
19. May A, Nachbar L, Pohl J, et al. Endoscopic interventions in the small bowel using double balloon enteroscopy: feasibility and limitations. Am J Gastroenterol 2007;102:527–35.
20. Lee BI, Choi H, Choi KY, et al. Retrieval of a retained capsule endoscope by double-balloon enteroscopy. Gastrointest Endosc 2005;62:463–5.
21. Haruta H, Yamamoto H, Mizuta K, et al. A case of successful enteroscopic balloon dilation for late anastomotic stricture of choledochojejunostomy after living donor liver transplantation. Liver Transpl 2005;11:1608–10.
22. Aabakken L, Bretthauer M, Line PD. Double-balloon enteroscopy for endoscopic retrograde cholangiography in patients with a Roux-en-Y anastomosis. Endoscopy 2007;39:1068–71.
23. Kuga R, Safatle-Ribeiro AV, Faintuch J, et al. Endoscopic findings in the excluded stomach after Roux-en Y gastric bypass surgery. Arch Surg 2007;142:942–6.
24. Kaltenbach T, Soetikno R, Friedland S. Use of a double balloon enteroscope facilitates caecal intubation after incomplete colonoscopy with a standard colonoscope. Dig Liver Dis 2006;38:921–5.
25. Mönkemüller K, Knippig C, Rickes S, et al. Usefulness of the double-balloon enteroscope in colonoscopies performed in patients with previously failed colonoscopy. Scand J Gastroenterol 2007;42:277–8.
26. Pasha SF, Harrison ME, Das A, et al. Utility of double-balloon colonoscopy for completion of colon examination after incomplete colonoscopy with conventional colonoscope. Gastrointest Endosc 2007;65:848–53.
27. Ell C, May A. Mid-gastrointestinal bleeding: capsule endoscopy and push-and-pull enteroscopy give rise to a new medical term. Endoscopy 2006;38:73–5.
28. Hadithi M, Heine GD, Jacobs MA, et al. A prospective study comparing video capsule endoscopy with double-balloon enteroscopy in patients with obscure gastrointestinal bleeding. Am J Gastroenterol 2006;101:52–7.
29. Matsumoto T, Esaki M, Moriyama T, et al. Comparison of capsule endoscopy and enteroscopy with the double-balloon method in patients with obscure bleeding and polyposis. Endoscopy 2005;37:827–32.
30. Nakamura M, Niwa Y, Ohmiya N, et al. Preliminary comparison of capsule endoscopy and double-balloon enteroscopy in patients with suspected small-bowel bleeding. Endoscopy 2006;38:59–66.
31. Matsumoto T, Moriyama T, Esaki M, et al. Performance of antegrade double-balloon enteroscopy: comparison with push enteroscopy. Gastrointest Endosc 2005;62:392–8.
32. Plum N, May AD, Manner H, et al. [Peutz–Jeghers syndrome: endoscopic detection and treatment of small bowel polyps by double-balloon enteroscopy]. Z Gastroenterol 2007;45:1049–55 [in German].
33. Schwartz GD, Barkin JS. Small-bowel tumors detected by wireless capsule endoscopy. Dig Dis Sci 2007;52:1026–30.
34. Ross A, Mehdizadeh S, Tokar J, et al. Double balloon enteroscopy detects small bowel mass lesions missed by capsule endoscopy. Dig Dis Sci 2008;53:2140–3.
35. Hadithi M, Al-toma A, Oudejans J, et al. The value of double-balloon enteroscopy in patients with refractory celiac disease. Am J Gastroenterol 2007;102:987–96.

36. Mensink P, Haringsma J, Kucharzik T, et al. Complications of double balloon enteroscopy: a multicenter survey. Endoscopy 2007;39:613–5.
37. Möschler O, May AD, Müller MK, et al, DBE-Studiengruppe Deutschland. [Complications in double-balloon enteroscopy: results of the German DBE registry]. Z Gastroenterol 2008;46:266–70 [in German].
38. Kav T, Balaban Y, Bayraktar Y. The power suction maneuver in single-balloon enteroscopy. Endoscopy 2008;40:961–2.

Spiral Enteroscopy and Push Enteroscopy

Paul A. Akerman, MD[a,c,*], Daniel Cantero, MD[b]

KEYWORDS

- Enteroscopy • Spiral enteroscopy • Push enteroscopy
- Spiral • Overtube

SPIRAL ENTEROSCOPY

Spiral enteroscopy is a new technique for endoscopic evaluation of the small bowel. The concept was first proposed by Dr. Akerman and the first case was performed by Drs. Akerman and Cantero in 2006. The small bowel is uniquely designed to thwart the standard push techniques of endoscopy. Standard endoscopy uses linear application of force to advance through the gastrointestinal tract. Pushing the endoscope through the gastrointestinal tract relies on the resistance and fixed points of the bowel to allow passage of the endoscope. In humans, the small bowel is on a floppy mesentery. The mobile mesentery stretches and moves to absorb the linear movement of the endoscope when advancing in a standard push fashion. Early work with the Sonde enteroscope used the motility of the small bowel to pull the enteroscope through the small bowel. Although the entire small bowel could be traversed, the lack of ability to provide therapy, uncontrolled withdrawal, poor patient tolerance, and long procedure times have eliminated the Sonde enteroscope as a useful tool. The breakthrough for endoscopic visualization of the small bowel came with Yamamoto's application of the double balloon technique to the small bowel anatomy.[1,2] Yamamoto used the double balloon technique for a "hand over hand" approach to pleat the small bowel on the enteroscope. This technique took advantage of the mobility of the small bowel mesentery to pull the small bowel on the enteroscope. Spiral enteroscopy uses a different mechanism that takes advantage of the mobile small bowel and allows lengths of small bowel much longer than the enteroscope to be visualized.

Spiral enteroscopy applies the mechanical advantage of a screw to convert rotational force into linear force and pleat the small bowel on the enteroscope. The mechanical advantage of a screw is related by the equation: mechanical advantage = circumference/pitch. Therefore, the higher the spiral, the more pulling power, and the smaller the pitch, the greater the mechanical advantage of the spiral. Our initial

[a] Brown University, Providence, RI, USA
[b] National Hospital of Paraguay, Asuncion, Paraguay
[c] University Gastroenterology, 33 Staniford Street, Providence, RI 02905, USA
* Corresponding author. University Gastroenterology, 33 Staniford Street, Providence, RI 02905.
E-mail address: pakerman@lifespan.org (P.A. Akerman).

Gastrointest Endoscopy Clin N Am 19 (2009) 357–369
doi:10.1016/j.giec.2009.04.001
giendo.theclinics.com
1052-5157/09/$ – see front matter © 2009 Published by Elsevier Inc.

theory was that the spiral could be rotated in the lumen of the small bowel, and, once past the Ligament of Trietz (LOT), the small bowel could be pulled and pleated on the enteroscope. The theory was that the mesentery would fix the small bowel and act as a resisting force to rotation of the small bowel. The pulling force of the rotating spiral must be sufficient to pleat the small bowel but any rotational force must be less than the resistance to rotation of the small bowel to prevent damage to the small bowel.

Initial studies were performed using a prototype device and a pediatric colonoscope.[3,4] The prototype device was an overtube 130 cm long, 18.5 mm in diameter, with a 5.5 mm raised spiral and the spiral length was 21 cm. Twenty-seven patients were enrolled in our pilot study and 25/27 patients underwent successful spiral enteroscopy, defined as advancement through the small bowl by rotating the overtube. Two patients had esophageal narrowing that precluded examination. Average time of procedure was 36.5 minutes and an estimated average maximum depth of intubation of the small bowel past the LOT was 176 cm. There were no serious complications although 28% has a sore throat for less than 72 hours. To better understand the technique of spiral enteroscopy and estimate the depth of insertion, we developed an ex vivo model for spiral enteroscopy training.[5] The primary feature of the model is to fix the porcine intestine to an artificial mesentery. This study and the work with our model demonstrated proof of concept for spiral enteroscopy.

Current Device

The current device is called the Discovery SB overtube from Spirus Corporation (**Figs. 1** and **2**). The Discovery SB has been approved by the Food and Drug Administration (FDA) and has been granted a CE mark. The device specifications are: overall length 118 cm, internal diameter 9.8 mm, outer diameter 14.5 mm, spiral height 5.5 mm, and spiral length 22 cm. Significantly, the new version of the Discovery SB has a soft hollow spiral. The device has a variable stiffness distal end and a locking device that fixes the Discovery SB overtube to the endoscope but still allows rotation of the overtube at the other end. The proximal end of the Discovery SB has two foam handles to assist rotation. The Discovery SB is designed to accommodate an endoscope that is 9.4 mm in diameter or less. Specifically, the Discovery SB accommodates the 9.2 mm 200 cm Olympus SIF-Q180 and the 9.4 mm 200 cm Fujinon EN-450T5 enteroscopes. They are also known as single and double balloon enteroscopes, respectively.

Spiral Enteroscopy Technique

The Discovery SB overtube is a sterile single-use device. Two operators are usually required to perform the technique. Before use, the internal liner of the Discovery SB is well lubricated with the proprietary lubricant supplied with the device. After careful

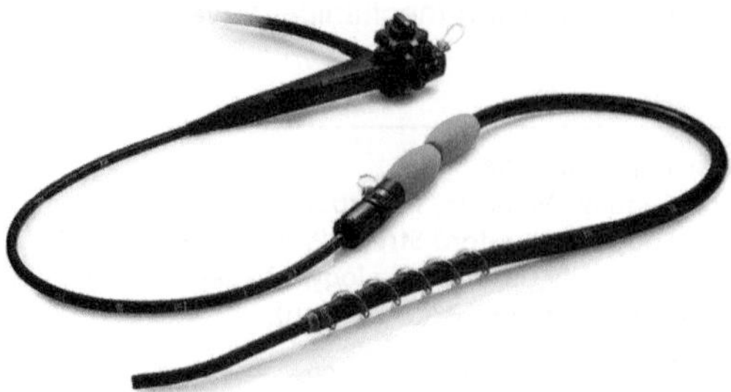

Fig. 1. The Discovery SB overtube and enteroscope.

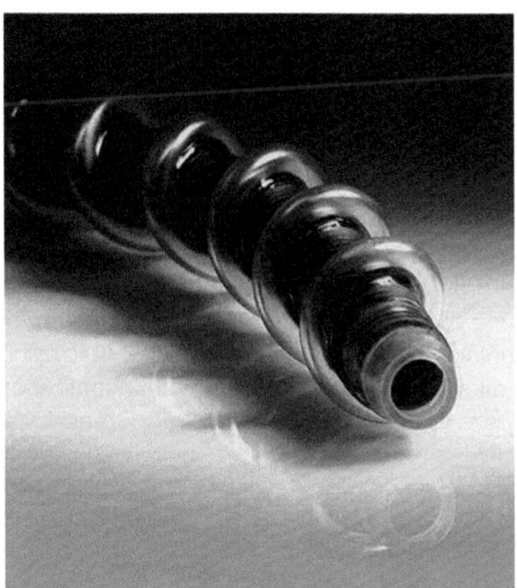

Fig. 2. The Discovery SB distal end with hollow spiral.

lubrication, the Discovery SB is installed on the enteroscope (Fujinon EN-450T5 or Olympus SIF-Q180). Typically the device is locked on the enteroscope at 145 cm to begin the procedure, leaving approximately 27 cm of enteroscope past the distal tip of the Discovery SB and ensuring that the enteroscope will retain its flexibility as it passes through the fixed portions of the upper gastrointestinal tract to the LOT.

The fixed Discovery SB and enteroscope are advanced slowly with gentle rotation of the overtube until the enteroscope typically reaches past the LOT. It is important to minimize insufflations of air and CO_2 may offer some advantages. Minimizing air reduces the formation of a loop in the stomach and allows better apposition of the spiral threads to the bowel wall to initiate spiral advancement.

To begin spiral enteroscopy advancement, the spiral must be past the LOT, whereby the mobile small bowel can be pleated on the enteroscope. The Discovery SB functions most efficiently if the overtube is straight and rotating easily to pleat the small bowel. Early resistance to rotation is almost always due to a loop in the stomach. A loop may be formed in the stomach from the gentle forward pressure when advancing the spiral past the LOT. Often it is helpful to slowly rotate the overtube while pulling back gently on the overtube. This causes a paradoxic forward motion of the enteroscope and often initiates spiral enteroscopy. If this maneuver is repeated with abdominal pressure and if it still does not work, shortening and straightening the Discovery SB is recommended. The Discovery SB is then unlocked from the enteroscope and the enteroscope is maximally advanced into the small bowel. Next, the overtube is advanced over the enteroscope with gentle slow rotation. This usually installs the spirals past the LOT and the overtube can be straightened and rotated to begin spiral advancement. It is a general principle that rapid or forceful rotation is never the solution to initiating spiral enteroscopy.

Once the maximal depth of insertion has been reached with spiral advancement, it is sometimes possible to pleat additional small bowel using the following maneuver. The enteroscope is unlocked and advanced to the maximal depth of insertion. A hook and suction maneuver is performed with the enteroscope. The Discovery SB is then rotated and the enteroscope is slowly withdrawn. This can be repeated several times as long as additional depths of small bowel are visualized. The enteroscope is never pulled back past the 130 cm mark on the enteroscope as the bending section of the enteroscope will then be in the overtube.

Once maximal depth of insertion is reached, the process of careful, controlled visualization begins. Typically, the enteroscope is fixed at 145 cm for withdrawal. At this point, a considerable distance of small bowel may be pleated on the overtube. The overtube is slowly rotated counterclockwise with periodic pauses to allow the small bowel to be carefully visualized. It is important to apply a slight forward pressure on the Discovery SB when performing counter clockwise withdrawal. This maintains position to avoid rapid withdrawal. Once counterclockwise rotation is no longer effective, we recommend allowing the overtube to come back to 60 cm at the bite block. The enteroscope is then unlocked and slowly drawn back through the proximal jejunum and duodenum. This allows a careful and complete visualization of these important areas. The enteroscope is then fixed to the Discovery SB and the device is withdrawn with slow counterclockwise rotation.

Spiral Enteroscopy Studies

Akerman and colleagues[6] performed the first study using the Discovery SB with the slim 200-cm enteroscopes, Olympus SIF Q180[7] and Fujinon EN-450T5.[8] Seventy-five patients were prospectively enrolled in the study. Average estimated depth of insertion of the enteroscope past the LOT was 243 cm for the Olympus enteroscope and 256 cm for the Fujinon enteroscope (*P* value .55). The average time to reach the maximum depth of insertion was 18.7 minutes and average total procedure time was 29 minutes in the Olympus enteroscope group and 16.2 and 26 minutes, respectively, in the Fujinon enteroscope group (*P* values .17 and .19). The diagnostic yield in this study was 32% in the Olympus group and 22% in the Fujinon group. The diagnostic yield is low but was attributed to the overall young age of the cohort and the lack of a pre-evaluation capsule study.

Morgan and colleagues[9] performed a prospective multicenter trial of spiral enteroscopy in the United States. One hundred and forty-eight patients were enrolled in 10 centers. The average age was 68 years and 60% of patients had significant co morbid conditions. Seventy-two percent of the patients had obscure gastrointestinal (GI) bleeding and this was the most common indication. Eighty-four percent of patients had prior capsule endoscopy. Fifty-five percent of patients had prior abdominal surgeries. Spiral enteroscopy was successful in 96% of patients. The average estimated maximum depth of insertion was 250 cm. Estimated depth of insertion by small bowel segment was jejunum (proximal 6%, middle 12%, distal 29%), ileum (proximal 44%, middle 6%, terminal ileum 1%). The average time was 45 minutes for therapeutic procedures and 34 minutes for nontherapeutic procedures. There were no serious complications, including no cases of pancreatitis, perforation, or death. Conclusions were that spiral enteroscopy is safe and effective and the total time of procedure and depth of insertion compare favorably with double balloon enteroscopy (DBE) and single balloon enteroscopy (SBE).

Esmail and colleagues[10] published a single center experience of spiral enteroscopy. Fifty-seven patients were included in this retrospective study. The mean age was 60 years. Forty percent had undergone previous abnormal capsule endoscopy studies. Twenty-five percent of patients had altered postsurgical GI anatomy. Fifty-four of 57 procedures were successful. The average estimated depth of insertion was 246 cm. The excluded stomach was reached in five of seven patients after Roux-en-Y gastric surgery. The average total procedure time was 28 minutes. The diagnostic yield was 51%. There were no reported cases of pancreatitis, perforation, or death.

Schembre and colleagues[11] reported on a retrospective study comparing DBE and spiral enteroscopy. Thirty-four cases of DBE and 19 cases of spiral enteroscopy were analyzed. The groups had similar demographics including age, prior capsule studies, and indications. The diagnostic yield was similar in the two groups: DBE 70% and spiral enteroscopy 65%. Average procedure time was 77 minutes for DBE and 59 minutes for spiral enteroscopy. A crossover study was performed in three patients. In one of these three patients, spiral enteroscopy exceeded the DBE tattoo site by an estimated 100 cm; one patient reached the same point of maximum insertion; and in one patient DBE was performed successfully after a failed spiral enteroscopy procedure. The conclusion of the study was that DBE and spiral enteroscopy had similar success rates for the detection and treatment of small bowel bleeding. DBE depth of insertion was perceived to be greater than spiral enteroscopy although spiral enteroscopy was somewhat faster than DBE. There were no serious complications in either group.

Buscaglia and colleagues[12] published a prospective study of the results of spiral enteroscopy during training of physicians in the spiral enteroscopy technique. Ninety patients were included in the study. Thirty-three physicians were trained in the procedure. The average age of the patients was 49 years. Spiral enteroscopy was successfully performed in 96% of the patients. Mean time to maximum insertion was 21 minutes and total procedure time was 34 minutes. Average estimated depth of insertion past the LOT was 262 cm. There were no serious complications. The conclusions were: spiral enteroscopy allows safe advancement into the distal small bowel, the maximal depth of insertion seems comparable to double balloon enteroscopy, and spiral enteroscopy took less time. The device was considered easy to use and operated effectively after as few as five training cases.

Depth of Intubation During Spiral Enteroscopy

Estimating the depth of intubation during enteroscopy is at best an educated guess by an experienced endoscopist and at worst a fool's errand. Despite this, significant time has been spent attempting to estimate the depth of insertion into the small bowel. In the double balloon experience, attempting to quantitate the gain of each cycle of the inflation and deflation has had some success but is not universally accepted.[13] Visual estimates of the depth of insertion into the small bowel by segment are, at best, only a rough estimate. For spiral enteroscopy, we have developed an endotrainer, which we believe has assisted in estimating depths of small bowel traversed although this is not proven.[5] Akerman and colleagues[6] published the results of three patients who were sent to surgery and had the distance to the maximal depth of insertion measured and compared with our endoscopic estimates: 100 cm/75 cm, 260 cm/240 cm, and 260 cm/300 cm. This gives some support to the accuracy of the estimates of the depth of insertion into the small bowel.

Four studies had almost identical estimated average depth of insertion: Akerman and colleagues[6] 252 cm, Morgan and colleagues[9] 250 cm, Esmail and colleagues[10] 246 cm, and Buscaglia and colleagues[12] 262 cm. It is likely that this represents the limits of the Discovery SB to pleat small bowel on the overtube. The Discovery SB overtube is 118 cm long but the handles and locking device limit the functional length to approximately 95 cm. The published depths of insertion into the small bowel with the Discovery SB device compare favorably with double balloon enteroscopy.

Chiorean and colleagues[14] published a report on the predictors of depth of insertion with spiral enteroscopy in a prospective multicenter trial in the United States. The depth of insertion was estimated by centimeters past the LOT and by the estimated small bowel segment. One hundred and forty-eight patients were included in the analysis. Prior abdominal surgery did not affect the depth of insertion past the LOT. Surgical type, including small bowel surgery, was not an independent predictor. Age, gender, body mass index (BMI), and Mallapatti score were not significant factors. The presence of at least one comorbid condition had a modest effect on insertion depth: 249 cm versus 260 cm.

Double Balloon Enteroscopy versus Spiral Enteroscopy

DBE and spiral enteroscopy are competing technologies. Schembre and Ross[11] published a comparison of DBE with spiral enteroscopy. In this retrospective study of 34 patient who underwent DBE and 23 patients who underwent spiral enteroscopy, the demographics and indications were similar in the two groups. The yields were comparable in DBE (70%) and spiral enteroscopy (65%). Depths of insertion were not estimated, although three patients were subjected to crossover studies. In one patient, spiral enteroscopy exceeded DBE by 100 cm; there was no difference in the depth of insertion in one patient, and spiral enteroscopy failed in one patient who then had successful DBE. In a personal communication from Upchurch and colleagues, retrospective analysis of 13 patients with DBE and 12 patients with spiral enteroscopy revealed faster times for the spiral enteroscopy versus DBE: 46 minutes versus 60 minutes. The estimated depth of insertion was numerically greater for spiral enteroscopy than DBE: 378 cm versus 302 cm.

Spiral enteroscopy procedure times seem to be shorter than the published procedure times for DBE. In five studies presented here, the average total procedure time was 28 minutes,[6] 45 minutes,[9] 28 minutes,[10] 59 minutes,[11] and 34 minutes.[12] Procedure times varied considerably depending on the number of therapies performed and the comorbidities of the patient. Although it is not clear which technique of small bowel enteroscopy traverses the longest distance of small bowel, there is strong evidence that for the distance travelled, spiral enteroscopy is faster. Clearly, prospective randomized studies are needed to compare DBE and spiral enteroscopy.

Retrograde Spiral Enteroscopy

Total small bowel visualization is rarely achieved in the United States in anterograde deep small bowel enteroscopy. In up to 40% of cases of anterograde deep small bowel intubation, a retrograde small bowel evaluation is indicated.[13] The anatomy of the colon can make traversing the small bowel difficult in a retrograde fashion. In addition, the 90-degree right-angle turn from the cecum into the terminal ileum is a challenge for all retrograde enteroscopy techniques.

We have performed three studies using different spiral overtube devices and endoscopes. Using the Discovery SB with the Olympus SIF Q-180,[15–18] the average time to reach the cecum was 8.3 minutes and the average time to maximum small bowel insertion was 27.5 minutes. The average total procedure time was 35 minutes. The estimated average depth of insertion was 136 cm. Spiral enteroscopy was successfully initiated in only 40% of patients but, in these cases, the depth of insertion was superior (average 170 cm). In a study of 11 patients, retrograde small bowel enteroscopy was performed using the Vista-SB overtube (outer diameter 18.5 mm) and the Olympus SIF Q-140 260 cm enteroscope.[15] Average total procedure time was 29 minutes and the estimated maximum depth of insertion was 125 cm. In a third study, the Vista SB and the pediatric colonoscope was used in eight patients.[18] The average procedure time was 39 minutes and the estimated average depth of small bowel insertion was 113 cm. In conclusion, retrograde small bowel enteroscopy may be successfully performed with a variety of spiral devices and endoscopes. The optimal spiral overtube and endoscope are yet to be determined.

Complications of Spiral Enteroscopy

Serious complications of deep small bowel enteroscopy occur infrequently but have been reported for DBE to be between 0.3% and 3.4% for perforations and 0.0% to 0.5% for pancreatitis.[13,19] In all the studies published to date for spiral enteroscopy, there were no serious complications in 303 patients. Specifically, there were no reported episodes of pancreatitis, perforations, or severe bleeding postprocedure. In a review of 1750 patients who underwent spiral enteroscopy, six perforations (0.34%) occurred during spiral enteroscopy.[20] All six patients underwent surgical repair and did well postoperatively. There were no episodes of uncontrolled bleeding, pancreatitis, small bowel ischemia, or nontransient intussusceptions.

Future Developments in Spiral Enteroscopy

Development of an inflatable spiral would offer considerable benefits: advancement of the spirals past the LOT may be simplified; rapid withdrawal of the Discovery SB would likely also be improved. A variable height inflatable spiral would potentially be useful to adjust the efficiency of the spiral as needed to improve spiral advancement. A prototype inflatable spiral device has been developed and initial studies are promising.[21]

The ability to pleat small bowel with the Discovery SB is limited by the length of the overtube. Lengthening the overtube decreases the length of enteroscope available to push through the Discovery SB and increases the likelihood of developing a loop in the overtube. Production of loops increases resistance to rotation. In theory, a spiral that rotated only at the distal end of the overtube or scope would not be limited by the length of the device and could advance through the entire small bowel. Prototype work is currently underway to develop such a device.

Summary

Spiral enteroscopy is a new technique for deep small bowel intubation. Currently, more than 2000 cases have been performed worldwide. The Discovery SB has been approved by the Food and Drug Administration and has been granted a CE mark. The technique is safe and effective for the management and detection of small bowel pathology. Recent studies of spiral enteroscopy have demonstrated diagnostic yield, total time of procedure, and depth of insertion that compare favorably with double and single balloon enteroscopy. Spiral enteroscopy can be performed in postgastric surgery patients including Roux-en-Y patients requiring endoscopic retrograde cholangiopancreatography. Retrograde spiral enteroscopy can also be performed successfully. The strengths of spiral enteroscopy are rapid advancement in the small bowel and controlled, stable withdrawal that facilitates therapy. Future studies will be needed to compare competing technologies.

PUSH ENTEROSCOPY

Push enteroscopy can be performed with a dedicated enteroscope of extended length (200–250 cm) with or without an overtube. The pediatric colonoscope and standard colonoscope can also be used for push enteroscopy. Push enteroscopy with a standard colonoscope or pediatric colonoscope is probably the most common type of enteroscopy performed. No additional equipment or training is required and anesthesia needs are similar to standard upper endoscopy. There is also no additional risk with the pediatric colonoscope.[22,23] With use of the dedicated enteroscope, extended length accessories may be needed. Anesthesia requirements are usually similar to standard upper endoscopy. When using the overtube for the dedicated enteroscope, the following technique using fluoroscopic guidance is recommended. Backload the well-lubricated overtube on the enteroscope and then advance the enteroscope to the proximal jejunum. With gentle back pressure of the enteroscope, advance the overtube to the third part of the duodenum. Once the overtube is in place, the assistant holds the overtube in place and the enteroscope is advanced into the jejunum.

The dedicated enteroscope, with and without the overtube, allows increased depth of insertion into the small bowel. Push enteroscopy with the standard and pediatric colonoscope reaches 25 to 50 cm past the LOT on average. Use of the dedicated enteroscope without the overtube reaches 25 to 75 cm past the LOT and, with the overtube, estimated depths of insertion are 40 to 100 cm past the LOT.[5,7,8,15–18,21,24,25] The colonoscope has the advantage of larger channel size, forward washing capability, and uses standard accessories. The dedicated enteroscope allows deeper depths of insertion[26] but with the additional risk of complications mostly secondary to use of the overtube.[27–35] Choice of endoscope and technique is guided by the individual patient.

Indications

The most common indication for enteroscopy is obscure gastrointestinal bleeding. Approximately 5% of patients with gastrointestinal hemorrhage and 38% of patients with chronic iron deficiency anemia do not have a bleeding site identified after routine upper endoscopy and colonoscopy.[36] Other indications include suspected celiac disease, abnormal small bowel imaging, suspected enteropathy from nonsteroidal antiinflammatory drugs, inflammatory bowel disease, polyposis syndromes, unexplained diarrhea, and malabsorption syndromes.

Current Role of Push Enteroscopy in the Management of Small Bowel Disease

Capsule endoscopy is superior to push enteroscopy in the evaluation of obscure gastrointestinal bleeding. In most cases, capsule endoscopy is recommended before enteroscopy in the management and workup of obscure gastrointestinal bleeding.[37–42] In a large meta-analysis,[43] the diagnostic yield of push enteroscopy was 28% and for capsule endoscopy 63%. The yield for clinically significant findings was 26% for push enteroscopy and 56% for capsule endoscopy. There was no statistical difference in the detection of tumors between the two techniques. In another study, although capsule endoscopy had more positive findings, the number of definitive findings was low.[44] If the capsule finding is in the first 10% of the timeline of small bowel visualization, some experienced investigators believe the finding may be reached with push enteroscopy.[45,46]

In certain circumstances, push enteroscopy may be the preferred modality for diagnosis and treatment of small bowel diseases. In 25% to 75% of cases referred for small bowel bleeding, the bleeding site may be within the reach of standard upper endoscopy.[47] These areas of the stomach and duodenum are often better seen with push endoscopy than capsule endoscopy. In one study, capsule endoscopy had a miss rate of 8%. All of these findings were found with push enteroscopy.[41] Active proximal small bowel bleeding that can be reached with the colonoscope may be more easily managed due to the forward wash capabilities of the colonoscope, larger working channel, and ability to use all standard accessories. Celiac disease, suspected clinically and serologically despite an indeterminate duodenal biopsy, may be diagnosed with jejunal biopsy.[48] In cases of malabsorption, 17% to 37% of patients may have a diagnosis made at push enteroscopy.[47] Most small bowel tumors are within the reach of push enteroscopy and one large meta-analysis of capsule studies versus push enteroscopy showed no statistical difference in the detection of small bowel tumors.[43]

Overall, DBE has a significantly higher yield than push enteroscopy for obscure gastrointestinal bleeding: 60% to 70% versus 25% to 34%.[24,49] A cost-effectiveness strategy for obscure gastrointestinal bleeding demonstrated superiority of initial workup with DBE over all other modalities including push and capsule endoscopy.[50] In nonbleeding patients requiring small bowel enteroscopy, one study showed no statistical advantage to performing DBE versus push enteroscopy.[51] In patients with chronic renal failure and melena, one study demonstrated statistical equivalence for diagnostic yield and therapeutic efficacy for push enteroscopy and DBE. Push enteroscopy may also be superior to capsule endoscopy for duodenal polyps and visualization of the ampulla.[36] Push enteroscopy and DBE have little value in the surveillance of Crohn disease.[52]

Therapeutic Enteroscopy

Small bowel tumors constitute approximately 5% of gastrointestinal tumors and are most commonly found in the duodenum and proximal jejunum.[53–55] When expandable metal stenting and dilation are required, push enteroscopy with a colonoscope may have advantages over spiral enteroscopy, DBE, and SBE. Similarly, push enteroscopy using a pediatric or standard colonoscope may have advantages when dilating small bowel strictures secondary to Crohn disease. One study had a success rate for dilation of Crohn strictures of 68% and a complication rate of 10%.[56–58]

Long-term follow-up for therapeutic success in treating angiodysplasia with push enteroscopy has shown a decreased transfusion requirement in treated patients.[59] Push enteroscopy was also found to be cost-effective in the long-term treatment of angiodysplasia[60] Push enteroscopy using the pediatric colonoscope has a diagnostic yield for obscure gastrointestinal bleeding ranging from 13% to 38%.[61] In some studies, using a dedicated enteroscope had diagnostic yield of 60%.[25] Although the use of an overtube with the dedicated enteroscope may increase diagnostic yield, there is an increased risk of complications.[27,62–64] Overall, push enteroscopy has proved to be an effective and safe choice for the diagnosis and treatment of small bowel disease. If double balloon, single balloon, and spiral enteroscopy are not available, push enteroscopy is a reasonable alternative that gives significant potential benefit to the patient with minimal risk.

Complications of Push Enteroscopy

Complications from push enteroscopy with a pediatric and standard colonoscope are rare. There have been no reported complications from oral passage of colonoscopes.[47] Most of the complications from dedicated push enteroscopes have been attributed to the passage of the overtube. Complications include gastric, duodenal, and jejunal perforations.[64] Other complications include mucosal stripping, swelling of the parotid gland, and pancreatitis.[63,65] The overall complication rate from push enteroscopy is approximately 1%.[36]

Summary

Push enteroscopy is a readily available, safe, and effective technique for detecting and treating proximal gut pathology. If performed without an overtube, complications are rare. Use of a dedicated push enteroscope with an overtube is generally reserved for specific indications, whereby the moderate increase in depth of insertion into the small bowel is required. Push enteroscopy may be the preferred endoscopic method in specific indications such as a negative capsule study in a patient with gastrointestinal bleeding, suspected proximal small bowel tumor, the presence of melena in chronic renal failure, polyposis syndromes, malabsorption, and suspected celiac sprue. If capsule endoscopy and deep small bowel enteroscopy are not available, push enteroscopy is a reasonable option with low risk and moderate yield. Push enteroscopy will remain an important part of the armamentarium of the modern endoscopist.

REFERENCES

1. Yamamoto H, Sekine Y, Sato Y, et al. Total enteroscopy with a nonsurgical steerable double-balloon method. Gastrointest Endosc 2001;53(2):216–22.
2. May A, Nachbar L, Schneider M, et al. Push and pull enteroscopy using the double-balloon technique: method of assessing depth of insertion and training of the enteroscopy technique using the Erlangen endotrainer. Endoscopy 2005; 37:66–70.
3. Akerman P, Agrawal D, Chen W, et al. Spiral enteroscopy: a novel method of enteroscopy by using the Endo-Ease Discovery SB overtube and a pediatric colonoscope. Gastrointest Endosc 2009;69(2):327–32.
4. Schembre D, Ross A. Spiral enteroscopy: a new twist on overtube-assisted endoscopy. Gastrointest Endosc 2009;69(2):333–6.
5. Akerman P, Cantero D, Bookwalter W, et al. A new in vitro porcine model for spiral enteroscopy training: The Akerman Enteroscopy Trainer. Gastrointest Endosc 2008;67(5):AB264.
6. Akerman P, Agrawal D, Cantero D, et al. Spiral enteroscopy with the new DSB overtube: a novel technique for deep peroral small-bowel intubation. Endoscopy 2008;40:974–8.
7. Akerman P, Cantero D, Avila J, et al. A pilot study of spiral enteroscopy using a new design 48F Discovery SB overtube and the Olympus 200 cm × 9.2 mm enteroscope. Gastro Endoscopy 2008;67(5):AB264.
8. Akerman P, Cantero D, Avila J, et al. A pilot study of spiral enteroscopy using a new design 48F Discovery SB overtube and the Fujinon 200 cm × 9.4 mm enteroscope. Gastro Endoscopy 2008;67(5):AB264.
9. Morgan DR, Upchurch BR, Draganov PV, et al. Spiral enteroscopy: prospective multicenter US trial in patients with small bowel disorders. Gastrointestinal Endoscopy 2009;69:AB127–8.
10. Esmail S, Odstrcil EA, Mallat D, et al. A single center retrospective review of spiral enteroscopy. Gastrointestinal Endoscopy 2009;69:197.
11. Schembre D, Ross A. Yield of antegrade double balloon versus spiral enteroscopy for obscure gastrointestinal bleeding. Abstract DDW 2009;69.
12. Buscaglia J, Dunbar K, Okolo P, et al. The Spiral Enterosocpy Training Initiative: results of a prospective study evaluation the discovery SB™ overtube device during small bowel enteroscopy (with video). Endoscopy 2009;41:194–9.
13. May A, Nachbar L, Pohl J, et al. Endoscopic interventions in the small bowel using double-balloon enteroscopy: feasibility and limitations. Am J Gastroenterol 2007;102:527–35.
14. Chiorean MV, Upchurch BR, Draganov PV, et al. Spiral enteroscopy: predictors of depth of insertion from the prospective multicenter U.S. study. Gastrointestinal Endoscopy 2009;69:AB191.
15. Akerman P, Cantero D, Pangtay J, et al. Retrograde small bowel enteroscopy using the Olympus SIF-140 260 cm enteroscope and the Vista-SB spiral overtube. Gastrointestinal Endoscopy 2009;69:AB201.
16. Cantero D, Akerman P, Pangtay J. Retrograde spiral enteroscopy using the Fujinon EN-450T5 and Olympus SIF-180 200 cm enteroscopes with the Discovery SB overtube. Gastrointestinal Endoscopy 2009;69:AB192.

17. Akerman P, Cantero D, Agrawal D, et al. Novel method of enteroscopy via anal approach using EndoEase Discovery SB overtube. Gastro Endoscopy 2007; 65(5):AB277.
18. Akerman P, Cantero D, Agrawal D, et al. Novel method of enteroscopy using Endoease Discovery SB overtube. Gastro Endoscopy 2007;65(5):AB125.
19. Mensink PB, Haringsma J, Kucharzik T, et al. Complications of double balloon enteroscopy: a multicenter survey. Endoscopy 2007;3:613.
20. Akerman P, Cantero D. Severe complications of spiral enteroscopy in the first 1750 patients. Abstract DDW 2009.
21. Akerman P, Cantero D, Pangtay J. Development of a new inflatable spiral is a potentially important advancement in spiral enteroscopy. Abstract DDW 2009.
22. Goff JS. Peroral colonoscopy: technique, depth, and yield of lesions. Gastrointest Endosc Clin N Am 1996;6:753.
23. Parker H, Agayoff J. Enteroscopy and small bowel biopsy utilizing a peroral colonoscope. Gastrointest Endosc 1983;29:139.
24. May A, Nachbar L, Schneider M, et al. Prospective comparison of push enteroscopy and push-and-pull enteroscopy in patients with suspected small-bowel bleeding. Am J Gastroenterol 2006;101(9):2016–24.
25. Chong J, Tagle M, Barin J, et al. Small bowel push-type fiberoptic enteroscopy for patients with occult gastrointestinal bleeding or suspected small bowel pathology. Am J Gastroenterol 1994;89:2143.
26. Eisen G, Dominitz JA, Faigel D, et al. Enteroscopy. Gastrointest Endosc 2001;53: 871–3.
27. Landi B, Cellier C, Fayemendy L, et al. Duodenal perforation occurring during push enteroscopy. Gastrointest Endosc 1996;43(6):631.
28. Benz C, Jakobs R, Riemann JF. Do we need the overtube for push-enteroscopy? Endoscopy 2001;33:658–61.
29. Sharma B, Bhasin D, Makharia G, et al. Diagnostic value of push-type enteroscopy: a report from India. Am J Gastroenterol 2000;95:137–40.
30. Foutch P, Sawyer R, Sanowski R. Push-enteroscopy for diagnosis of patients with gastrointestinal bleeding of obscure origin. Gastrointest Endosc 1990;36:337–41.
31. Taylor A, Buttigieg R, McDonald I, et al. Prospective assessment of the diagnostic and therapeutic impact of small-bowel push enteroscopy. Endoscopy 2003;35: 951–6.
32. Ell C, Remke S, May A, et al. The first prospective controlled trial comparing wireless capsule endoscopy with push enteroscopy in chronic gastrointestinal bleeding. Endoscopy 2002;34:685–9.
33. Mata A, Bordas JM, Feu F, et al. Wireless capsule endoscopy in patients with obscure gastrointestinal bleeding: a comparative study with push enteroscopy. Aliment Pharmacol Ther 2004;20:189–94.
34. Taylor A, Chen R, Desmond P. Use of an overtube for enteroscopy: does it increase depth of insertion? A prospective study of enteroscopy with and without an overtube. Endoscopy 2001;33:227–30.
35. Gay G, Loudu P, Bichet G, et al. Parotid gland and submaxillary enlargement after push video enteroscopy. Endoscopy 1996;28:328.
36. DiSario J, Petersen B, Tierney W, et al. Enteroscopes – technology status evaluation report. Gastrointest Endosc 2007;66(5):872–80.
37. Leighton J, Sharma V, Hentz J, et al. Capsule endoscopy versus push enteroscopy for evaluation of obscure gastrointestinal bleeding with 1-year outcomes. Dig Dis Sci 2006;51(5):891–9.

38. Redondo-Cerezo E, Sanchez-Manjavacas N, Gomez-Ruiz C. Capsule endoscopy vs push enteroscopy: which one should we perform first? Gastroenterology 2005;129(4):1358.
39. Marmo R, Rotondano G, Piscopos R, et al. Meta-analysis: capsule enteroscopy vs. conventional modalities in diagnosis of small bowel diseases. Aliment Pharmacol Ther 2005;22(7):595–604.
40. Lepere C, Cuillerier E, Van Gossum A, et al. Predictive factors of positive findings in patients explored by push enteroscopy for unexplained GI bleeding. Gastrointest Endosc 2005;61(6):709–14.
41. Sidhu R, McAlindon M, Kapur K, et al. Should push enteroscopy be reserved for therapeutic intervention after capsule endoscopy. Experience from a tertiary centre in the United Kingdom. Gastroenterology 2007;133(2):729.
42. Monkemuller K, Bellutti M, Fry L. Enteroscopy. Gastrointest Endosc 2008;22(5): 789–811.
43. Leighton J, Treuster SM, Sharma V. Capsule: a meta-analysis for use with obscure gastrointestinal bleeding. Gastrointest Endosc Clin N Am 2006;16:229–50.
44. Adler D, Knipschield M, Gostout C. A prospective comparison of capsule endoscopy and push enteroscopy in patients with GI bleeding of obscure origin. Gastrointest Endosc 2004;59(4):492–8.
45. Lewis B. Obscure GI bleeding in the world of capsule endoscopy, push, and double balloon enteroscopies. Gastrointest Endosc 2007;66(3):S66–8.
46. May A. Current status of double balloon enteroscopy with focus on the Wiesbaden results. Gastrointest Endosc 2007;66(3):S12–4.
47. Oates B, Morris A. Enteroscopy. Curr Opin Gastroenterol 2000;16(2):121–5.
48. Horoldt B, McAlindon M, Stephenson T, et al. Making the diagnosis of celiac disease: is there a role for push enteroscopy? Eur J Gastroenterol Hepatol 2004;16(11):1143–6.
49. de Leusse A, Vahedi K, Edery J, et al. Capsule endoscopy or push enteroscopy for first-line exploration of obscure gastrointestinal bleeding? Gastroenterology 2007;132(3):855–62.
50. Gerson L, Kamal A. Cost-effectiveness analysis of management strategies for obscure GI bleeding. Gastrointest Endosc 2008;68(5):920–36.
51. Matsumoto T, Moriyama T, Esaki M, et al. Performance of antegrade double-balloon enteroscopy: comparison with push enteroscopy. Gastrointest Endosc 2005;62(3):392–8.
52. Best W, Becktel J, Singleton J. Rederived values of the eight coefficients of the Crohn's disease activity index (CDAI). Gastroenterology 1979;l77:L843–6.
53. Lewis B, Kornbluth A, Waye J. Small bowel tumours: yield of enteroscopy. Gut 1991;32:763–5.
54. Kleinerman J, Yardumian K, Tamaki H. Primary carcinoma of the duodenum. Ann Intern Med 1950;32:451–8.
55. Benz C, Jakobs R, Riemann JF. Does the insertion depth in push enteroscopy depend on the working length of the enteroscope? Endoscopy 2002;34:543–5.
56. Couckuyt H, Gevers A, Coremans G, et al. Efficacy and safety of hydrostatic balloon dilatation of ileocolonic Crohn's stricture: a prospective longterm analysis. Gut 1995;36:577–80.
57. Blomberg B, Rolny P, Jarnerog G. Endoscopic treatment of anastomotic strictures in Crohn's disease. Endoscopy 1991;12:195–8.
58. Davies G, Benson M, Gertner D, et al. Diagnostic and therapeutic push type enteroscopy in clinical use. Gut 1995;37:346–52.

59. Ashkin M, Lewis B. Push enteroscopic cauterization: long-term follow-up of 83 patients with bleeding small intestinal angiodysplasia. Gastrointest Endosc 1996;43:580.
60. Morris A, Mokhashi M, Straiton M, et al. Push enteroscopy and heater probe therapy for small bowel bleeding. Gastrointest Endosc 1996;44:384.
61. Berner J, Mauer K, Lewis B. Push and Sonde enteroscopy for the diagnosis of obscure gastrointestinal bleeding. Am J Gastroenterol 1994;89:2139.
62. American Society for Gastrointestinal Endoscopy. Status evaluation: enteroscopy. Gastrointest Endosc 1990;3:337.
63. Yang R, Laine L. Mucosal stripping: a complication of push enteroscopy. Gastrointest Endosc 1995;41:156.
64. Landi B, Tkoub M, Gaudric M, et al. Diagnostic yield of push enteroscopy in relation to indications. Gut 1998;42:421–5.
65. MacKenzie JF. Push enteroscopy. Gastrointest Endosc Clin N Am 1999;9(1):71–92.

Intraoperative Enteroscopy

Hans-Joachim Schulz, MD*, Harald Schmidt, MD

KEYWORDS

- Intraoperative enteroscopy • Small intestine
- Obscure bleeding • Peutz-Jegher's syndrome
- Small bowel tumor

Current options for the diagnosis and management of small bowel lesions include push enteroscopy, video capsule endoscopy (VCE), single-balloon enteroscopy (SBE), double-balloon enteroscopy (DBE) and intraoperative enteroscopy (IOE). In the past, IOE, which exposes the patient to complications related to laparotomy or laparoscopy, was the only reliable procedure for exploration of the entire small bowel.[1]

Exploratory laparotomy without IOE is not recommended because it subjects the patient to all the risks of surgery without the benefit of a complete endoscopic examination for the detection of subtle mucosal lesions that can be missed by palpation and transillumination alone. The potential of IOE has been attested to through case reports,[2–4] small series reports,[5–11] larger series of patients from a single institution,[12,13,15–17] and multicenter studies.[14] These studies have demonstrated the usefulness and limitations of IOE in a variety of difficult gastrointestinal problems. The indications for IOE have been reduced in recent years because of the development of VCE and DBE.

INDICATIONS

IOE is now accepted as the ultimate procedure for completely evaluating the small bowel.[8,9] However, improvements in imaging procedures (CT, magnetic resonance imaging [MRI], angiography) and the introduction of VCE and balloon enteroscopy (BE) have restricted the indications for IOE to the following diagnostic and therapeutic situations:

1. Obscure GI bleeding
   - Massive "mid-gut" GI bleeding or "mid-gut" GI bleeding in urgent situations when VCE or BE are not available
   - Lesions not accessible by BE
   - Lesions difficult or impossible to treat by BE

Oskar-Ziethen-Hospital, Sana Clinic Lichtenberg, Medical Clinic I, Berlin University-Teaching Hospital (Charité), Fanninger Street 32, 10365 Berlin, Germany
* Corresponding author.
E-mail address: hj.schulz@sana-kl.de (H-J. Schulz).

Gastrointest Endoscopy Clin N Am 19 (2009) 371–379
doi:10.1016/j.giec.2009.04.011 **giendo.theclinics.com**
1052-5157/09/$ – see front matter © 2009 Elsevier Inc. All rights reserved.

2. Difficult GI problems, for example, in cases of suspected lymphoma, suspected active small bowel endocrine tumor, or suspected malignant tumors.[17]
3. Crohn disease: IOE is useful for identifying mucosal changes and the degree of strictures that require surgical intervention.[18–20]
4. In Peutz-Jeghers syndrome IOE improves polyp clearance without the need for additional enterotomies and may help to reduce the frequency of laparotomies.[21]

Although most patients who have undergone operative enteroscopy have been adults, operative enteroscopy has been performed in children as young as 4 years.[21]

TECHNIQUE

The technique of IOE varies in several potentially important respects, such as the approach to intraabdominal access (laparotomy versus laparoscopy), the endoscope used, and the technique of endoscope insertion.

The standard procedure consists of a laparotomy followed by one enterotomy (usually in the middle of the small intestine) or two small incisions through which the endoscope (a standard colonoscope, preferably pediatric, a push enteroscope, or even a standard gastroscope) is introduced. IOE through an enterotomy offers the best option for inspecting the entire small bowel and for decreasing trauma to the bowel.[13–17,20,22,23] In 1968, Sweeting used a fiberoptic esophagoscope passed through two separate operative enterotomies to examine the entire small bowel mucosa of a patient with hereditary familial teleangiectasia.

The technique of IOE combining laparotomy and peroral endoscopic inspection was reported by several investigators[5–8,10–13,24] who performed intraoperative video-panendoscopies with an endoscope inserted transorally for jejunal examination and with another endoscope introduced transanally for ileal examination.

Laparoscopically assisted total enteroscopies have also been described.[25–27] Recently, Ross described a laparoscopically assisted double-balloon enteroscopy.[28] Agarwal described a special technique of laparo-enteroscopy using the laparoscope to perform IOE.[29]

Peroral/Peranal Technique

Transoral and transanal methods are less likely to achieve full visualization of the small intestine; many reports describe failure to reach the terminal ileum in a significant number of patients.[8,9,16,30] The limited working length of endoscopes prevent the entire small bowel from being visualized by the peroral approach.

After the abdomen is opened and generally explored, the endoscope is introduced orally. With the laparoscopically assisted modification, the endoscope is inserted perorally as far as possible into the small intestine. Care is taken to limit insufflation of intestinal loops. The intestine is gently grasped with two endo-Babcock clamps to allow the endoscope to slide more easily.[26] Another difficulty with this technique is looping of the enteroscope in the stomach, which can be avoided by the use of an overtube. Compared with the standard procedure the method is time-consuming and sometimes difficult to perform. Some cases require an additional enterotomy to prevent overdistension of the mesentery when reaching the terminal ileum.

Standard Method

The most invasive but effective technique of IOE is open surgery combined with enterotomy. The enterotomy method allows a more complete and controlled visualization of the entire small intestinal mucosa. After standard explorative laparotomy the bowel is inspected for external changes (eg, vascular malformation), the presence of any palpable lesions or mural thickening, indicating Crohn disease. Small bowel mobilization and adhesiolysis can be performed. In patients with extensive adhesions or areas of extreme fixation more than one enterotomy can be used to maximize mucosal inspections and avoid overdistension and subsequent laceration of the mesentery.

Endoscopes

Usually a pediatric video colonoscope (135 cm) or a video enteroscope (220 cm) is used to perform IOE. Care has to be taken to avoid infection of the surgical field. The thoroughly cleaned and disinfected instrument is prepared with gas sterilization or a nonsterilized endoscope covered by a sterile plastic sleeve is inserted through an enterotomy opening.[22,23,31] The small bowel is than examined segmentally. With an occlusion clamp lightly applied at fixed distances, overdistension of the stomach or the more distal bowel can be prevented.[8] Noncrushing occluding clamps can also be positioned at the ileocecal valve distally and at the duodeno-jejunal junction.

Primarily we examine our patients proximally to the duodeno-jejunal junction or up to the duodenum. Then we inspect the distal jejunum and ileum down to the ileocecal valve. It is essential to examine the mucosa as the endoscope is being advanced and to aspirate the inflated segment thoroughly but gently before progressing distally.

The endoscopic views are supplemented by simultaneously viewing the mucosa from the outside of the transilluminated bowel wall to detect bleeding or vascular malformations (mucosa transillumination). Abnormalities seen on transillumination are also assessed internally to distinguish vascular lesions from any hematomas caused by operative trauma.

In patients with Peutz-Jeghers syndrome enteroscopy is usually performed through an enterotomy at the site of planned surgical polypectomy. Endoscopic examination of the bowel is performed on withdrawal of the scope.[21]

TREATMENT

Treatment may be performed endoscopically, or the affected small bowel segments may be identified endoscopically and then treated surgically, usually in the form of a segmental resection.[11,13,16,19,21]

LIMITING FACTORS FOR IOE

Limiting factors for IOE are comorbidities and the requirement of general anesthesia in the elderly. Dense adhesions with a shortened mesentery and massive hemorrhage with blood obscuring the intestinal lumen may limit the full use of the endoscope during IOE.[5]

OBSCURE GI BLEEDING

Identifying the source of obscure GI bleeding presents a diagnostic challenge.[32] It has been estimated that approximately 5% of GI bleeding occurs between the ligament of Treitz and the cecal valve.[33,34] IOE during laparotomy is typically used as a last resort in patients with obscure GI bleeding requiring multiple transfusions or repeated hospitalizations.[1]

In contrast to other conventional procedures, including enteroclysis, angiography, and various forms of small bowel endoscopy, the ability of IOE to identify potential bleeding lesions has been impressive, ranging from 70% to 100% (**Table 1**). Detailed data from our two cooperating German centers are given in **Table 2**.

Table 1
Intraoperative enteroscopy in obscure GI bleeding: diagnostic yield

Author	Patients (n)	Diagnostic Yield
Bowden et al 1980[5]	18	89
Lau et al 1987[6]	15	80
Flickinger et al 1989[7]	14	93
Lewis et al 1991[9]	23	87
Desa et al 1991[8]	12	83
Ress et al 1992[11]	44	70
Szold et al 1992[12]	30	93
Lopez et al 1996[35]	16	88
Dourad et al 2000[13]	20	80
Kendrick et al 2001[16]	70	74
Jakobs et al 2006[15]	81	84
Kopáčova et al 2007[17]	41	90

In a prospective 2-center study comparing wireless capsule endoscopy with IOE in 47 consecutive patients with obscure GI bleeding, the diagnostic yield of IOE varied with the type of bleeding.[35] In patients with ongoing obscure overt bleeding, the diagnostic yield was high (positive findings in 100%) and was greater than in patients with previous overt bleeding (positive findings in 70.8%) or with obscure occult bleeding (positive findings in 50%; **Table 3**). Vascular lesions and polyps may be treated endoscopically or marked with a suture for local or segmental resection.

Angiodysplasia were treated by argon plasma coagulation therapy or by resection depending on the size of the lesions. Resection was performed in cases of tumor, large polyps, Meckel diverticulum, or multiple/large diverticula (**Table 4**).

Table 2
Intraoperative enteroscopy in obscure GI bleeding at 2 cooperating centers (n = 123)

Center	Ludwigshafen[a]	Berlin[b]	Total Number of Patients (%)
n	81	42	123
Mid-age (y)	–	–	65
Complete enteroscopy	81/81	42/42	123/123
Severe complications	1/81	1/42	2/123 (1.6)
Mortality	0/81	1/42[c]	1/123 (0.8)
Pathologic results	68/81	34/42	102/123 (83)
Angiodysplasia	44/68	20/34	64/102
Ulcers	9/68	5/34	14/102
Tumor/polyp	6/68	5/34	11/102
Diverticula (Meckel, multiple)	7/68	2/34	9/102
Other (anastomotic vessels, fistula)	2/68	2/34	4/102

[a] *Data from* Jakobs R, Hartmann D, Benz C, et al. Diagnosis of obscure gastrointestinal bleeding by intraoperative enteroscopy in 81 consecutive patients. World J Gastroenterol 2006;12(2):313–16.
[b] Schulz HJ, Schmidt H, own unpublished results.
[c] One death after surgical resection.

Table 3
Diagnostic yield of intraoperative enteroscopy according to type of bleeding

	Type of Lesion, n (%)		
Type of Bleeding	**Positive**	**Suspicious**	**Negative**
Overt ongoing (n = 11)	11 (100)	0 (0)	0 (0)
Overt previous (n = 12)	17 (70.8)	3 (12.5)	4 (16.7)
Occult (n = 12)	6 (50)	3 (25)	3 (25)

LONG-TERM RESULTS

The bleeding rate after IOE was 30% at a mean follow-up of 19 months[13] or 25.5% with a mean follow-up of 346.3 days (range 253–814 d).[35]

In our study, nine patients with multiple angiodysplasia required the following treatment after IOE: blood transfusions in four patients, endoscopic interventions in five patients. In two patients the bleeding could not be stopped definitively (**Fig. 1**). Intestinal bleeding remains the most common indication for diagnostic enteroscopy and the therapeutic approach depends on the severity of bleeding and the patient's condition (age, comorbidity, medications such as anticoagulants).

An initial DBE is a cost-effective approach for patients with obscure bleeding. However, capsule-directed DBE may be associated with better long-term outcomes.[36] In nonsevere bleeding VCE findings are helpful to decide between BE and IOE (**Fig. 2**).

SMALL BOWEL ENDOCRINE TUMORS

In patients with a clinical suspicion of active bleeding, small bowel endocrine tumors found endoscopically (five carcinoids) could be easily resected by surgical means.[17]

CROHN DISEASE

Surgical strategies can be optimized based on IOE findings. The luminal status, including the degree of stricture and ulcer activity, may be helpful for decision making during surgery for patients with Crohn disease.[23]

Table 4
Intraoperative enteroscopy guided therapy: results from 2 cooperating centers (n = 83)

	Number of Procedures
Angiodysplasia	
APC	31
APC + surgical suture	26
Surgical resection	9
Tumor/polyp	
Surgical resection	8
Large diverticula	
Surgical resection	9

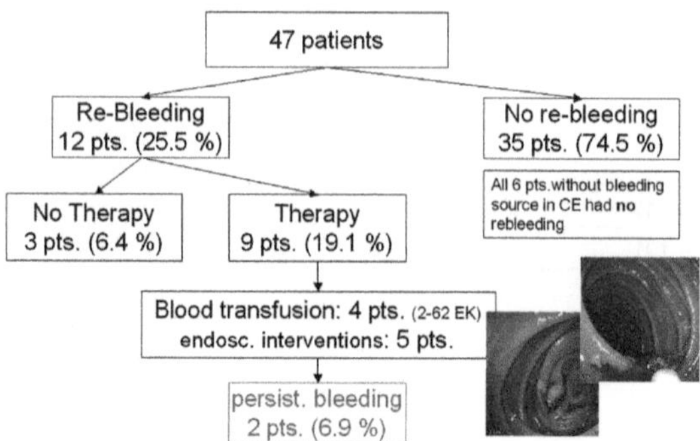

Fig. 1. Intraoperative enteroscopy in obscure GI bleeding: long-term results. (*Data from* Hartmann D, Schmidt H, Bolz G, et al. A prospective two-center study comparing wireless capsule endoscopy with intraoperative enteroscopy in patients with obscure GI bleeding. Gastrointest Endosc 2005;61(7):826–32; and Schmidt H, Hartmann D, Kinzel F, et al. Prospective controlled multicentic trial comparing capsule enteroscopy: long term results in patients with chronic gastrointestinal bleeding. Gastrointest Endosc 2004;59:16.)

PEUTZ-JEGHERS SYNDROME

Intraoperative evaluation of the small intestine has became the standard at several hospitals.[21,37] IOE improves polyp clearance without the need for additional enterotomies and may help to reduce the frequency of laparotomies. DBE and a laparoscopically assisted DBE are minimally invasive, single-step procedures that can be used for small bowel polyp surveillance and treatment of patients with Peutz-Jeghers syndrome.

COMPLICATIONS

Complication rates have ranged from 0% to 52% and include mucosal laceration, intramural hematomas, mesenteric hemorrhage, perforation (mini-perforations after adhesiolysis; these are difficult to find and to close), prolonged paralytic ileus, intestinal ischemia, intestinal obstruction, wound infection, and postoperative pulmonary infection.[8,9,24,38–40]

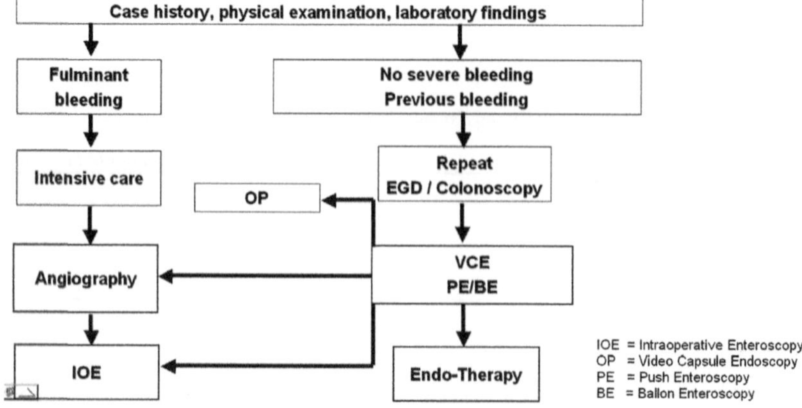

Fig. 2. Management of intestinal bleeding.

Using a transoral or transanal method of insertion requires excessive pleating or telescoping of the bowel onto the endoscope, which may cause complications such as mucosal or serosal tears with an incidence as high as 52%. Significant intraoperative complications are reported in 3%, postoperative complications occurred in 26%, and 30-day mortality in 6%.[16] Although most studies do not report mortality, mortality related to the procedure or to postoperative complications has been reported to be as much as 11%.[8,9] In our study one patient died of peritonitis after small bowel resection and the development of an anastomotic fistula.

SUMMARY

Current options for the diagnosis and management of small bowel lesions include PE, VCE, SBE, DBE, and IOE. IOE, the ultimate diagnostic and therapeutic modality for small bowel disorders, is a major surgical and endoscopic procedure. It should be reserved for cases that cannot be managed with others modalities because of the difficulties of the procedure and significant morbidity. The indication for IOE have diminished in recent years because of the development of VCE and DBE. IOE is reserved for patients with massive mid-gut bleeding, lesions not accessible by balloon enteroscopy, and lesions difficult or impossible to treat by balloon enteroscopy. There are special indications in Crohn disease and in Peutz-Jeghers syndrome.

REFERENCES

1. Cave DR, Cooley JS. Intra-operative enteroscopy. Indications and techniques. Gastrointest Endosc Clin N Am 1996;6(4):793–802.
2. Lucas CE, Sugawa C. Diagnostic endoscopy during laparotomy for acute hemorrhage from the upper part of the gastrointestinal tract. Surg Gynecol Obstet 1972; 135(2):285–6.
3. Bombeck CT. Intraoperative esophagoscopy, gastroscopy, colonoscopy, and endoscopy of the small bowel. Surg Clin North Am 1975;55(1):135–42.
4. Greenberg GR, Phillips MJ, Tovee EB, et al. Fiberoptic endoscopy during laparotomy in the diagnosis of small intestinal bleeding. Gastroenterology 1976; 71(1):133–5.
5. Bowden TA Jr, Hooks VH III, Mansberger AR Jr. Intraoperative gastrointestinal endoscopy. Ann Surg 1980;191(6):680–7.
6. Lau WY. Intraoperative enteroscopy – indications and limitations. Gastrointest Endosc 1990;36(3):268–71.
7. Flickinger EG, Stanforth AC, Sinar DR, et al. Intraoperative video panendoscopy for diagnosing sites of chronic intestinal bleeding. Am J Surg 1989;157(1): 137–44.
8. Desa LA, Ohri SK, Hutton KA, et al. Role of intraoperative enteroscopy in obscure gastrointestinal bleeding of small bowel origin. Br J Surg 1991;78(2):192–5.
9. Lewis BS, Wenger JS, Waye JD. Small bowel enteroscopy and intraoperative enteroscopy for obscure gastrointestinal bleeding. Am J Gastroenterol 1991; 86(2):171–4.
10. Mathus-Vliegen EM, Tytgat GN. Intraoperative endoscopy: technique, indications, and results. Gastrointest Endosc 1986;32(6):381–4.
11. Ress AM, Benacci JC, Sarr MG. Efficacy of intraoperative enteroscopy in diagnosis and prevention of recurrent, occult gastrointestinal bleeding. Am J Surg 1992;163(1):98–9.
12. Szold A, Katz LB, Lewis BS. Surgical approach to occult gastrointestinal bleeding. Am J Surg 1992;163(1):90–3.

13. Douard R, Wind P, Panis Y, et al. Intraoperative enteroscopy for diagnosis and management of unexplained gastrointestinal bleeding. Am J Surg 2000;180(3): 181–4.
14. Hartmann D, Schmidt H, Bolz G, et al. A prospective two-center study comparing wireless capsule endoscopy with intraoperative enteroscopy in patients with obscure GI bleeding. Gastrointest Endosc 2005;61(7):826–32.
15. Jakobs R, Hartmann D, Benz C, et al. Diagnosis of obscure gastrointestinal bleeding by intraoperative enteroscopy in 81 consecutive patients. World J Gastroenterol 2006;12(2):313–6.
16. Kendrick ML, Buttar NS, Anderson MA, et al. Contribution of intraoperative enteroscopy in the management of obscure gastrointestinal bleeding. J Gastrointest Surg 2001;5(2):162–7.
17. Kopacova M, Bures J, Vykouril L, et al. Intraoperative enteroscopy: ten years' experience at a single tertiary center. Surg Endosc 2007;21(7):1111–6.
18. Arima S, Yoshimura S, Futami K, et al. The postoperative recurrence of Crohn's disease: an analysis of 37 patients with Crohn's disease who underwent endoscopy during initial surgery. Surg Today 1992;22(4):346–50.
19. Esaki M, Matsumoto T, Hizawa K, et al. Intraoperative enteroscopy detects more lesions but is not predictive of postoperative recurrence in Crohn's disease. Surg Endosc 2001;15(5):455–9.
20. Hotokezaka M, Jimi SI, Hidaka H, et al. Role of intraoperative enteroscopy for surgical decision making with Crohn's disease. Surg Endosc 2007;21(7): 1238–42.
21. Edwards DP, Khosraviani K, Stafferton R, et al. Long-term results of polyp clearance by intraoperative enteroscopy in the Peutz-Jeghers syndrome. Dis Colon Rectum 2003;46(1):48–50.
22. Smedh K, Olaison G, Nystrom PO, et al. Intraoperative enteroscopy in Crohn's disease. Br J Surg 1993;80(7):897–900.
23. Almer S, Granerus G, Strom M, et al. Leukocyte scintigraphy compared to intraoperative small bowel enteroscopy and laparotomy findings in Crohn's disease. Inflamm Bowel Dis 2007;13(2):164–74.
24. Lopez MJ, Cooley JS, Petros JG, et al. Complete intraoperative small-bowel endoscopy in the evaluation of occult gastrointestinal bleeding using the sonde enteroscope. Arch Surg 1996;131(3):272–7.
25. Reddy ND, Rao VG. Laparoscopically assisted panenteroscopy for snare excision. Gastrointest Endosc 1996;44(2):208–9.
26. Ingrosso M, Prete F, Pisani A, et al. Laparoscopically assisted total enteroscopy: a new approach to small intestinal diseases. Gastrointest Endosc 1999;49(5): 651–3.
27. Sriram PV, Rao GV, Reddy DN. Laparoscopically assisted panenteroscopy. Gastrointest Endosc 2001;54(6):805–6.
28. Ross AS, Dye C, Prachand VN. Laparoscopic-assisted double-balloon enteroscopy for small-bowel polyp surveillance and treatment in patients with Peutz-Jeghers syndrome. Gastrointest Endosc 2006;64(6):984–8.
29. Agarwal A. Use of the laparoscope to perform intraoperative enteroscopy. Surg Endosc 1999;13(11):1143–4.
30. Zaman A, Sheppard B, Katon RM. Total peroral intraoperative enteroscopy for obscure GI bleeding using a dedicated push enteroscope: diagnostic yield and patient outcome. Gastrointest Endosc 1999;50(4):506–10.
31. Lachter J, Krausz MM. Novel use of a plastic overtube facilitates intraoperative enteroscopy in Crohn's disease. Hepatogastroenterology 2003;50(53):1446–8.

32. Leighton JA, Goldstein J, Hirota W, et al. Obscure gastrointestinal bleeding. Gastrointest Endosc 2003;58(5):650–5.
33. Katz LB. The role of surgery in occult gastrointestinal bleeding. Semin Gastrointest Dis 1999;10:78–81.
34. Eisen GM, Dominitz JA, Faigel DO, et al. Enteroscopy. Gastrointest Endosc 2001; 53(7):871–3.
35. Hartmann D, Schmidt H, Schilling D, et al. Follow-up of patients with obscure gastrointestinal bleeding after capsule endoscopy and intraoperative enteroscopy. Hepatogastroenterology 2007;54(75):780–3.
36. Gerson L, Kamal A. Cost-effectiveness analysis of management strategies for obscure GI bleeding. Gastrointest Endosc 2008;68(5):920–36.
37. Pennazio M, Rossini FP. Small bowel polyps in Peutz-Jeghers syndrome: management by combined push enteroscopy and intraoperative enteroscopy. Gastrointest Endosc 2000;51(3):304–8.
38. Whelan RL, Buls JG, Goldberg SM, et al. Intraoperative endoscopy. University of Minesota experience. Am Surg 1989;55:281–6.
39. Krisham RS, Kent RB III. Enterovaginal fistula as a complication of intraoperative small bowel endoscopy. Surg Laparosc Endosc 1998;8:388–9.
40. Schmidt H, Hartmann D, Kinzel F, et al. Prospective controlled multicentic trial comparing capsule enteroscopy: long term results in patients with chronic gastrointestinal bleeding. Gastrointest Endosc 2004;59:166.

Techniques, Tricks, and Complications of Enteroscopy

Simon K. Lo, MD

KEYWORDS

• Enteroscopy • Technique • Complication
• Trick • Spiral • Overtube

Small bowel endoscopy has made tremendous advances over the last 8 years. The introduction of capsule endoscopy, double-balloon enteroscopy, single-balloon enteroscopy and spiral overtube-assisted enteroscopy have completely removed the mystery in investigating the small intestine. For convenience, spiral overtube-assisted enteroscopy is referred to as spiral enteroscopy in this article. Many readers do not have first-hand experience with these new procedures, which are challenging and time-consuming to perform. A brief overview on the technical issues and complications related to these small bowel endoscopy procedures is presented.

PUSH ENTEROSCOPY

Technique

A variety of long-length endoscopes have been used for this purpose, including the standard colonoscope, pediatric colonoscope, and standard push enteroscope. Special skill is not typically required for this procedure. Most endoscopists experienced in colonoscopy are capable of navigating their scope into the proximal jejunum, but rarely reach the mid-jejunum. The specially designed push enteroscopes are typically 250 cm in length and may be used in combination with an overtube, which is felt by some endoscopists to improve the depth of scope insertion.[1] The extra length of a push enteroscope probably allows a slightly farther reach within the jejunum; however, it is also associated with increased friction when passing an accessory through the instrument channel.

The author has received a traveling grant from Given Imaging Inc., an honorarium from Olympus America Inc., and an honorarium from Spirus Medical.

Division of Digestive Diseases, Department of Medicine, Cedars-Sinai Medical Center, David Geffen School of Medicine at UCLA, 8700 Beverly Boulevard, Room 7511, Los Angeles, CA 90048, USA

E-mail address: simon.lo@cshs.org

Gastrointest Endoscopy Clin N Am 19 (2009) 381–388
doi:10.1016/j.giec.2009.04.013 giendo.theclinics.com
1052-5157/09/$ – see front matter © 2009 Elsevier Inc. All rights reserved.

Tricks

The technique of push enteroscopy is basic and there is little in the way of improving the performance. Nonetheless, it is important to keep the scope straight and minimize air collection in the gastric fundus. If a lot of the scope is inside the stomach, it implies coiling within the fundus, which would reduce the efficiency of scope advancement and cause trauma to the gastric mucosa. After reaching the descending duodenum, gentle shortening of the scope allows better forward passage and reduces the chance of fundic coiling. From that point on, intermittent to and fro motion is necessary to facilitate scope advancement. A wire stiffener can occasionally be used to reduce scope bending and shift the pushing force to the front of the enteroscope. Alternatively, tightening the dial of a variable stiffness enteroscope (Olympus America, Inc.) may enhance the pushing ability of the scope. A small study has reported improved depth of small bowel examination with the variable stiffness push enteroscope over its conventional counterpart, regardless of usage of an overtube.[2]

Complications

Push enteroscopy is a safe procedure that has been used as a routine examination of the proximal small bowel for many years. Few reports of significant complications can be found in the recent literature. Nonetheless, one report cited a 1% complication rate, with a case of a piriform sinus perforation and another case of a small bowel perforation.[3] Because most push enteroscopes are stiff and bulky, care must be taken to avoid trauma to the thin-walled duodenum and jejunum.

DOUBLE-BALLOON ENTEROSCOPY

Technique

This is perhaps the most complicated and physically demanding endoscopy to perform, particularly for the retrograde procedure. Double-balloon enteroscopy is a two-person procedure that requires an assistant to manage the overtube. An upper double-balloon enteroscopy begins with taping the overtube, with its balloon fully collapsed, to the proximal end of the shaft of the endoscope. After the scope has reached the prepyloric antrum, the tape is removed and the overtube is advanced over the scope until it reaches a wide white band (155 cm point from the tip of the endoscope) on the endoscope. The scope is then inserted until the overtube keeps it from going further. The scope balloon is inflated to anchor against the jejunal wall to allow forward sliding of the overtube. If the distal end of the overtube has clearly gone past the duodenum, its balloon can be inflated to anchor down the overtube. With both balloons up and close together, the tube and scope are pulled back simultaneously until there is resistance. This withdrawal maneuver represents the first pleating of intestinal folds over the overtube. With the overtube gripping the jejunum with its balloon, the scope's balloon is deflated and the scope is advanced again until it hits the proximal end of the overtube. The scope can then be used to anchor against the jejunum, with its balloon inflated, to help slide the deflated overtube forward. Once the overtube has reached the white band, its balloon is inflated with the push of a button on the control device. The scope and overtube are then pulled back together to pleat the small bowel further. This cycle of forward advancement and pull back (**Box 1**) is repeated until the scope is no longer able to gain ground despite forward motions. After reaching the desired depth of insertion, the scope may be withdrawn by reversing the maneuvers for the insertion cycle.

Box 1
The 7 steps of each insertion cycle of double-balloon enteroscopy

1. insert scope
2. inflate scope balloon
3. deflate overtube balloon
4. advance overtube
5. inflate overtube
6. pull back scope and overtube
7. deflate scope balloon

Tricks

The basic technique is standardized and is so repetitive that it may seem difficult to add to the basic maneuvers. Although it is easy to learn to perform double-balloon enteroscopy, it takes extensive practice and acquisition of some fine skills to become an expert in this procedure. Similar to the performance of colonoscopy, air distention of the intestine must be keep to the absolute minimum to pleat effectively and travel far. In contrast to the colon with a wide lumen, the small bowel has a small caliber and is easily collapsed with suctioning. Thus, it is difficult to recapture the air within the small intestine. It is advantageous to employ CO_2 gas rather than room air for bowel insufflation because of its rapid diffusion across the mucosa. A recent study showed that CO_2 insufflation significantly extended intubation depth and reduced postprocedure discomfort.[4]

Double-balloon enteroscopes are thin and long and are difficult to insert through the overtube. Keeping the overtube filled with water, to reduce friction between the scope and the overtube, is essential to a smooth procedure. Beginners may find a through-the-scope stiffening wire beneficial to add to the insertion rigidity of the enteroscope. Negotiating around tight corners seems to be more effective by rotating the shaft than adjusting the right-left dial of the enteroscope. It is important to keep the scope short because rotation is easier to carry out when the scope is kept straight. Effective pleating of the intestine also tends to reduce the redundancy ahead of the scope and enhance its forward movement during scope passage. During pleating-pull back, it is helpful to simultaneously rotate the scope slightly to find the lumen. Even though it is recommended to stick to the alternating push-pull cycle, it is sometimes necessary to skip a pull back step if there is no forward progress following the usual maneuvers. Abdominal compression in the central or left lower quadrant is also an effective technique when other maneuvers have failed to move the scope forward.

After reaching the farthest or desired location, many endoscopists inject tattoo ink to mark the spot for future reference. The thin wall of the small intestine predisposes to leakage of ink outside of the serosa and spill into the peritoneum causing abdominal pain. This problem can be avoided by first injecting saline into the wall of the intestine. Once a saline blister has been raised, tattoo ink can then be delivered into the tissue without worrying about spilling it outside of the intestinal wall.

Performing therapy and taking biopsy specimens are usually a frustrating experience. Targeting a lesion is a difficult task, as is finding a lesion that has been seen during an earlier part of the examination. It is absolutely crucial to tattoo an area nearby a lesion as soon as it is noted, as motility and the lack of landmarks within the long, featureless intestine can easily make a small lesion disappear. Inserting a needle catheter, biopsy forceps or argon plasma probe is often extremely difficult because of friction created by the long and skinny instrument channel. Using a standard instrument jelly may not be sufficient to overcome the friction. Vegetable oil is an excellent lubricant for this purpose. When attempting a hemostasis procedure, it is easier to use argon plasma than a bipolar circumactive probe (BICAP) because it does not require precise placement of the instrument. Straightening and rotation of the scope is usually necessary to improve aim on a lesion. Insertion of an endoscopic clip can be challenging, but a version of the clip (Resolution Clip; Boston Scientific, Natick, Massachusetts) can be stripped of its outer plastic catheter and passed through the scope "naked" to take advantage of the smaller caliber device.

Retrograde scope passage through the ileocecal value and the distal ileum can be a challenging task.[5] Advancement of the thin scope from the descending colon into the ileum pushes the shaft into the cecum and flips the scope toward a different direction from the ileum. This cecal-looping effect can paradoxically pull the scope back out of the ileocecal valve. To overcome this technical problem, the cecum should be decompressed to reduce the space for looping. The overtube is shortened and its balloon is maximally inflated to keep the scope in a straight position. During passage into the ileum, air should not be used to open up the lumen for visualization. A small amount of water may be infused through the scope to help explore the lumen to guide passage. Additional maneuvers to ensure success in reaching the terminal ileum include external compression of the right lower quadrant, rotating the patient onto his/her back and inserting a wire or dilating balloon across the ileocecal valve.

Complications

When double-balloon enteroscopy was first introduced, there were concerns that the balloons would induce perforation, intussusceptions, and prolonged ileus. Although perforation does seem to occur more frequently in patients with surgical anastomosis,[6] intussusception and prolonged ileus have not been reported. Nonetheless, an international, multicenter, report has identified a surprisingly high rate (0.3%) of pancreatitis.[7] The reason for pancreatitis is still unknown,[8] but this complication seems to be linked only to orally inserted double-balloon enteroscopy. Excessive traction during the pull backs has been speculated to be the cause of this complication. Even though many experts do not believe that direct injury to the major papilla is the source, the usual recommendation is to avoid inflating the balloons within the duodenum. Cases of mucosal and peritoneal bleeding have also been reported with diagnostic double-balloon enteroscopy.[9] Abdominal pain used to be reported in 5% to 10% of the cases. However, the use of CO_2 gas seems to have coincided with a dramatic reduction in postprocedure abdominal discomfort.

SINGLE-BALLOON ENTEROSCOPY

Technique

Single-balloon enteroscopy was designed to mimic the functions of double-balloon enteroscopy. The single-balloon system looks just like double-balloon enteroscopy except for the lack of a balloon at the tip of the endoscope. The technique employed to advance the device is similar to that for the double balloon, but simpler. The maneuvers to perform oral insertion, separate the overtube from the endoscope, and pass the scope into the proximal jejunum are identical to that for the double-balloon system. Because there is no scope balloon, the tip of the enteroscope is deflected and air is removed to provide the traction needed to slide the overtube forward. Once the overtube has reached the desired distance, the 150 cm mark on the endoscope, the overtube balloon is inflated to anchor against the intestinal wall. The scope, along with the overtube, is then pulled back until increased tension is felt. The scope is then inserted while the balloon keeps the overtube in position. When the scope can advance no further, the overtube balloon is inflated. The overtube and scope are pulled back together again. This cycle of insertion and pleating continues until the scope can no longer gain ground despite efforts to move it forward (**Box 2**). The withdrawal cycle is a complete reversal of the insertion cycle. As shown in **Boxes 1** and **2**, single-balloon enteroscopy is simpler to perform than double-balloon enteroscopy.

Tricks

The balloon in this system is made of silicon, which takes time to expand and contract. To take full advantage of the traction created by the overtube, roughly 10 seconds should be allowed for the balloon to get fully inflated. The same amount of time is needed for the balloon to deflate. On the other hand, the scope must create traction by suctioning and tip angulation. Therefore, it is critically important that air insufflation is kept to the minimum during the study. As in the case of double-balloon enteroscopy, CO_2 use may reduce the chance of overinflating the intestine and, at the same time, eliminate abdominal pain as a result of gaseous distention of the abdomen. Many endoscopists find it helpful to use water, instead of air, to expand the intestinal lumen for scope passage. It is assumed that it takes a larger volume of air than water to distend the lumen ahead of the endoscope because of the tendency of air to spread fast in different directions. The techniques used to insert instruments and target lesions are similar to those for double-balloon enteroscopy. Once again, it is helpful to use vegetable oil to lubricate the long and narrow instrument channel to facilitate passage of accessories.

Complications

There are few reports on the clinical experience of single-balloon enteroscopy. It is generally considered safe and perhaps similar to double-balloon enteroscopy. Because the balloon is made of silicone, allergy to latex is not an issue for this device. Pancreatitis is considered to be one of the most common complications of diagnostic double-balloon enteroscopy, no pancreatitis has been linked to the single-balloon procedure to date. A perforation was reported to occur in the ileal pouch of a patient with a previous history of ulcerative colitis.[10] A mucosal tear, requiring endoscopic clip closure, was noted in a patient with Crohn disease.[11] Transient postprocedure fever has also been reported.

Box 2
The 6 steps of each insertion cycle of single-balloon enteroscopy

1. **insert scope**
2. **deflate overtube balloon**
3. **suction and deflect scope tip**
4. **advance overtube**
5. **inflate overtube**
6. **pull back scope and overtube**

SPIRAL ENTEROSCOPY

Technique

This is a two-person procedure, with a physician or a nurse rotating the overtube and an endoscopist keeping the lumen in view throughout the procedure.[12] The overtube for spiral enteroscopy is equipped with a soft spiral element attached to the outside surface of the distal 20 cm of the tube. Before performing the procedure, the channel of the overtube must be thoroughly lubricated with a special lubricant gel. The lumen of the spiral tube is small and can only accommodate a standard double- or single-balloon enteroscope. When locked tightly onto a coupler at the proximal end of the overtube at the 140 cm mark, the scope is inserted into the esophagus. From this point on, all forward and backward movements of the scope must be done with gentle rotation of the overtube except when the overtube coupler has been unlocked.

Engagement of the spiral in the duodenum may be difficult, and it requires patience and backing up of the scope and the overtube, if necessary. Once the overtube has cleared the ligament of Treitz, further advancement by clockwise spiral is typically easy and fast, as long as the luminal view is in sight. When the spiraling motion is met with significant resistance, the scope can be freed up from the overtube by loosening up the coupler and passing through the overtube as far as possible. Withdrawal of the enteroscope is accomplished by coupling the scope to the overtube and rotating the tube in the counterclockwise direction. When the withdrawing overtube reaches the stomach at around 55 cm, it should be unlocked from the enteroscope to allow a careful endoscopic examination of the ligament of Treitz and the duodenum. Afterward, the scope is again coupled to the overtube and the entire device is removed by continuation of the counterclockwise motion until it is outside the esophagus.

Tricks

This is a procedure that requires total cooperation of the patient. Deep sedation with propofol or general anesthesia is strongly recommended. If general anesthesia is performed, the space in the esophagus for passage of the distal end of the overtube may be limited. Temporary deflating the endotracheal balloon to free up some room is recommended. As in the other forms of enteroscopy, excessive air insufflation may prevent engagement of the spiral and promote looping within the stomach and should be avoided. The difficulty in engaging the spiral in the duodenum may also be minimized by reducing the looping with external abdominal compression or gentle withdrawal while the overtube is being rotated clockwise. If these maneuvers fail to engage the spiral inside the duodenum, the endoscope can be unlocked and advanced beyond the ligament of Treitz. Once the scope has reached the jejunum, it should be pulled back without losing ground, while the overtube is gently spun forward. If multiple attempts at the different maneuvers fail to advance the spiral enteroscope, the procedure should be aborted to avoid unwanted trauma. Inspection during the withdrawal phase is best done by performing the counterclockwise spiraling in a deliberate manner because of the tendency of the wound-up intestine to spring free from the overtube. For the same reason, the overtube should be kept at the same level from the mouth during the initial withdrawal process. Sedation should not be lightened up even toward the end of the procedure, as a semi-awake patient can pull on the fully engaged overtube and sustain injury.

Complications

As this is a new procedure, there is no widespread experience to date. Nonetheless, a recent report described 41% of minor complications; all were related to esophageal mucosal trauma or sore throat.[13] Although no major complications have been reported in the literature thus far, the rotational force used to drive the enteroscope may potentially split the mucosa and cause perforation if tissue is intussuscepted between the overtube and the bowel wall.

INTRAOPERATIVE ENTEROSCOPY

Technique

Many forms of intraoperative enteroscopy have been described. The most common version is done in conjunction with an open laparotomy. Once the small intestine has been exposed, a long enteroscope is inserted orally and passed into the small intestine. The surgeon then helps the passage by pleating the small bowel over the enteroscope, advancing until the ileocecal valve is reached. Alternatively, an enterotomy is created in the mid small intestine. Either a long-length enteroscope or a pediatric colonoscope is inserted through the enterotomy in the retrograde direction until the ligament of Treitz is reached. The scope is then redirected antegrade down the small bowel until the ileocecal valve is identified. In recent years, laparoscopy-assisted intraoperative enteroscopy has been performed with success.[14] Some surgeons choose to adopt modifications of laparoscopic intraoperative enteroscopy that include examination by an enterotomy,[15] hand-assisted scope passage, and even orally inserted double-balloon enteroscopy.[16]

Tricks

Performing successful intraoperative enteroscopy requires good understanding and cooperation between the endoscopist and the surgeon. It is important to minimize air insufflation to prevent excessive bloating of the small bowel and the colon. An additional measure to prevent overinflation is to place a clamp across the small bowel distally. CO_2 may be used to insufflate the small bowel instead of room air to speed up absorption across the small bowel mucosa. When an open laparotomy is performed, the exposed small bowel should be covered with a wet surgical towel to reduce the translumination effect, which can distract the endoscopist.

Complications

Intra- and postoperative complications in the era of laparotomy-assisted enteroscopy were common,[17,18] with serosal laceration and prolonged ileus being the main problems. Air embolism during a laparotomy-assisted endoscopy has been reported[19] and it led to the use of CO_2 for endoscopic insufflation. Abdominal abscess and peritonitis have also been encountered.

SUMMARY

This latest group of endoscopic procedures are more time-consuming and labor-intensive to perform than the traditional forms of endoscopy. Many endoscopists consider them specialty items and are deferring them to their colleagues in tertiary centers. As indications expand and demands grow, these procedures are likely going to spread to the general gastroenterology communities. It is important that all gastroenterologists are well acquainted with how these procedures are done and familiar with their potential complications.

REFERENCES

1. Taylor AC, Chen RY, Desmond PV. Use of an overtube for enteroscopy – does it increase depth of insertion? A prospective study of enteroscopy with and without an overtube. Endoscopy 2001;33:227–30.
2. Harewood GC, Gostout CJ, Farrell MA, et al. Prospective controlled assessment of variable stiffness enteroscopy. Gastrointest Endosc 2003;58:267–71.
3. Lin S, Branch MS, Shetzline M. The importance of indication in the diagnostic value of push enteroscopy. Endoscopy 2003;35:315–21.
4. Domagk D, Bretthauer M, Lenz P, et al. Carbon dioxide insufflation improves intubation depth in double-balloon enteroscopy: a randomized, controlled, double-blind trial. Endoscopy 2007;39:1064–7.
5. Mehdizadeh S, Han NJ, Cheng DW, et al. Success rate of retrograde double-balloon enteroscopy. Gastrointest Endosc 2007;65:633–9.
6. Gerson LB, Flodin JT, Miyabayashi K. Balloon-assisted enteroscopy: technology and troubleshooting. Gastrointest Endosc 2008;68:1158–67.
7. Mensink PB, Haringsma J, Kucharzik T, et al. Complications of double balloon enteroscopy: a multicenter survey. Endoscopy 2007;39:613–5.
8. Lo SK, Simpson PW. Pancreatitis associated with double-balloon enteroscopy: how common is it? Gastrointest Endosc 2007;66:1139–41.
9. Cheng DW, Han NJ, Mehdizadeh S, et al. Intraperitoneal bleeding after oral double-balloon enteroscopy: a case report and review of the literature. Gastrointest Endosc 2007;66:627–9.
10. Kawamura T, Yasuda K, Tanaka K, et al. Clinical evaluation of a newly developed single-balloon enteroscope. Gastrointest Endosc 2008;68:1112–6.
11. Tsujikawa T, Saitoh Y, Andoh A, et al. Novel single-balloon enteroscopy for diagnosis and treatment of the small intestine: preliminary experiences. Endoscopy 2008;40:11–5.
12. Schembre DB, Ross AS. Spiral enteroscopy: a new twist on overtube-assisted endoscopy. Gastrointest Endosc 2009;69:333–6.
13. Akerman PA, Agrawal D, Chen W, et al. Spiral enteroscopy: a novel method of enteroscopy by using the Endo-Ease Discovery SB overtube and a pediatric colonoscope. Gastrointest Endosc 2009;69:327–32.
14. Ingrosso M, Prete F, Pisani A, et al. Laparoscopically assisted total enteroscopy: a new approach to small intestinal diseases. Gastrointest Endosc 1999;49:651–3.
15. Sriram PV, Rao GV, Reddy DN. Laparoscopically assisted panenteroscopy. Gastrointest Endosc 2001;54:805–6.
16. Ross AS, Dye C, Prachand VN. Laparoscopic-assisted double-balloon enteroscopy for small-bowel polyp surveillance and treatment in patients with Peutz-Jeghers syndrome. Gastrointest Endosc 2006;64:984–8.
17. Zaman A, Sheppard B, Katon RM. Total peroral intraoperative enteroscopy for obscure GI bleeding using a dedicated push enteroscope: diagnostic yield and patient outcome. Gastrointest Endosc 1999;50:506–10.
18. Desa LA, Ohri SK, Hutton KA, et al. Role of intraoperative enteroscopy in obscure gastrointestinal bleeding of small bowel origin. Br J Surg 1991;78:192–5.
19. Holzman RS, Yoo L, Fox VL, et al. Air embolism during intraoperative endoscopic localization and surgical resection for blue rubber bleb nevus syndrome. Anesthesiology 2005;102:1279–80.

Enteroscopy and its Relationship to Radiological Small Bowel Imaging

Stijn J.B. Van Weyenberg, MD[a], Jan Hein T.M. Van Waesberghe, MD, PhD[b], Christian Ell, MD, PhD[c], Jürgen Pohl, MD, PhD[c,*]

KEYWORDS

• Crohn disease • Small bowel polyposis • Celiac disease
• Small intestinal cancer • Radiology • Enteroscopy

For several decades small bowel radiology was the only nonoperative modality to investigate the total small bowel. The introduction of video capsule endoscopy (VCE) and balloon-assisted enteroscopy, like double-balloon endoscopy (DBE) and single-balloon endoscopy (SBE), have allowed endoscopic evaluation of the small intestine. Despite these recent major advances in small bowel endoscopy, radiological imaging remains important for patients with suspected or established small bowel disease. The advantages of radiological imaging include its low invasiveness and the possibility of investigating extraluminal abnormalities as well as intraluminal changes. However, in most conditions, obtaining biopsy specimens for histologic analysis by enteroscopy remains mandatory and small bowel radiology is usually used to select patients who require enteroscopy. Important factors when considering radiological imaging of the small bowel include patient exposure to potentially carcinogenic radiation and the diagnostic accuracy of tests. A problem with the interpretation of studies on radiological small bowel imaging, is that many compare the results of a new modality with a suboptimal reference test, like conventional enteroclysis. Complete balloon-assisted enteroscopy and operative findings are in our view the standard of reference in small bowel investigation. However, there is only a limited amount of literature using enteroscopy as the reference test.

In addition, excellent diagnostic accuracies of many new imaging modalities are only achieved when these tests are performed and interpreted by experts in the field,

[a] Department of Gastroenterology and Hepatology, VU University Medical Center PO Box 7057, 1007 MB, Amsterdam, The Netherlands
[b] Department of Radiology, VU University Medical Center, PO Box 7057, 1007 MB, Amsterdam, The Netherlands
[c] Department of Internal Medicine II, Dr. Horst Schmidt Klinik (Medical School of the University of Mainz), Ludwig Erhardt Strasse 100, Wiesbaden, Germany
* Corresponding author.
E-mail address: pohljuergen@web.de (J. Pohl).

Gastrointest Endoscopy Clin N Am 19 (2009) 389–407
doi:10.1016/j.giec.2009.04.008 giendo.theclinics.com
1052-5157/09/$ – see front matter © 2009 Elsevier Inc. All rights reserved.

usually in highly selected patient populations. Therefore, it is unlikely that in daily practice, the same sensitivity and specificity can be achieved.

In this article the current techniques of radiological small bowel imaging and findings in the most prevalent small bowel disorders are reviewed, with special emphasis on the relationship between endoscopic and radiological methods. It is important for gastroenterologists to be aware of the progress that has been achieved in small bowel radiology. However, in many hospitals around the world the expertise in and the availability of newer methods like magnetic resonance imaging is limited.

PART 1: METHODS OF RADIOLOGICAL SMALL BOWEL IMAGING

General Issues

The ideal small bowel imaging method should be noninvasive, not require potentially toxic (intravenous) contrast agents, not use ionizing radiation, and be able to visualize the total small intestinal lumen, bowel wall, and surrounding structures. In addition, the ideal modality should be widely available, result in images that are easy to interpret, and be cost-effective. Although many of these aspects are true for many radiological modalities, there is no modality that fulfills all the criteria of the ideal examination (**Table 1**). Most patients undergo VCE or enteroscopy because of mid-gastrointestinal blood loss. In most of these patients, especially those in Western countries, the cause will be angioectasia. These lesions are usually small and flat. Therefore, no radiological modality will be able to detect such lesions. VCE and DBE are clearly superior for detecting intramucosal flat lesions, and should therefore be considered first for patients with mid-gastrointestinal bleeding.

Conventional Radiology and Contrast Studies

Small bowel follow through and conventional enteroclysis

Small bowel follow through (SBFT) requires the ingestion of at least 0.5 L of 40% to 50% barium suspension by mouth. As the barium progresses through the small bowel, fluoroscopy is performed and serial images are obtained (**Fig. 1**). Often manual palpation is necessary to separate individual small bowel loops to help identify abnormalities.[1] The main advantage of SBFT is the ease of performance. The disadvantages include poor definition of small bowel fold pattern, poor distention and separation of individual segments, and the use of ionizing radiation.

In general, SBFT has been replaced by enteroclysis, which is considered to be more accurate.[2] Enteroclysis is performed by administering a low-density barium suspension through a fluoroscopically placed nasojejunal catheter. The administration of the contrast medium directly into the small bowel is usually followed by administration of methylcellulose suspension or air to enable optimal distension of individual small bowel loops.[1,2] As with SBFT, fluoroscopy is performed and serial images are obtained. In general, small bowel enteroclysis, especially if performed using double contrast, enables a more detailed examination of the small bowel lumen and wall. Compared with cross-sectional imaging, the information about trans- and extraluminal abnormalities is limited. The need for nasojejunal intubation makes small bowel enteroclysis more invasive than SBFT, CT enterography, and magnetic resonance (MR) enterography.

Ultrasound

Although ultrasound investigation of the abdomen is often hampered by the presence of intestinal gas and by collapse of the small intestinal lumen, this can be overcome by filling the small bowel with anechoic fluid. The main advantages of ultrasound include its wide availability and low cost. In addition, ultrasound enables better functional

Table 1
Comparison between radiological and endoscopic small bowel imaging methods

Modality	Invasiveness	Enteral Contrast	IV Contrast	Radiation Exposure	Total SB	Luminal Detail	Wall Detail	Surrounding Structures	Availability	Ease of Interpretation	Costs
Plain abdominal radiograph	–	–	–	+	+	–	–	–	+++	+++	+
SBFT	+	+	–	+++	+++	++	++	–	+++	++	++
SB enteroclysis	++	+	–	+++	+++	+++	+++	–	++	++	++
Ultrasound	–	–	–	–	–	+	++	++	+++	+	+
CT enterography	+	+	+	+++	+++	++	++	+++	++	++	++
CT enteroclysis	++	+	+	+++	+++	+++	+++	+++	++	++	++
MR enterography	+	+	+	–	+++	++	++	+++	+	++	++
MR enteroclysis	++	+	+	+ (tube)	+++	+++	+++	+++	+	++	++
VCE	+	–	–	–	++	+++	–	–	+	++	++
Push enteroscopy	+++	–	–	– (if no fluoroscopy)	–	+++	–	–	+	++	+
Balloon-assisted enteroscopy[a]	+++	–	–	– (if no fluoroscopy)	+ (usually in 2 sessions)	+++	–	–	+	++	+++

Abbreviations: CT, computed tomography; DBE, double-balloon endoscopy; IV, intravenous; SB, small bowel; MR, magnetic resonance; SBFT, small bowel follow through; VCE, video capsule endoscopy.

[a] Applies to double-balloon and single-balloon endoscopy and other nonsurgical enteroscopy methods.

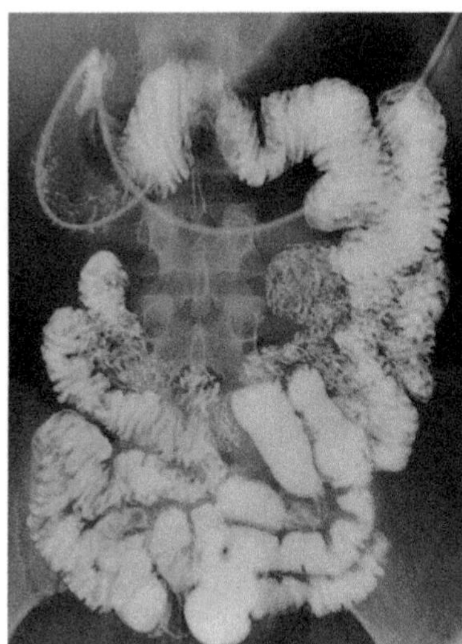

Fig. 1. Normal conventional enteroclysis.

evaluation than many other small bowel imaging modalities.[3] The diagnostic accuracy of sono-enteroclysis has been reported to be comparable to that of barium enteroclysis.[3] However, in general, it is most often only used in patients with (suspected) Crohn disease and to demonstrate the presence of small bowel obstruction or paralytic ileus.[4]

Cross-sectional Imaging

Computed tomography

In routine settings, opacification of the small bowel during CT is achieved by administering oral contrast agent by mouth. A possible drawback of this method is that the small intestinal lumen might remain collapsed and the bowel wall is not visualized in detail. This situation can be overcome by increasing the dose of orally ingested contrast medium (CT enterography) or by administering methylcellulose (neutral enteral contrast) or barium (positive enteral contrast) directly into the small bowel using an enteroclysis catheter (CT enteroclysis).[5]

Magnetic resonance imaging

The development of fast imaging sequences has enabled small bowel imaging by MRI (**Fig. 2**). As in CT imaging of the small bowel, luminal distention is a prerequisite for adequate depiction of luminal abnormalities. Several luminal contrast agents can be used: Positive contrast agents (such as gadolinium chelate) produce high signal intensities on T1-weighted and T2-weighted sequences, whereas negative contrast agents (such as perfluoro-octyl bromide) produce low signal intensity on T1-weighted and T2-weighted sequences. Biphasic contrast agents (like polyethyleneglycol and methylcellulose) produce different patterns of contrast depending on the sequence used.[6] The luminal contrast agent can be delivered by mouth (MR enterography) or by means of a nasojejunal catheter, positioned using fluoroscopic guidance (MR enteroclysis). The main advantages of MRI are the lack of exposure to ionizing radiation and excellent soft-tissue contrast.[7]

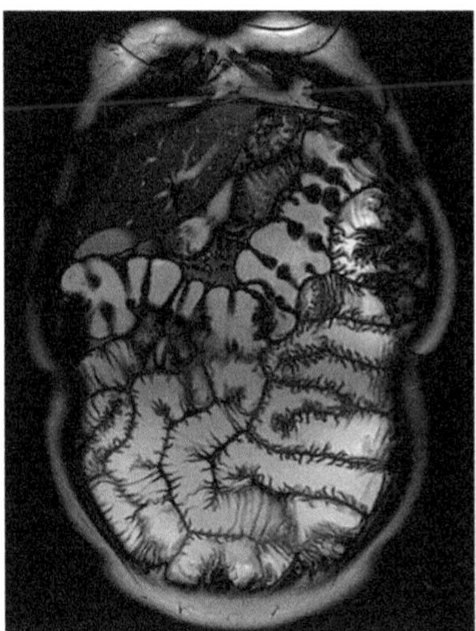

Fig. 2. Normal magnetic resonance enteroclysis.

In expert hands, MR enteroclysis is probably the best radiological modality for examination of the small bowel, especially if repeated examinations are expected. Drawbacks include limited availability, high cost, and the need for jejunal intubation.

PART 2: RADIOLOGICAL FINDINGS IN SELECTED SMALL BOWEL DISEASES

Crohn Disease

General considerations

It is estimated that 0.6% to 3% of the cumulative risk of cancer in the general population can be attributed to the medical use of radiography.[8] The increased risk of radiation-induced cancer may be of particular concern in patients with Crohn disease, who are often exposed to radiological imaging starting in childhood. In 15.5% of patients with Crohn disease, the cumulative effective dose exceeded 75 mSv, which can be translated to an excess risk of cancer mortality of 7.3%.[9] Factors associated with high cumulative exposure in patients with Crohn disease are age <17 years at diagnosis, small bowel involvement, penetrating disease, and requirement for intravenous steroids, infliximab, or multiple surgeries.[9]

As in all patients in whom radiological imaging with ionizing radiation is considered, the potential benefits should be weighed against the potential long-term risks, and imaging modalities that do not expose the patient to ionizing radiation (such as ultrasound or MRI) should be considered.

The main problems when interpreting research results of radiological imaging in Crohn disease are the often heterogeneous study populations (especially when patients with suspected Crohn disease are studied) and the lack of a solid reference test. These problems often apply to studies comparing the use of VCE and small bowel radiology.

Suspected Crohn disease

When the results of ileocolonoscopy and esophagogastroduodenoscopy are normal but a high suspicion of Crohn disease is still present, several modalities can be used to examine the small bowel. There is much debate about the best modality to use in such situations, because (wireless) endoscopic examinations, like radiological studies, have their advantages and disadvantages. In our view, histologic confirmation of suspected lesions (either visualized with VCE or radiological imaging) should be pursued. It is difficult to compare the diagnostic accuracy of VCE with that of radiological methods, because most studies comparing VCE with small bowel radiology in patients with Crohn disease do not relate VCE or radiology findings to an accepted reference standard. Therefore, usually the "diagnostic yield" is reported, which includes all abnormalities encountered during VCE examination, without histologic proof of Crohn disease being present. Therefore, only the sensitivity of these methods can be assessed.

Although the risk of capsule retention in patients with suspected Crohn disease seems low, some gastroenterologists prefer to perform radiological evaluation of the small bowel before VCE to exclude the presence of small bowel stenosis.[10,11]

A meta-analysis comparing the yield of radiological imaging and VCE included 5 studies comparing small bowel radiographs (either SBFT or conventional enteroclysis) in patients with suspected Crohn disease. The total yield for the radiological studies was 13%, whereas the yield for VCE was 43%, a difference that failed to reach statistical significance.[12] In addition, patients with radiological evidence of stenotic disease were excluded in several of the studies and the inclusion criteria varied widely between the studies.

Conventional enteroclysis and SBFT are the traditional modalities to examine the small bowel in patients with suspected Crohn disease, and are still used as the standard of reference in almost all studies comparing radiological modalities. The sensitivity and specificity of state-of-the-art conventional enteroclysis performed by experts have been reported to be 100% and 98.3%, respectively.[13] In comparison with double-contrast enteroclysis, the sensitivity, specificity, and diagnostic accuracy of multidetector CT enteroclysis are 92%, 83%, and 90%, respectively.[14] However, in another recent comparison between conventional enteroclysis and CT enteroclysis in 50 patients with histologically proven Crohn disease, conventional enteroclysis showed normal findings in 42 patients, whereas CT enteroclysis showed abnormalities in 44 patients. No differences between conventional enteroclysis and CT enteroclysis were found for mucosal changes, stenosis, and prestenotic dilatation. However, CT was able to depict extraluminal complications like fistula, abscesses, and lymphadenopathy better than conventional enteroclysis. CT enteroclysis was also superior in detecting skip lesions.[15]

When comparing the amount of exposure to radiation, multidetector CT is less attractive; the mean effective dose of multidetector CT has been reported to be 16.1 mSv, whereas the effective doses for SBFT were 1.37 mSv (right lower quadrant), 2.02 mSv (central abdomen) and 3.83 mSv (pelvis).[16] To avoid these amounts of radiation exposure, reliable alternatives for SBFT, conventional enteroclysis, and CT examinations of the small bowel are needed.

A meta-analysis of studies on the use of ultrasound to diagnose Crohn disease reported sensitivity and specificity between 75%–94% and 67%–100%, respectively.[17] Compared with a reference standard consisting of a combination of clinical and conventional enteroclysis findings, the specificity and sensitivity of ultrasound in the diagnosis of Crohn disease have been reported to be 88.4% and 93.3%, respectively.[18] However, ultrasound was less reliable in patients with early stage Crohn disease of the small bowel (sensitivity 66.7%). Therefore, if ultrasound is used as the initial modality to examine the small bowel in patients with suspected Crohn disease, a negative result warrants further evaluation.

Compared with conventional enteroclysis, MR enteroclysis might be less sensitive in detecting superficial ulceration, fold distortion, and fold thickening.[19] No difference was found in the sensitivity of MRE for the detection of deep ulcers, cobblestoning pattern, stenosis, and prestenotic dilatation. However, additional information provided by MR imaging includes fibrofatty proliferation and mesenteric lymphadenopathy (**Fig. 3**). It is not clear whether MR investigations in patients with suspected Crohn disease should be performed with oral contrast, or with contrast delivered by a nasojejunal catheter. It is clear that patients prefer MR investigation without a nasojejunal catheter.[20] In one study, MR enteroclysis, when compared with MR enterography, was better for visualizing superficial abnormalities, whereas no differences were found in depicting mural stenosis or fistulae, which suggests that MR enteroclysis could be superior to MR enterography in patients with suspected Crohn disease.[21]

Only one study compared DBE with radiological examination of the small bowel in patients with suspected small bowel Crohn disease.[22] Antegrade DBE revealed pathologic results in five patients. MR enteroclysis and DBE agreed for 75% of all lesions found.

In conclusion, the lack of exposure to ionizing radiation and the possibility of detecting extraluminal abnormalities all favor MR or ultrasound as the initial radiological investigation in suspected small intestinal Crohn disease. However, conventional enteroclysis has probably still the best accuracy in detecting early stage small bowel Crohn disease. In our view, VCE is more reliable than radiology to investigate suspected Crohn disease, in the absence of symptoms suggestive of stenotic disease. However, in view of the major impact the diagnosis of Crohn disease might have, histologic confirmation by enteroscopy should be considered.

Monitoring established Crohn disease and post-operative recurrence

In patients with established Crohn disease, the risk of video capsule retention has been reported to be as high as 13%, even in the absence of clinical symptoms suggestive of small bowel stenosis.[10] Small bowel series were performed previous

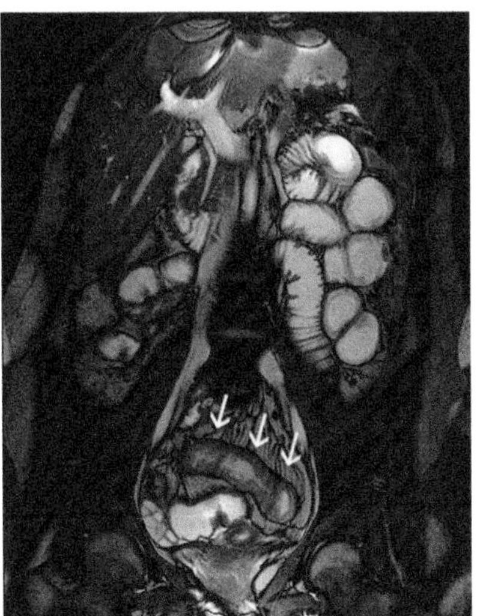

Fig. 3. Magnetic resonance enteroclysis in a 17-year old female patient with Crohn's disease. Note the irregular thickening of the wall of the terminal ileum (*arrows*). Additionally, mild hyperemia of the surrounding mesenteric fat can be observed.

to VCE in all patients. No significant small bowel stenoses were reported and small bowel series were reported to be normal in 82% of these patients. Because normal findings during small bowel radiology do not prevent capsule retention, established Crohn disease is considered by some to be a contraindication for VCE. In addition, to monitor the effect of medical therapy, which is often expensive and associated with major side-effects, one can argue that nonspecific capsule and radiological findings are sometimes not sufficient, and histologic proof (obtained by means of enteroscopy) of the effectiveness of medical therapy is mandatory.

Triester and colleagues reported a higher yield for VCE capsule compared with conventional enteroclysis (78% versus 32%), and CT enterography (68% versus 38%).[12] However, patients with radiological evidence of small bowel stenosis were excluded. Therefore, these results are only valid for patients with proven nonstricturing small bowel Crohn disease.

In our view conventional enteroclysis it is not informative enough to monitor therapy in patients with Crohn disease, because Crohn disease-related complications, such as fistula and abscesses, cannot be depicted reliably. The reported sensitivities and specificities of CT enterography and CT enteroclysis are 73% to 82% and 70% to 98%, respectively, and these techniques are superior for mural, serosal, and mesenteric abnormalities such as bowel wall thickening, fibrofatty proliferation of mesenteric fat, mesenteric abscess, and mesenteric lymphadenopathy. Such information is important for monitoring disease activity.[23] A recent study of 41 patients with known Crohn disease showed CT enterography to have the same accuracy for mural disease as conventional enteroclysis.[24] However, CT enterography provided additional information on colonic involvement, mesenteric involvement, and extraintestinal complications.

The sensitivity and specificity of MRI (enterography or enteroclysis) are comparable with those of conventional enteroclysis for diagnosing advanced small bowel Crohn disease.[25] Inter- and intraobserver agreement is good or excellent for most pathologic signs.

CT enteroclysis/enterography and MR enterography/enteroclysis have been used to estimate disease activity in patients with Crohn disease. Mural enhancement after intravenous administration of contrast agents and wall thickening seem to correlate with endoscopic and clinical scoring systems for disease activity.[26–29] However, most studies on this subject focus on Crohn disease of the terminal ileum. Little is known on CT and MRI to evaluate disease activity in the more proximal small bowel, not accessible during conventional ileocolonoscopy.

Cross-sectional imaging in patients with established Crohn disease seems to be preferred over conventional enteroclysis. The role of VCE in this category is still unclear. DBE should be considered early in the diagnostic pathway to assess mucosal healing.

Small Bowel Tumors and Small Bowel Polyposis Syndromes

Small bowel cancers are rare. The risk of adenocarcinoma of the small bowel is increased in patients with Crohn disease, celiac disease, and small bowel polyposis syndromes (**Fig. 4**). Circumstantial evidence suggests an adenoma–carcinoma sequence.[30] Gastrointestinal stromal tumors (GISTs) are small, well-circumscribed lesions, usually with central ulceration or umbilication; they can be benign or malignant. Although most GISTs occur sporadically, some are associated with neurofibromatosis type 1. Neuroendocrine tumors are the only tumors that occur predominantly in the small intestine. They are more likely to occur in the ileum than in the jejunum (**Fig. 5**).

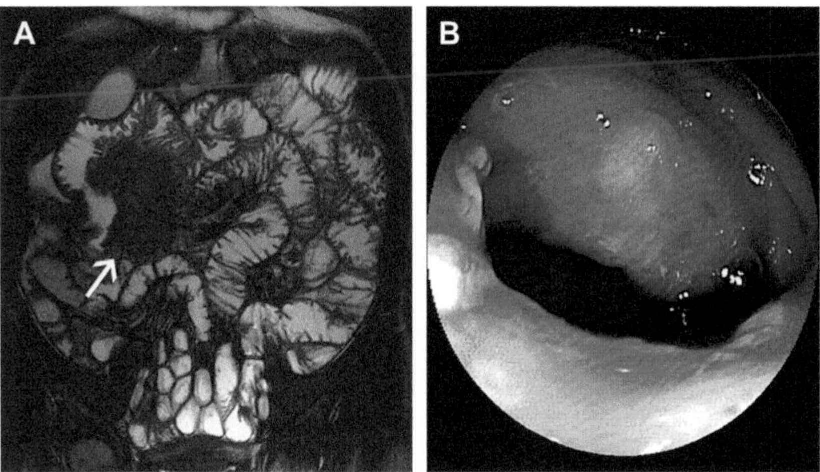

Fig. 4. 49-year old female with recently diagnosed celiac disease and persisting weight loss. (*A*) Magnetic resonance enteroclysis shows irregular thickening of the wall of a proximal jejunal loop, with an adjacent eccentric mass (*arrow*). (*B*) Double balloon endoscopy image of the tumor. Histological examination proved the lesion to be adenocarcinoma.

Approximately one third of all gastrointestinal lymphoma occur in the small bowel.[31] The most prevalent histologic types are summarized in **Box 1**. Four major forms of small bowel involvement can be seen: primary small bowel lymphoma, enteropathy-associated T cell lymphoma, mesenteric nodal lymphoma, and a disseminated lymphoma.[32] Several radiographic patterns can be observed: a polypoid form, multiple nodules, an infiltrating form, an endoexoenteric form with excavation and fistulization, and a mesenteric invasive form with extraluminal masses. However, the correlation between radiological appearance and histology is poor.[31]

In a review of 55 cases of small bowel metastasis, metastases from lobular breast cancer (47.2%), lung cancer (11.1%), and malignant melanoma (8.3%) were most

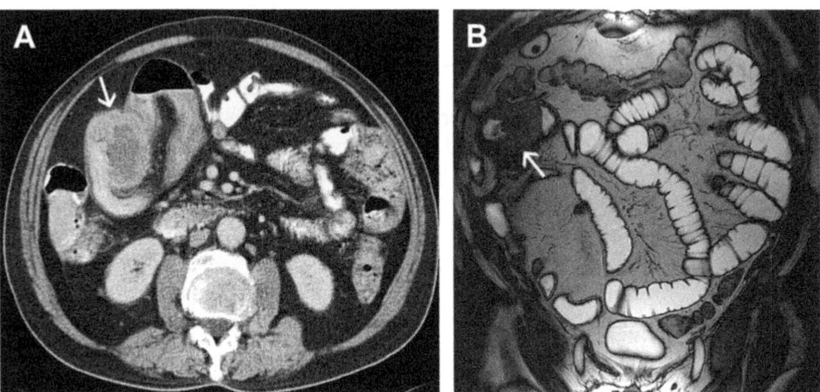

Fig. 5. 68-year old male patient with a neuro-endocrine tumor of the ileum. (*A*) Abdominal CT-image shows a mass in the right lower quadrant of the abdomen (*arrow*), probably originating from an adjacent ileal loop. (*B*) Magnetic resonance enteroclysis clearly shows the relation between the ileum and the mass (*arrow*).

Box 1
Features of Crohn disease using magnetic resonance imaging

Luminal and mural findings

- Ulceration
- Cobblestoning
- Wall thickening
- Stenosis
- Fold thickening
- Distortion of the valvulae conniventes
- Mucosal nodularity

Extraluminal findings

- Fibrofatty proliferation in the mesentery
- Fistula
- Abscesses
- Phlegmons
- Mesenteric lymphadenopathy

Markers of disease activity

- Mucosal hyperemia
- Intramural edema
- Transmural ulceration
- Wall thickening and enhancement
- Vascular engorgement (comb sign)
- Enhancement of mesenteric lymph nodes

Data from Gourtsoyiannis NC, Papanikolaou N, Karantanas A. Magnetic resonance imaging evaluation of small intestinal Crohn's disease. Best Pract Res Clin Gastroenterol 2006;20(1):137–56.

frequent.[33] Small intestinal metastases should be considered in patients with known malignancies who experience small bowel obstruction, gastrointestinal blood loss, or abdominal pain (**Fig. 6**).

Due to the rarity of small bowel tumors, primary and metastatic, information on the diagnostic accuracy of radiological and endoscopic techniques is limited.

The diagnostic accuracy of SBFT in the diagnosis of small intestinal malignancies has been reported to be around 60%, whereas that of conventional enteroclysis has been reported to be as high as 95% if performed by experts.[34,35] Contrast and water-enhanced multidetector CT enterography has a reported sensitivity and specificity of 85% and 97%, respectively, in the detection of malignant and benign small intestinal tumors.[36] Negative results of transabdominal ultrasound in patients with suspected small bowel tumors warrant further examination, because the reported sensitivity is only 26%. However, the 99% specificity of transabdominal ultrasound for the detection of small bowel tumors might allow ultrasound to be considered as the first screening modality, because of its low invasiveness and low cost.[37]

A study performed in the VU University Medical Center on the diagnostic accuracy of MR enteroclysis shows even more promising results: The overall sensitivity and

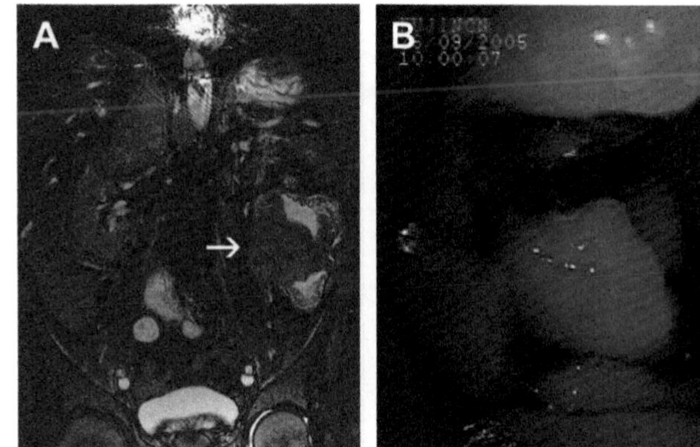

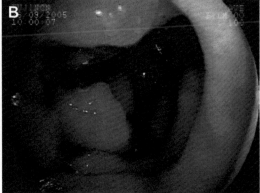

Fig. 6. 65-year old patients with jejunal metastasis of non-small-cell lung cancer. (*A*) Magnetic resonance enteroclysis shows an irregular tumor in the jejunum. (*B*) Corresponding DBE-image.

specificity of MR enteroclysis in the detection of small bowel tumors was between 91% and 94% and between 95% and 97%, respectively.[38] In this study, 12 patients with known small bowel polyposis syndromes (mostly Peutz Jeghers syndrome) were included, which might have led to overestimation of diagnostic accuracy. However, when these patients were excluded in a subgroup analysis, the diagnostic accuracy remained high (94%). Interobserver agreement was excellent, with a kappa value of 93%.

Although the potential negative effect of exposure to ionizing radiation is probably of little relevance in patients who need to undergo small bowel imaging only once to exclude or investigate suspected small bowel malignancies, it might be of importance in patients who need to undergo repeated examinations in the follow-up of small bowel polyposis syndromes.

Even if radiological or wireless capsule examination shows a clear tumor, enteroscopy remains mandatory. Not only does enteroscopy facilitate histologic analysis of the tumor, it also is useful to tattoo a lesion to guide surgical resection, if indicated.

In patients with familial adenomatous polyposis syndrome (FAP), DBE and VCE have been proposed as tools to investigate the presence of small bowel adenoma.[39] VCE seems less reliable in detecting duodenal adenoma.[40,41] There is limited experience with CT enterography as a tool to examine the duodenum of patients with FAP.[42,43] However, this seems less reliable than esophagogastroduodenoscopy, especially in defining the number of polyps, because fine carpeting of miniscule duodenal polyps is poorly visualized with CT. VCE is probably superior to conventional enteroclysis in detecting small adenoma or hamartoma distal to the duodenum.[44] However, the clinical relevance of these small polyps is uncertain.

In patients with suspected small bowel tumors MR enteroclysis might be used as the first modality of choice. If the presence of a tumor is confirmed, DBE is used to allow histologic determination. In addition, MR enteroclysis helps in the choice of the preferred route of insertion of the DBE endoscope. In patients with small bowel polyposis syndromes, MR enteroclysis is used to estimate the number, location, and size of small bowel polyps. In patients with Peutz Jeghers syndrome, we only perform DBE if polyps larger than 2 cm are present and if the patient experiences symptoms suggestive of (intermittent) small bowel obstruction (**Fig. 7**). These polyps are then removed using snare coagulation.

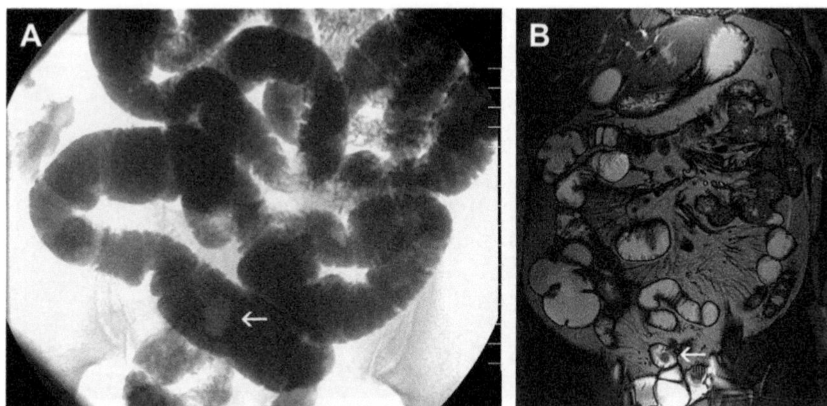

Fig. 7. 20-year old male patient with Peutz-Jeghers syndrome. (*A*) Conventional enteroclysis revealed a polyp in the proximal ileum (*arrow*). (*B*) Corresponding magnetic resonance enteroclysis image of the polyp (*arrow*).

Celiac Disease

The sensitivity and specificity of serologic tests (transtissue glutaminase and anti-endomysial antibodies) and histologic examination of biopsies obtained in the duodenum are high.[45] Therefore, small bowel imaging is not likely to have additional value in a novel diagnosis of celiac disease. However, several radiological abnormalities can be encountered (**Box 2**) (**Figs. 8** and **9**).[46]

Box 2
Radiological features of celiac disease

Luminal findings

- Bowel dilatation and small bowel atony
- Increased number of ileal folds[a]
- Decreased number of jejunal folds[a]
- Small intestinal wall thickening
- Intussusception
- Stenosis and prestenotic dilation[b]
- Small intestinal masses[b]

Extraluminal findings

- Mesenteric lymphadenopathy
- Mesenteric vascular engorgement
- Hyposplenism
- Ascites

[a] The combined presence of a decreased number of jejunal folds and an increased number of ileal folds is referred to as jejunoileal fold pattern reversal.
[b] Might indicate refractory celiac disease or enteropathy-associated T cell lymphoma.
Data from Paolantonio P, Tomei E, Rengo M, et al: Adult celiac disease: MRI findings. Abdom Imaging 2007;32:433.

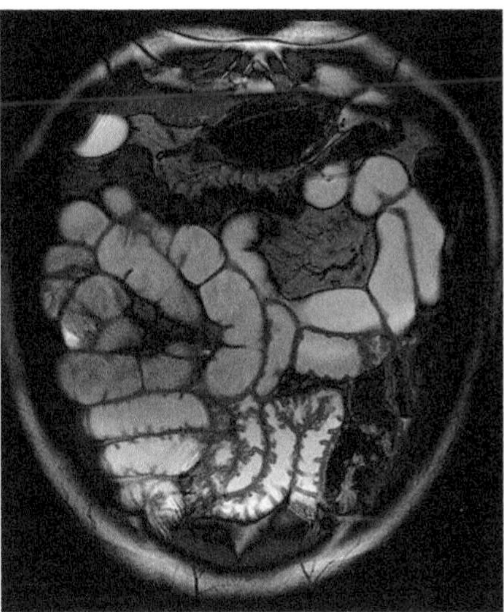

Fig. 8. Magnetic resonance enteroclysis image of a 66-year old male patient with refractory celiac disease. The decrease of jejunal folds (left upper abdominal quadrant) and the increase of ileal folds (right lower abdominal quadrant) results in jejunoileal foldpattern reversal.

In patients who do not respond well to a gluten-free diet, refractory celiac disease should be suspected. This condition warrants a more aggressive diagnostic pathway, because one subtype (type II) is associated with high mortality, mainly due to its association with ulcerative jejunitis and enteropathy-associated T cell lymphoma (EATL). These entities often present in regions of the small bowel that are not within reach of a conventional gastroscope.

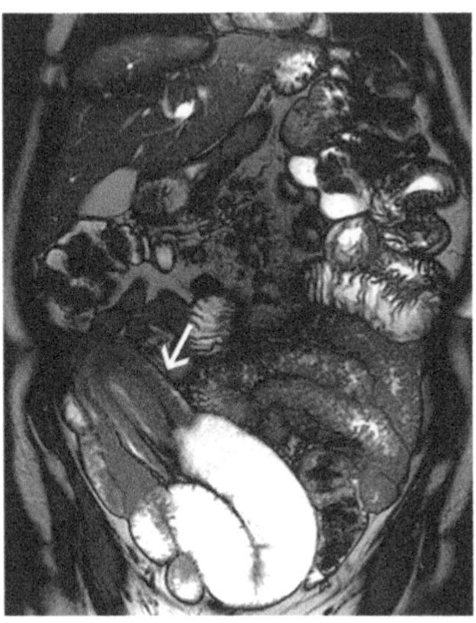

Fig. 9. Magnetic resonance enteroclysis image of a patient with intussusception. The bowel-in-bowel appearance with proximal dilation is clearly visible (*arrow*).

SBFT, conventional enteroclysis, and ultrasound have not been studied in patients with refractory celiac disease. A study on the use of CT with oral contrast in patients with suspected refractory celiac disease showed more bowel wall thickening, lymphadenopathy, and intussusception, less increase in the number of small mesenteric vessels and a smaller splenic volume in patients with refractory celiac disease type II or EATL compared with patients with uncomplicated celiac disease or refractory celiac disease type I. No discrimination between uncomplicated celiac disease and refractory celiac disease type I was possible.[47] The use of MRE in patients with suspected celiac disease has not yet been clarified. Preliminary results from the VU University Medical Center show that the presence of less than six jejunal folds per 5 cm and bowel wall thickness of 9 mm or greater were only observed in patients with refractory celiac disease type II.[48] In addition, factors possibly associated with the development of ulcerative jejunitis and lymphoma, such as small splenic volume and infiltration of the mesenteric fat, can be assessed.

Because small bowel histology is mandatory in patients with suspected refractory disease, DBE should always be performed to assess the presence of ulcerative jejunitis. Magnetic resonance might be helpful in assessing extraintestinal complications of refractory celiac disease. However, DBE will always be a more reliable tool to diagnose ulcerative jejunitis and nonprotruding lymphoma.[45]

Small Bowel Diverticular Disease, Including Meckel's Diverticulum

The incidence of diverticula in the small intestine distal to the duodenum is reported to be between 0.06% and 2.3%.[49,50] Usually, these diverticula are asymptomatic. Complications include bacterial overgrowth, bleeding, and inflammation. Several radiological imaging methods have been described for the diagnosis of small bowel diverticulitis.[51] Plain abdominal radiography is usually not helpful, although small bowel diverticula may be visible as air-filled pockets and intraperitoneal air can be identified. SBFT or conventional enteroclysis can visualize small bowel diverticula, but usually does not provide information on mural, serosal, or mesenteric involvement.[52] Although abdominal ultrasound is able to visualize extraluminal air and hyperechoic fat, it does not inform about the extent of small bowel diverticula[53,54] Abdominal CT might allow a specific diagnosis of small bowel diverticulitis, however in the absence of clearly depicted small bowel diverticula, inflammation in and around small bowel loops cannot be distinguished from other conditions such as small bowel Crohn disease and small bowel malignancies. MR and CT enteroclysis have the benefit of being able to depict small bowel diverticula (because distension of the small bowel prevents collapse of diverticular segments) and the extraluminal abnormalities encountered with inflammation (**Fig. 10**).

Meckel's diverticula result from failure of the omphalomesenteric duct to regress and occur in approximately 2% of all adults. Complications include bleeding and intussusception.[55] In our experience, VCE is a disappointing modality to investigate the small bowel for Meckel's diverticulum. Although we have seen clear images of a Meckel's diverticulum occasionally, the absence of bowel distention prevents a clear depiction of Meckel's diverticula in most patients. Meckel's diverticula are usually not seen with SBFT or conventional enteroclysis, although the latter seems a little more sensitive.[56] On ultrasound or cross-sectional imaging, Meckel's diverticula are frequently difficult to discriminate from normal small bowel loops.[55] Scintigraphy with [^{99m}Tc]Na-pertechnetate has limited sensitivity in adults, but might be more reliable in children.[57] Retrograde DBE has been described as a tool to visualize Meckel's diverticula and its complications.[58] In addition, hemostatic procedures can be performed in case of bleeding. Although no studies comparing radiological imaging

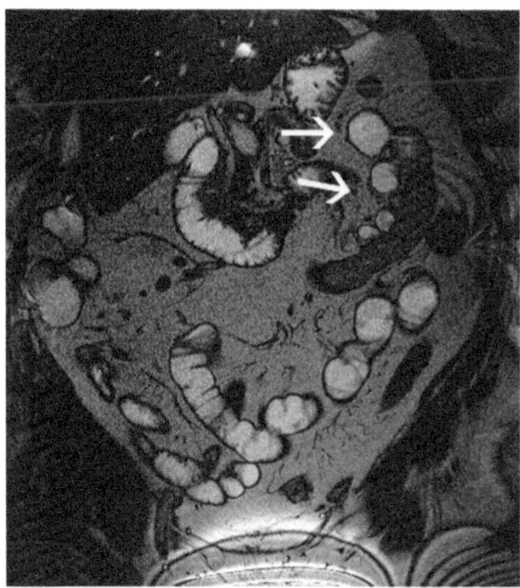

Fig. 10. Magnetic resonance enteroclysis of a 68-year old patient with small bowel diverticulosis, several weeks after she presented with signs of diverticulitis. Several ileal diverticula can be observed (*arrows*).

with DBE have been performed, DBE does seem more reliable. Therefore, with obscure gastrointestinal blood loss, retrograde DBE should be considered early in the diagnostic pathway, especially in young adults.

PART 3: ENTEROSCOPY AND RADIOLOGICAL IMAGING: SUPPLEMENTARY TECHNIQUES

Small bowel endoscopy and radiological imaging of the small bowel are supplementary techniques. One of the drawbacks of radiological imaging is that it is usually not informative on flat mucosal lesions, as most vascular lesions are. Therefore its role as a primary investigation in patients with mid-gastrointestinal bleeding is limited, because VCE is more informative for vascular lesions. The major advantage of radiological examination, especially cross-sectional techniques, is its ability to visualize mural and extramural abnormalities.

It is difficult to suggest standardized diagnostic protocols for evaluating suspected small bowel diseases, because there are many factors to be considered when choosing the optimal sequence of diagnostic tests. Several strategies can be followed. In general, in acute mid-gastrointestinal bleeding, we refrain from VCE and proceed directly to DBE because the need for endoscopic intervention is high in these patients. Usually, we start with the antegrade approach, because active bleeding might interfere with endoscopic progress during the retrograde approach. However, in young patients with acute mid-gastrointestinal bleeding, the retrograde approach might be preferable given the high likelihood of a Meckel's diverticulum. In patients with chronic mid-gastrointestinal bleeding, some centers prefer to plan antegrade DBE followed by retrograde DBE to achieve total enteroscopy, whereas other centers prefer VCE to be able to choose the optimal route of insertion to avoid 2 enteroscopy sessions. Usually, in mid-gastrointestinal bleeding, the role of radiology is limited to patients with additional symptoms suggesting small bowel obstruction or a history of cancer. Radiology findings might indicate lesions that allow gastroenterologists to perform a targeted enteroscopy.

The optimal strategy depends on the endoscopic skills of the gastroenterologist, the experience of the radiology department in small bowel imaging and on reimbursement of the various examinations by local health care authorities.

Only one study has been performed to investigate the effect of small bowel imaging on the yield of DBE.[59] In this retrospective study of 124 patients undergoing DBE, conventional enteroclysis was performed in 76 patients and was abnormal in 45 patients. Positive DBE findings were more likely to occur in patients who had abnormal enteroclysis than in patients with normal enteroclysis results or in whom enteroclysis was performed. Although the retrospective nature of this study made it prone to inclusion and confirmation bias, it is clear that pre-DBE small intestinal imaging might be useful to select patients for DBE. However, only 1 of 16 patients with vascular lesions as the final diagnosis had abnormal enteroclysis results. This finding emphasizes the limited value of radiological modalities in patients with MGIB. In our view, negative radiological results should lead to referral for VCE or DBE.

In conclusion, similar to the major developments that have been achieved in small bowel endoscopy, small bowel radiology is a rapid changing field. Although the already high diagnostic accuracy of advanced cross-sectional small bowel imaging will probably increase even more, endoscopic methods will remain indispensable for diagnosing nonprotruding mucosal lesions and obtaining histologic confirmation of suspected small bowel lesions. Solid prospective studies comparing radiological methods with VCE and enteroscopy, using either enteroscopy or operative findings as the standard of reference, are needed. To design and interpret such studies, it is important for gastroenterologists to be able to speak the same language as radiologists, and vice versa. It is of the upmost importance for physicians interested in small intestinal diseases to realize that there is no need for competitive comparison between radiological imaging, VCE, and DBE. The combination of endoscopic, radiological, and surgical knowledge, used to explore new boundaries, will lead to new developments in gastroenterology.

REFERENCES

1. Levine MS, Rubesin SE, Laufer I. Pattern approach for diseases of mesenteric small bowel on barium studies. Radiology 2008;249:445–60.
2. Maglinte DD, Lappas JC, Kelvin FM, et al. Small bowel radiography: how, when, and why? Radiology 1987;163:297–305.
3. Nagi B, Rana SS, Kochhar R, et al. Sonoenteroclysis: a new technique for the diagnosis of small bowel diseases. Abdom Imaging 2006;31:417–24.
4. Valette PJ, Rioux M, Pilleul F, et al. Ultrasonography of chronic inflammatory bowel diseases. Eur Radiol 2001;11:1859–66.
5. Gourtsoyiannis N, Papanikolaou N, Daskalogiannaki M. The duodenum and small intestine. In: Adam A, Dixon AK, Grainger RG, editors. Adam: Grainger & Allison's diagnostic radiology. 5th edition. Churchill Livingstone; 2008.
6. Laghi A, Paolantonio P, Iafrate F, et al. Oral contrast agents for magnetic resonance imaging of the bowel. Top Magn Reson Imaging 2002;13:389–96.
7. Papanikolaou N, Prassopoulos P, Grammatikakis I, et al. Technical challenges and clinical applications of magnetic resonance enteroclysis. Top Magn Reson Imaging 2002;13:397–408.
8. Berrington de Gonzalez A, Darby S. Risk of cancer from diagnostic X-rays: estimates for the UK and 14 other countries. Lancet 2004;363:345–51.
9. Desmond AN, O'Regan K, Curran C, et al. Crohn's disease: factors associated with exposure to high levels of diagnostic radiation. Gut 2008;57:1524–9.

10. Cheifetz AS, Kornbluth AA, Legnani P, et al. The risk of retention of the capsule endoscope in patients with known or suspected Crohn's disease. Am J Gastroenterol 2006;101:2218–22.
11. Solem CA, Loftus EV Jr, Fletcher JG, et al. Small-bowel imaging in Crohn's disease: a prospective, blinded, 4-way comparison trial. Gastrointest Endosc 2008;68:255–66.
12. Triester SL, Leighton JA, Leontiadis GI, et al. A meta-analysis of the yield of capsule endoscopy compared to other diagnostic modalities in patients with non-stricturing small bowel Crohn's disease. Am J Gastroenterol 2006;101:954–64.
13. Maglinte DD, Chernish SM, Kelvin FM, et al. Crohn disease of the small intestine: accuracy and relevance of enteroclysis. Radiology 1992;184:541–5.
14. Minordi LM, Vecchioli A, Poloni G, et al. CT enteroclysis: multidetector technique (MDCT) versus single-detector technique (SDCT) in patients with suspected small-bowel Crohn's disease. Radiol Med 2007;112:1188.
15. Sailer J, Peloschek P, Schober E, et al. Diagnostic value of CT enteroclysis compared with conventional enteroclysis in patients with Crohn's disease. AJR Am J Roentgenol 2005;185:1575–81.
16. Jaffe TA, Gaca AM, Delaney S, et al. Radiation doses from small-bowel follow-through and abdominopelvic MDCT in Crohn's disease. AJR Am J Roentgenol 2007;189:1015–22.
17. Fraquelli M, Colli A, Casazza G, et al. Role of US in detection of Crohn disease: meta-analysis. Radiology 2005;236:95–101.
18. Tarjan Z, Toth G, Gyorke T, et al. Ultrasound in Crohn's disease of the small bowel. Eur J Radiol 2000;35:176–82.
19. Gourtsoyiannis NC, Grammatikakis J, Papamastorakis G, et al. Imaging of small intestinal Crohn's disease: comparison between MR enteroclysis and conventional enteroclysis. Eur Radiol 2006;16:1915–25.
20. Negaard A, Sandvik L, Berstad AE, et al. MRI of the small bowel with oral contrast or nasojejunal intubation in Crohn's disease: randomized comparison of patient acceptance. Scand J Gastroenterol 2008;43:44–51.
21. Masselli G, Casciani E, Polettini E, et al. Comparison of MR enteroclysis with MR enterography and conventional enteroclysis in patients with Crohn's disease. Eur Radiol 2008;18:438–47.
22. Seiderer J, Herrmann K, Diepolder H, et al. Double-balloon enteroscopy versus magnetic resonance enteroclysis in diagnosing suspected small-bowel Crohn's disease: results of a pilot study. Scand J Gastroenterol 2007;42:1376–85.
23. Goldberg HI, Gore RM, Margulis AR, et al. Computed tomography in the evaluation of Crohn disease. AJR Am J Roentgenol 1983;140:277–82.
24. Amitai MM, Arazi-Kleinman T, Hertz M, et al. Multislice CT compared to small bowel follow-through in the evaluation of patients with Crohn disease. Clin Imaging 2008;32:355–61.
25. Gourtsoyiannis N, Papanikolaou N, Grammatikakis J, et al. MR enteroclysis: technical considerations and clinical applications. Eur Radiol 2002;12:2651–68.
26. Bodily KD, Fletcher JG, Solem CA, et al. Crohn disease: mural attenuation and thickness at contrast-enhanced CT enterography – correlation with endoscopic and histologic findings of inflammation. Radiology 2006;238:505–16.
27. Hassan C, Cerro P, Zullo A, et al. Computed tomography enteroclysis in comparison with ileoscopy in patients with Crohn's disease. Int J Colorectal Dis 2003;18:121–5.
28. Koh DM, Miao Y, Chinn RJ, et al. MR imaging evaluation of the activity of Crohn's disease. AJR Am J Roentgenol 2001;177:1325–32.

29. Maccioni F, Bruni A, Viscido A, et al. MR imaging in patients with Crohn disease: value of T2- versus T1-weighted gadolinium-enhanced MR sequences with use of an oral superparamagnetic contrast agent. Radiology 2006;238:517–30.
30. Sellner F. Investigations on the significance of the adenoma-carcinoma sequence in the small bowel. Cancer 1990;66:702–15.
31. Gollub MJ. Imaging of gastrointestinal lymphoma. Radiol Clin North Am 2008;46: 287–312.
32. Levine MS, Rubesin SE, Pantongrag-Brown L, et al. Non-Hodgkin's lymphoma of the gastrointestinal tract: radiographic findings. AJR Am J Roentgenol 1997;168: 165–72.
33. Idelevich E, Kashtan H, Mavor E, et al. Small bowel obstruction caused by secondary tumors. Surg Oncol 2006;15:29–32.
34. Bessette JR, Maglinte DD, Kelvin FM, et al. Primary malignant tumors in the small bowel: a comparison of the small-bowel enema and conventional follow-through examination. AJR Am J Roentgenol 1989;153:741–4.
35. Maglinte DD, Burney BT, Miller RE. Lesions missed on small-bowel follow-through: analysis and recommendations. Radiology 1982;144:737–9.
36. Pilleul F, Penigaud M, Milot L, et al. Possible small-bowel neoplasms: contrast-enhanced and water-enhanced multidetector CT enteroclysis. Radiology 2006; 241:796–801.
37. Fukumoto A, Tanaka S, Imagawa H, et al. Usefulness and limitations of transabdominal ultrasonography for detecting small-bowel tumors. Scand J Gastroenterol 2009;44:332–8.
38. Van Weyenberg SJB, Craanen ME, Jacobs MAJM, et al. Magnetic resonance enteroclysis in the diagnosis of small bowel bowel neoplasms: a retrospective diagnostic accuracy study. Gastroenterology 2008;4:A578.
39. Monkemuller K, Fry LC, Ebert M, et al. Feasibility of double-balloon enteroscopy-assisted chromoendoscopy of the small bowel in patients with familial adenomatous polyposis. Endoscopy 2007;39:52–7.
40. Iaquinto G, Fornasarig M, Quaia M, et al. Capsule endoscopy is useful and safe for small-bowel surveillance in familial adenomatous polyposis. Gastrointest Endosc 2008;67:61–7.
41. Wong RF, Tuteja AK, Haslem DS, et al. Video capsule endoscopy compared with standard endoscopy for the evaluation of small-bowel polyps in persons with familial adenomatous polyposis (with video). Gastrointest Endosc 2006; 64:530–7.
42. Sata N, Endo K, Shimura K, et al. A new 3-D diagnosis strategy for duodenal malignant lesions using multidetector row CT, CT virtual duodenoscopy, duodenography, and 3-D multicholangiography. Abdom Imaging 2007;32:66–72.
43. Taylor SA, Halligan S, Moore L, et al. Multidetector-row CT duodenography in familial adenomatous polyposis: a pilot study. Clin Radiol 2004;59:939–45.
44. Mata A, Llach J, Castells A, et al. A prospective trial comparing wireless capsule endoscopy and barium contrast series for small-bowel surveillance in hereditary GI polyposis syndromes. Gastrointest Endosc 2005;61:721–5.
45. Van Weyenberg SJB, Jarbandhan SVA, Mulder CJJ, et al. Double balloon endoscopy in celiac disease. Tech Gastrointest Endosc 2008;10:87–93.
46. Paolantonio P, Tomei E, Rengo M, et al. Adult celiac disease: MRI findings. Abdom Imaging 2007;32:433–40.
47. Mallant M, Hadithi M, Al-Toma AB, et al. Abdominal computed tomography in refractory coeliac disease and enteropathy associated T-cell lymphoma. World J Gastroenterol 2007;13:1696–700.

48. Van Weyenberg SJB, Mallant M, Al-Toma AB, et al. Magnetic resonance enteroclysis in adult coeliac disease: findings and comparisons between subtypes with different prognosis. Gut 2007;56:A56.
49. Coulier B, Maldague P, Bourgeois A, et al. Diverticulitis of the small bowel: CT diagnosis. Abdom Imaging 2007;32:228–33.
50. Sibille A, Willocx R. Jejunal diverticulitis. Am J Gastroenterol 1992;87:655–8.
51. Songne B, Costaglioli B, Michot F, et al. Management of surgical complications of small-bowel diverticulosis. Gastroenterol Clin Biol 2005;29:415–8.
52. Christiansen T, Thommesen P. Duodenal diverticula demonstrated by barium examination. Acta Radiol Diagn (Stockh) 1986;27:419–20.
53. Gore RM, Ghahremani GG, Kirsch MD, et al. Diverticulitis of the duodenum: clinical and radiological manifestations of seven cases. Am J Gastroenterol 1991;86: 981–5.
54. Kelekis AD, Poletti PA. Jejunal diverticulitis with localized perforation diagnosed by ultrasound: a case report. Eur Radiol 2002;3(Suppl 12):S78–81.
55. Elsayes KM, Menias CO, Harvin HJ, et al. Imaging manifestations of Meckel's diverticulum. AJR Am J Roentgenol 2007;189:81–8.
56. Maglinte DD, Elmore MF, Isenberg M, et al. Meckel diverticulum: radiologic demonstration by enteroclysis. AJR Am J Roentgenol 1980;134:925–32.
57. Poulsen KA, Qvist N. Sodium pertechnetate scintigraphy in detection of Meckel's diverticulum: is it usable? Eur J Pediatr Surg 2000;10:228–32.
58. Shinozaki S, Yamamoto H, Ohnishi H, et al. Endoscopic observation of Meckel's diverticulum by double balloon endoscopy: report of five cases. J Gastroenterol Hepatol 2008;23:e308–11.
59. Matsumoto T, Esaki M, Yada S, et al. Is small-bowel radiography necessary before double-balloon endoscopy? AJR Am J Roentgenol 2008;191:175–81.

Enteroscopy in the Diagnosis and Management of Obscure Gastrointestinal Bleeding

Marco Pennazio, MD

KEYWORDS

- Capsule endoscopy • Enteroscopy
- Double-balloon endoscopy
- Obscure gastrointestinal bleeding
- Diagnosis • Outcome

Gastrointestinal (GI) bleeding is one of the major health care problems encountered by gastroenterologists. In most patients the source of bleeding is readily identified by endoscopy and less frequently by radiological methods. Obscure gastrointestinal bleeding (OGIB) accounts for approximately 5% of all GI bleeds. It is defined as bleeding from the GI tract that persists or recurs without an obvious cause after upper and lower GI endoscopy and radiological evaluation of the small bowel, such as small-bowel follow-through (SBFT) or enteroclysis. It can be categorized into obscure overt and obscure occult bleeding, based on the presence or absence of clinically evident bleeding.[1] It has long been recognized that patients with OGIB are a special population requiring numerous hospital admissions; substantial time is generally required before a final diagnosis is reached.[2] After bleeding is recognized as recurrent, the focus of care shifts to identifying the site and cause of the bleeding; only then can appropriate therapy be instituted. Although a significant number of patients with OGIB have bleeding lesions in the esophagus, stomach, or colon that were overlooked during the initial workup, the source of bleeding is frequently located in the small bowel; bleeding may be due to several conditions, including vascular lesions, tumors, and inflammatory lesions (**Table 1**). Small-bowel bleeding with the source located

---

Conflict of interest: Marco Pennazio is member of the speakers board of Given Imaging Inc. (Yoqneam, Israel).

Small Bowel Disease Section, 2nd Division of Gastroenterology, Department of Medicine, San Giovanni Battista University Teaching Hospital, Via Cavour 31, 10123 Turin, Italy

E-mail address: pennazio.marco@gmail.com

Gastrointest Endoscopy Clin N Am 19 (2009) 409–426
doi:10.1016/j.giec.2009.04.002

1052-5157/09/$ – see front matter © 2009 Elsevier Inc. All rights reserved.

Table 1
Causes of small-bowel bleeding

Vascular Lesions (70–80%)	Tumors (5–10%)	Other Causes (10–25%)
Angioectasia	Adenoma[b]	Crohn disease
Dieulafoy lesion	Hamartoma[c]	Drug-induced small-bowel injury
Teleangiectasia[a]	Lipoma	Ulcers in celiac disease
Varices	Adenocarcinoma	Chronic ulcerative jejuno-ileitis
Phlebectasia	Lymphoma	Vasculitis
Aorto-enteric fistula	GISTs	Radiation enteritis
Aneurysms	Carcinoid tumors	Ischemic injury
	Vascular tumors[d]	Meckel diverticulum
	Neurofibroma[e]	Diverticulosis
	Metastases	Zollinger-Ellison syndrome
		Endometriosis
		Pancreaticus hemosuccus/ hemobilia
		Infectious causes
		von Willebrand disease

[a] Associated syndromes: Osler-Weber-Rendu disease, CREST syndrome, Turner's syndrome.
[b] Familial adenomatous polyposis.
[c] Peutz-Jeghers syndrome.
[d] Blue rubber bleb nevus syndrome, Klippel-Trenaunay-Weber syndrome.
[e] Von Recklinghausen disease.

Data from Pennazio M. Approach to the patient with GI bleeding. In: Faigel DO, Cave DR, editors. Capsule endoscopy. London: Elsevier; 2007. p. 113–28.

between the papilla and the ileocecal valve is also defined as mid-gastrointestinal bleeding.[3]

Diagnosing OGIB has always been challenging. Traditional radiological techniques, including small-bowel follow-through (SBFT) and small-bowel enteroclysis, have a limited role in patients with OGIB patients because they often miss small or flat lesions. CT enterography (CTE) or magnetic resonance enterography (MRE) can be helpful in identifying large masses in the small bowel or extraintestinal disease. Mesenteric angiography, helical CT angiography, and bleeding scans can be useful, but only in patients with ongoing overt bleeding.[1,4] Compared with other diagnostic tools, enteroscopy has the advantage of visualizing the intestinal mucosa directly, and revealing subtle mucosal changes such as vascular abnormalities that do not alter the mucosal surface and are thus undetectable on contrast studies. Until the end of the 20th century, most of the small intestine was inaccessible to endoscopic imaging and therapy without surgery. Mucosal visualization of the small bowel was limited to the reach of the push enteroscope (PE) (with the exception of invasive and expensive intraoperative enteroscopy [IOE]). PE does not enable distal portions of the small intestine to be visualized but permits tissue sampling, polypectomy, and treatment of bleeding lesions of the proximal jejunum up to about 100 cm beyond the ligament of Treitz.

The advent of capsule endoscopy (CE) has revolutionized small-bowel imaging not only opening up "Pandora's box" but also stimulating the development of other imaging techniques aimed at studying the small bowel. A key advantage of CE is that the entire small bowel can be imaged endoscopically with minimal discomfort for the patient in a noninvasive way. The main limitations of CE are that the capsule cannot be maneuvered, the lack of therapeutic capabilities, and the risk of retention by strictures. In an attempt to design a new scope that would allow a large part of the small-bowel mucosa to be visualized, overcoming the limits of PE, CE, and IOE, a new method of push-and-pull enteroscopy using a double-balloon technique (DBE) has been developed.[5] Recently, another enteroscopy device with only 1 balloon at the tip of the overtube, known as the single-balloon enteroscopy (SBE) system, has been introduced.[6,7] Any endoscopic technique that includes balloon-assisted progression, such as DBE or SBE, is also defined as balloon-assisted enteroscopy (BAE).[8,9] BAE allows deep (in some cases complete) intubation of the entire small bowel, combining the oral and anal approaches, with the advantage that biopsies and endoscopic interventions can be performed in all parts of the small bowel without laparotomy. However, BAE is a complex, time-consuming examination and should be performed only by trained and experienced endoscopists.

This article reviews the data on enteroscopy, with particular emphasis on the use of CE and BAE for the diagnosis and management of patients with OGIB.

INTRAOPERATIVE ENTEROSCOPY

IOE was traditionally the gold standard for small-bowel imaging but its use has been declining since the development of BAE. The diagnostic yield of IOE in patients with OGIB has ranged from 58% to 100%.[1,4] IOE is a difficult and time-consuming technique, often traumatic to the bowel. Complication rates ranging from 0% to 52% have been reported and include mucosal lacerations and perforations; mortality related to the procedure or to postoperative complications has been as high as 17%.[4] Furthermore, finding a lesion does not always equate with cessation of bleeding. In one study of 25 patients, the re-bleeding rate after IOE was 30% at a mean follow-up of 19 months.[10] IOE is now considered a last resort in patients with OGIB or when BAE cannot be performed successfully due to the presence of abdominal adhesions or other technical factors.[1]

PUSH ENTEROSCOPY

PE has long been the established endoscopic method for examining the proximal small bowel because of its biopsy and therapeutic capabilities. The diagnostic yield of PE in patients with OGIB ranges from 20% to 80%.[11] However, many lesions found during PE are within the reach of a standard endoscope.[1,4] Lesions commonly missed in the upper tract include gastric or duodenal angioectasias, Dieulafoy lesions, Cameron lesions, peptic ulcers, neoplasms, esophageal or gastric varices, and gastric antral vascular ectasias. Lesions most often missed in the colon include angioectasias and neoplasms. Thus, the true diagnostic yield of PE for the workup of OGIB in the small bowel may be more realistically in the 15% to 40% range. Overt bleeding has been found to be a predictive factor of positive findings at PE.[12,13] PE has been reported to change management in 40% to 75% of patients,[14–17] particularly in patients with overt bleeding.[17] Little is known of the long-term outcome in patients with OGIB who undergo investigation by means of PE, and published studies are conflicting; one such study found that recurrent bleeding occurs in about one-third of these patients, with a trend toward more frequent re-bleeding in patients with angioectasias.[18] Cauterization of actively bleeding angioectasias through a push enteroscope was also found to be effective in improving clinical outcomes by reducing the transfusion requirement and improving quality of life.[16,19–21] However, other investigators have come to divergent conclusions.[22,23]

CAPSULE ENDOSCOPY

Diagnostic Yield of Capsule Endoscopy

CE is a valuable diagnostic modality for evaluating OGIB patients. Large studies, which considered only lesions with high bleeding potential to be diagnostic, report that a definite bleeding source is identified in approximately 50% to 60% of patients undergoing CE.[1,2] As far as the factors potentially affecting the diagnostic yield of CE are concerned, the presence of active bleeding at the time of examination or of a short interval between the last episode of acute bleeding and CE,[24–28] low hemoglobin levels and high transfusion requirement[29,30] have been found to be associated with a high diagnostic yield.

One of the major difficulties in ascertaining the true diagnostic value of CE, and establishing whether it really could replace other techniques, is the lack of a valid reference test through which capsule results could be confirmed. Only one prospective study compared CE with what has been considered the gold standard in small-bowel visualization, IOE. The calculated sensitivity of CE was 95%, specificity was 75%, and positive and negative predictive values were 95% and 86%, respectively.[31] In this excellent study, the gold standard was 100% positive for ongoing bleeding, but only 70.8% positive for previous overt bleeding and only 50% positive for occult bleeding. Through long-term follow-up studies,[24,32,33] the accuracy of diagnostic interpretation of CE has been calculated by obtaining a final diagnosis during the follow-up period (**Table 2**). The positive predictive value of CE is inversely correlated to its overall diagnostic yield, demonstrating that not all lesions found by CE should be regarded as relevant sources of bleeding.

Capsule Endoscopy Versus Other Diagnostic Modalities

Two meta-analyses have clearly demonstrated that, in patients with OGIB, CE is superior to traditional radiological techniques (SBFT and enteroclysis) and to PE. The latter comparison has also been confirmed recently in a specific prospective randomized controlled study.[34] The first meta-analysis analyzed 20 prospective studies, totaling 537 patients, and compared CE to one or more alternative diagnostic modalities for evaluating the small bowel in patients with OGIB.[35] For clinically significant findings, the yields for CE and PE were 56% and 26% ($P<.00001$), respectively; for CE and barium radiography the yields were 42% and 6%, respectively ($P<.00001$). The number needed to test (NNT) with CE to yield one additional clinically relevant finding over either of the two other diagnostic modalities, was 3. The diagnostic advantages

Table 2
Sensitivity, specificity, positive and negative predictive value of capsule endoscopy and double-balloon enteroscopy diagnosis

	Sensitivity (%)	Specificity (%)	Positive Predictive Value (%)	Negative Predictive Value (%)
Capsule endoscopy				
Pennazio[24]	88.9	95	97	82.6
Hartmann[31]	95	75	95	86
Delvaux[32]			94.4	100
Saurin[33]	92	48		
Double-balloon enteroscopy				
Tanaka[66]	92.7	96.4	98.1	87.1

with CE were most pronounced in diagnosing vascular and inflammatory-type mucosal lesions. Another similar meta-analysis[36] showed that, in the OGIB bleeding subgroup comprising 289 patients, the pooled "diagnostic rate difference" between CE and other diagnostic tests (ie, PE, SBFT, or enteroclysis) was 36.9% ($P<.0001$). Compared with PE, CE significantly increased the probability of a positive finding, with a calculated number needed to diagnose (NND) of three. A recent study also showed that CE detects more small-bowel lesions than angiographic modalities.[37]

ISSUES RELATED TO CAPSULE ENDOSCOPY FOR OBSCURE GASTROINTESTINAL BLEEDING

Some of the intrinsic technical characteristics of the system may hamper diagnosis in patients with OGIB. First, the lack of remote control and the inability to take biopsies may significantly decrease the specificity of CE findings, because the diagnosis can be based only on the endoscopic appearance. Second, it is difficult to localize and size small-bowel lesions precisely with the current technology. This problem may have important clinical consequences because the size and location of the lesions are key points to ultimately define the clinical significance of CE findings and direct further management. In addition, incomplete small-bowel visualization without any anatomic abnormality may occur in 15% to 20% of examinations.[38] This factor, together with suboptimal small-bowel cleanliness in some examinations, may decrease the negative predictive value of the test. Third, capsule retention is a rare but serious complication of CE because it can significantly modify the subsequent management of the patient. However, retention of the capsule endoscope seems to be infrequent in patients with OGIB (1%–1.5% of cases),[39,40] and in most cases in which the capsule is retained, significant and previously unknown diseases are identified at surgery. Although screening methods should always be taken into consideration when small-bowel strictures are suspected, to avoid capsule retention,[41] it must also be borne in mind that BAE may be a valid alternative to CE in these high-risk patients. BAE may also allow capsule retrieval, obviating the need for surgery in some cases.[42]

Despite the indisputable progress that the introduction of CE has brought to visualizing lesions of the small bowel, a substantial number of patients with OGIB still remain without a diagnosis. Outcome data suggest that a negative CE study may portend a favorable patient outcome because re-bleeding rates in these patients seem to be low.[43] Forty-nine patients who underwent CE for OGIB were followed up for a mean period of 19 months;[44] the overall long-term re-bleeding rate was 32.7%. The cumulative re-bleeding rate was significantly lower in patients with negative CE (5.6%) than in patients with positive CE (48.4%). In another study, 42 patients with OGIB were followed up for a mean period of 17 months after CE. The overall re-bleeding rate was 28%, and there was a statistically significant difference in re-bleeding rates between patients with a positive study (42%) and those with a negative study (11%). Anticoagulant use was also associated with an increased risk of re-bleeding.[45] It has thus been proposed that further invasive investigations be deferred in patients with negative CE until clinical re-bleeding occurs.[46] Such a conservative approach with regular follow-up seems to be justified provided that the capsule study has been performed under optimal conditions (complete small-bowel examination, adequate luminal view quality), as close to the bleeding episode as possible in cases of overt bleeding, and interpreted by an experienced reader. In case of persistent bleeding after a negative capsule examination, the best management strategy remains unclear. Repeat CE was shown to have a yield of between 35% and 75% in two small studies.[47,48] A recent study of 76 OGIB patients found that those with a nondiagnostic test would definitely benefit from second-look CE if the bleeding presentation changed from occult to overt, or if the hemoglobin value dropped by 4 g/dL or more.[49] However, the eventuality of false negative testing with CE must not be underestimated, because this may delay diagnosis and potentially worsen the outcome. A pooled analysis comparing CE to dated modalities, such as PE, SBFT, and colonoscopy by ileoscopy, found that CE missed 11% of lesions and 19% of neoplastic processes.[50] Reports of submucosal lesions or masses missed by CE but detected by new alternative imaging techniques, such as BAE, CTE, or MRE, have already begun to appear, and most missed lesions were in the proximal small bowel.[51–56] Therefore, given the risk of overlooking lesions at CE, it is not only critical to follow up patients carefully, and if there is clinical evidence of ongoing bleeding or persistent anemia, repeat CE, BAE or cross-sectional studies should also be considered. However, prospective, randomized, controlled trials comparing these modalities in the subgroup of patients with nondiagnostic first capsule study are necessary to clarify the most appropriate management.

BALLOON-ASSISTED ENTEROSCOPY

Diagnostic and Therapeutic Yield of Balloon-Assisted Enteroscopy

Because SBE has only recently been introduced onto the market, most clinical data are still based on DBE. Large published studies show that the diagnostic yield of DBE in OGIB ranges from 50% to 75% (**Table 3**).[57–66] Small-bowel ulcers of various causes and tumors are the commonest diagnostic findings in series studied in Far Eastern countries, whereas in European and North/South American studies the commonest diagnostic finding is angioectasia. A history of frequent bleeding episodes over a long period has been reported to be a predictive factor for positive DBE.[67] A recent study of 108 patients with OGIB[66] suggested that timely DBE is critical to identify the source of bleeding in these patients; yields were significantly higher when the indication was overt ongoing OGIB (100%) than with overt previous (48.4%) or occult OGIB (42.1%). The same study showed that the sensitivity, specificity, and positive and negative predictive values of DBE in the diagnosis of lesions responsible for small-intestinal bleeding were 92.7%, 96.4%, 98.1%, and 87.1%, respectively. These diagnostic values for DBE are similar to those reported for CE examination (**Table 2**).

Table 3
Summary of the largest double-balloon enteroscopy studies for obscure gastrointestinal bleeding

Author[ref.]	No. of Patients	Diagnostic Yield (%)	Endoscopic Therapeutic Yield (%)
Yamamoto[57]	66	50 (76)	20
Heine[58]	168	123 (73)	36
Monkemüller[59]	104	53 (51)	70
May[60]	52	38 (73)	50
Kaffes[61]	60	45 (75)	57
Sun[62]	152	115 (76)	12
Mehdizadeh[63]	130	66 (51)	27
Ohmiya[64]	479	277 (58)	20[a]
Madisch[65]	84	41 (49)	35
Tanaka[66]	96	52 (54)	12

[a] *Data from* 130 patients.

Apart from confirming diagnoses suspected at CE or radiological examination, one of the main advantages of DBE is the possibility of therapeutic approaches in most OGIB patients. Several reports have found endoscopic interventions by DBE to be possible in approximately one third of patients with OGIB (range 12%–70%) (**Table 3**). Argon plasma coagulation, injection therapy, endoscopic resection (**Fig. 1**A, B), and stricture dilation are some of the therapeutic options reported.

As far as SBE is concerned, preliminary studies on patients with suspected small-bowel disease[6,7] have found diagnostic and therapeutic yields to be similar to those achieved in initial experiences with DBE. However, the rate of whole small-bowel visualization was lower than with the DBE system. Prospective comparative studies will probably indicate whether SBE provides an advantage or whether performance is similar to that of the currently established DBE method. Other new enteroscopy methods, in which progression of the endoscope is assisted by a two-balloon add-on disposable element[68] or by a spiral overtube,[69] have recently been reported. In future studies, these apparently simple and rapid methods of performing deep enteroscopy should be compared with DBE or with SBE to clarify their potential.

Double-Balloon Enteroscopy Versus Other Diagnostic Modalities

A controlled prospective trial[60] on patients with suspected small-bowel bleeding showed that oral DBE is significantly superior to PE with regard to the length of small bowel visualized (230 cm versus 80 cm) and to the detection-rate of pathologic lesions (63% versus 44%). Moreover, in the same study, DBE identified additional lesions in deeper parts of the small bowel in 78% of patients who had positive findings at PE. Several studies have compared the diagnostic yields of CE and DBE in patients with OGIB; most have concluded that the diagnostic rates for the two methods are similar (**Table 4**).[63,70–75] A recent meta-analysis[76] based on 11 studies confirmed that CE and DBE have comparable diagnostic yields in small-bowel disease, including OGIB; the pooled overall yield for CE and DBE was 60% (n = 397) and 57% (n = 360).

ISSUES RELATED TO DOUBLE-BALLOON ENTEROSCOPY FOR OBSCURE GASTROINTESTINAL BLEEDING

DBE is useful for the diagnosis and management of patients with OGIB, but the technique is invasive and resource-intensive, can be associated with complications, and the learning curve is long.[77] Although the technical feasibility of DBE is clearly established, it remains a challenging procedure even for experienced endoscopists.

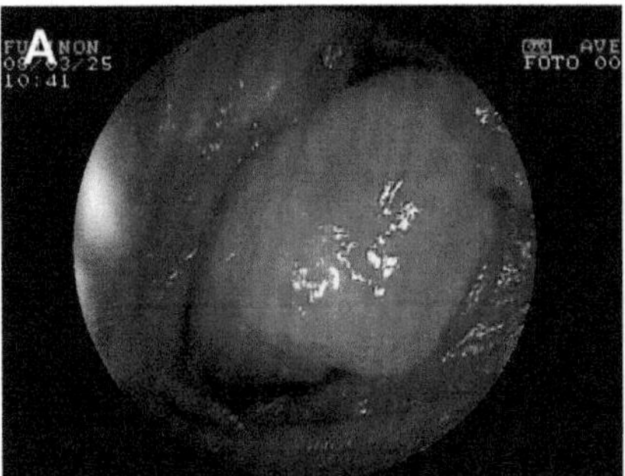

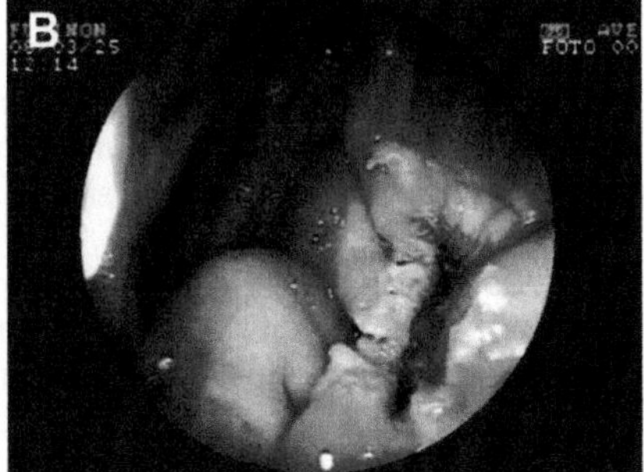

Fig. 1. (*A*) Large jejunal polyp in a patient with obscure overt bleeding. (*B*) After polypectomy by DBE.

Table 4
Studies comparing diagnostic yields of capsule endoscopy and double-balloon enteroscopy in patients with obscure gastrointestinal bleeding

Author[ref.]	No. of Patients	Results
Mehdizadeh[63]	115	CE ≈ DBE
May[70]	52	DBE > CE
Hadithi[71]	35	CE > DBE
Nakamura[72]	32	CE ≈ DBE
Matsumoto[73]	13	CE ≈ DBE
Kameda[74]	32	CE ≈ DBE
Arakawa[75]	74	CE ≈ DBE

Data from Pennazio M. Approach to the patient with GI bleeding. In: Faigel DO, Cave DR, editors. Capsule endoscopy. London: Elsevier; 2007. p. 113–28.

Complete enteroscopy by DBE is not generally required in most patients with OGIB, as the potential bleeding source can be identified without visualizing the entire small bowel.[58,65] Nonetheless, about one third of patients will require two separate DBEs to make a diagnosis, and this may significantly increase the workload at busy endoscopy centers. Unfortunately, it may not always be possible to perform complete enteroscopy, and particularly in patients with marked intestinal adhesions;[78] reported rates of total small-bowel intubation with DBE, most often combining oral and anal routes, range from 0% to 86%.[79] This means that lesions in the mid-small bowel, where access is often challenging, may be missed. For the same reason there may also be inadequate therapeutic control of bleeding lesions in patients receiving therapeutic DBE.

CE is currently the tool most frequently used to indicate the preferential endoscope insertion route for DBE. Although prospective, randomized, controlled studies validating the usefulness of CE-directed DBE in patients with OGIB are lacking, it has been suggested that, if the ratio of time to reach the lesion at CE to time to reach the cecum is <0.75, the oral route should be considered first to reach the lesion with DBE, The positive predictive value of CE in indicating the DBE route is 95%, with a negative predictive value of as high as 98%.[80] A CE-directed approach may thus avoid unnecessary combined DBE procedures.[81] If CE is unavailable or contraindicated, given the technical challenges associated with the anal route and most bleeding sources are located in the proximal two thirds of the small intestine, it is generally best to start with the oral route in most patients.[9]

An important issue is the safety of DBE. As more centers are reporting their experiences, and the results of a large number of DBE procedures are known, it is becoming increasingly clear that DBE carries a risk, especially during or after therapeutic interventions. Compared with conventional upper endoscopy and colonoscopy, DBE is associated with a significant complication rate. The complications most frequently reported to date have included pancreatitis, postpolypectomy bleeding, and intestinal perforation. A large, multicenter, international complication survey reported a total of 40 complications in 2362 DBE procedures (1.7%), 13 in 1728 diagnostic DBEs (0.8%), and 27 during 634 therapeutic procedures (4.3%).[82] Argon plasma coagulation of angioectasias seems to be a safe treatment, associated with a low complication rate of approximately 1%; complications such as bleeding or perforation may occur after polypectomy, especially of polyps larger than 3 cm. In this situation, the complication rate may reach 10%.[83] An increased risk of perforation during anal DBE in patients with prior ileoanal or ileocolonic anastomoses has recently been reported.[84] Safety data on SBE are still scarce, but may be comparable to those of DBE.

IMPACT ON PATIENT MANAGEMENT AND OUTCOMES

Capsule Endoscopy

As CE is a purely diagnostic procedure, improvements in bleeding parameters cannot be directly attributed to it. CE directs clinicians to the most appropriate definitive therapy. Published studies show that 25% to 60% of patients with OGIB received specific therapeutic interventions or changes in management based on a finding from CE.[85–91] Most studies with long-term follow-up data[24,30,32,43,49] support the usefulness of CE diagnosis for improving outcome; only a small number of studies have reached divergent conclusions.[92,93] Specifically, patient management dictated by CE results may lead to resolution of bleeding in approximately two thirds of patients.[24,30,94,95] Lesions with high bleeding potential are more likely to lead to therapeutic interventions and are associated with more frequent resolution of bleeding.[33,49,96] Other studies have reported a significant reduction in subsequent endoscopic procedures, blood transfusions, and hospitalizations after CE.[26]

A recent field of investigation examines the correlation between predicted and actual consequences of CE on patient management. In a prospective study on 128 patients with occult OGIB, small-bowel findings and appropriate clinical management were predicted on clinical grounds alone in approximately three quarters of patients. Although in this study CE altered clinical management in only a minority (26%) of patients referred for the procedure, it was especially useful in those under consideration for surgery, especially to exclude small-bowel neoplasia.[97] Similarly, another study showed that physicians performed well in estimating the consequences of CE on patient management, reflected by an overall match between anticipated and ultimate consequences in 78% of cases investigated.[98]

Double-Balloon Enteroscopy

The therapeutic impact of DBE may consist of a decision to start new treatment, change existing treatment, or to carry out surgical intervention or therapeutic endoscopy. DBE findings may influence subsequent management in about 40% to 50% of patients with OGIB.[99] A history of blood transfusions has been found to be a significant predictor of endoscopic therapy being performed during DBE.[61] A small number of studies have assessed the clinical impact of DBE. In a preliminary report, the therapeutic measures induced by DBE led to complete resolution of bleeding in 17 (89%) of 19 patients with OGIB, after a mean follow-up period of 8.5 months.[100] A large study of 152 patients with a mean follow-up of 16 months reported no re-bleeding on 89% of 95 patients with positive findings at DBE, but the analysis excluded 57 patients who had no findings at DBE or were lost to follow-up.[62] A targeted approach was applied to a group of 60 patients with OGIB and a positive finding at CE. The treatment performed as a result of DBE led to the cessation of bleeding in 80% of patients after a mean follow-up of 10 months.[61] In a similar study using combined CE and DBE in 45 patients, the re-bleeding rate was 5% in patients with positive diagnoses at CE or DBE, and 12% in negative cases.[101] Two recent studies report only a slight effect of DBE on re-bleeding; the first, on 108 patients, found that, although only 7.4% of patients had bleeding recurrence during the mean follow-up period of 28.5 months, the re-bleeding rate was not significantly different in patients with negative DBE findings (9.8%) from that in patients with positive DBE findings followed by specific treatments (7.7%).[66] Similarly, another prospective study on 84 patients with OGIB found that, at a mean follow-up of 2 months, the rate of re-bleeding in patients who had undergone interventions (20%) was similar to that in patients who had not (18%); however, about 40% of patients were lost to follow-up and total enteroscopy was accomplished in only 15%.[65]

Although these preliminary results are encouraging, they must be interpreted with caution for several reasons. First, most studies were retrospective. Second, in some reports most treatment modifications after CE did not reflect any specific impact of CE on changes in treatment modalities. Third, some studies found no difference in outcome between positive and negative CE cases, nor between those in which DBE found and treated a lesion or did not. Fourth, the follow-up periods may not be sufficiently long, because bleeding can recur even after longer time intervals. Most studies lack standardized treatment protocols for findings at CE or after DBE diagnosis.

In comparison with the end of the twentieth century, it is indisputable that, thanks to significant advances in enteroscopy such as CE and BAE, we can now benefit from better diagnostic and therapeutic efficacy for managing patients with OGIB. Nonetheless, the problem of managing patients with small-bowel angioectasias, the most frequent lesions found in patients with OGIB, is still unresolved. In many patients, successful therapy for these lesions remains a puzzling clinical challenge; this is confirmed by the findings of almost all outcome studies that re-bleeding is more frequent in patients with vascular lesions, especially diffuse lesions.[66,75,85,94,95] Although there seems to be spontaneous cessation of bleeding in approximately 40% of cases of angioectasias per year,[102] re-bleeding may be related to the inaccessible location of lesions, incomplete enteroscopic treatment, tiny vascular lesions between folds being overlooked, or the development of new lesions.[103] Because prior studies using PE have failed to demonstrate conclusively the efficacy of endoscopic therapy for vascular lesions,[16,18–23] a prospective controlled study with objective inclusion criteria, standardized therapeutic protocol, clear outcome measures, and adequate follow-up, formally evaluating the impact of BAE on clinical outcomes in this specific clinical setting, would be of considerable interest.

THE PLACE OF CAPSULE ENDOSCOPY AND BALLOON-ASSISTED ENTEROSCOPY IN THE MANAGEMENT ALGORITHM OF OBSCURE GASTROINTESTINAL BLEEDING

The specific approach to the diagnostic evaluation of any patient with OGIB will be dictated by the clinical setting, the availability of each technology, and local expertise.

Because there are as yet no randomized prospective studies on this issue, proposed algorithms for OGIB workup are based on feasibility and technical considerations (**Fig. 2**).[11,46,104] Endoscopic studies of the upper and lower GI tract should be repeated before evaluation of the small bowel, because of the significant miss rate on initial endoscopy. In 5% to 25% of patients with OGIB, investigation by PE,[105] CE,[106] or BAE[107] can identify significant treatable lesions within reach of conventional upper GI endoscopy and colonoscopy. The skill and experience of the initial endoscopist, as well as the quality and completeness of the initial evaluation, are factors that should be taken into consideration when deciding whether to repeat upper GI endoscopy or colonoscopy, although the diagnostic yield of repeat endoscopy may be enough to warrant a second look in any case.[1,4]

The diagnostic workup for subsequent small-bowel investigation should be individualized on the basis of clinical presentation.[108] Currently available data suggest that, in patients with obscure occult bleeding and intermittent obscure overt bleeding, provided that there is no suspected obstruction, CE should be the first diagnostic

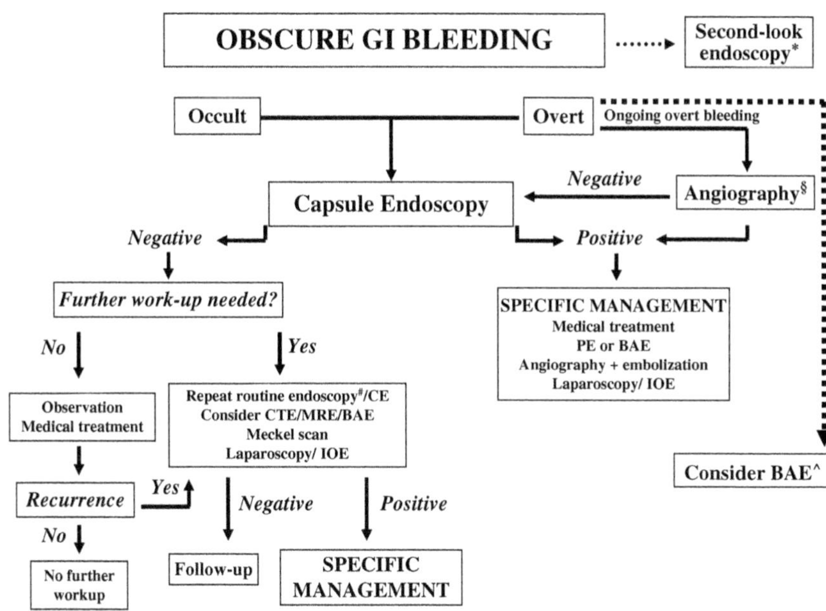

Fig. 2. Proposed algorithm for the diagnosis and management of obscure gastrointestinal bleeding. *Upper and lower gastrointestinal endoscopy should be repeated before investigation of the small bowel and will frequently identify lesions overlooked at the initial endoscopy. §Patients with significant active bleeding and unsuitable for flexible endoscopy. #Especially if it was not repeated before capsule endoscopy. ^If available, and especially in patients with known angioectasias in the upper or lower gastrointestinal tract. BAE, balloon-assisted enteroscopy; CE, capsule endoscopy; CTE, computed tomographic enterography; IOE, intraoperative enteroscopy; MRE, magnetic resonance enterography; PE, push enteroscopy. (*Adapted from* Pennazio M. Capsule endoscopy: where are we after 6 years of clinical use? Dig Liver Dis 2006;38(12):867–78; with permission.)

test to identify or exclude a bleeding intestinal lesion and thus direct subsequent management.[1,4,46,105,108–111] This is because of its noninvasive quality, tolerance, and ability to view the entire small bowel, and also to determine the initial route of BAE. Because of its therapeutic capabilities, BAE may be indicated in patients with a positive finding at CE requiring biopsy or therapeutic intervention. Because alternative imaging modalities such as BAE,[51–54,56] CTE,[112] or MRE[54] can also detect lesions that are missed by CE, they should be carefully considered in patients with strong clinical suspicion of a small-bowel lesion despite negative CE.

Patients with ongoing overt OGIB and with a high probability that treatment will be needed may also benefit from early BAE.[11] However, this approach is based mostly on expert opinion, as evidence for ongoing overt OGIB is still sparse. Moreover, it remains unclear whether such an approach is always feasible in routine clinical practice. Given the technical skill required to perform BAE, the ability to conduct the procedure adequately may, at present, be limited to referral centers; thus many patients with acute OGIB may not have prompt access to BAE, limiting its use. In cases of suspected active bleeding in the proximal jejunum, PE (and hopefully in future spiral enteroscopy) may be an easy-to-apply alternative;[11] in patients with significant active bleeding who are unsuitable for flexible endoscopy, mesenteric angiography should be considered. CE has also been shown to be a beneficial diagnostic tool for life-threatening OGIB in a small series of cases.[113] Prospective, randomized, controlled studies will be necessary to evaluate the most efficient and cost-effective strategy in this subgroup of patients.

SUMMARY

Improvements in endoscopic technology, that is, CE and BAE, have revolutionized our approach to the diagnosis and management of patients with OGIB. Intraoperative enteroscopy and conventional barium studies have largely been replaced by these two techniques; only the use of accurate methods of radiological investigation such as CTE or MRE can justify their continued use and make them complementary to CE and to BAE in the optimal investigation of OGIB.

Despite its limitations, CE may well be the most reasonable initial diagnostic strategy to evaluate most OGIB patients, leaving BAE in reserve as a complementary tool. New methods of performing deep enteroscopy, such as spiral or balloon-guided enteroscopy, will need to be compared against BAE, which is today's reference standard for nonsurgical enteroscopy in patients with OGIB. Appropriately designed prospective studies will be needed to clarify the impact of CE and of BAE on health care use and clinical outcome of patients with OGIB, especially those with angioectasias.

REFERENCES

1. Raju GS, Gerson L, Das A, et al. American Gastroenterological Association (AGA) Institute technical review on obscure gastrointestinal bleeding. Gastroenterology 2007;133(5):1697–717.
2. Pennazio M. Bleeding update. Gastrointest Endosc Clin N Am 2006;16(2): 251–66.
3. Ell C, May A. Mid-gastrointestinal bleeding: capsule endoscopy and push-and-pull enteroscopy give rise to a new medical term. Endoscopy 2006;38:673–5.
4. Pennazio M. Approach to the patient with GI bleeding. In: Faigel DO, Cave DR, editors. Capsule endoscopy. London: Elsevier; 2007. p. 113–28.
5. Yamamoto H, Sekine Y, Sato Y, et al. Total enteroscopy with a nonsurgical steerable double-balloon method. Gastrointest Endosc 2001;53(2):216–20.
6. Tsujikawa T, Saitoh Y, Andoh A, et al. Novel single-balloon enteroscopy for diagnosis and treatment of the small intestine: preliminary experiences. Endoscopy 2008;40(1):11–5.
7. Kawamura T, Yasuda K, Tanaka K, et al. Clinical evaluation of a newly developed single-balloon enteroscope. Gastrointest Endosc 2008;68(6):1112–6.
8. Mönkemüller K, Fry LC, Bellutti M, et al. Balloon-assisted enteroscopy: unifying double-balloon and single-balloon enteroscopy. Endoscopy 2008;40(6):537.
9. Gerson LB, Flodin JT, Miyabayashi K. Balloon-assisted enteroscopy: technology and troubleshooting. Gastrointest Endosc 2008;68(6):1158–67.
10. Douard R, Wind P, Panis Y, et al. Intraoperative enteroscopy for diagnosis and management of unexplained gastrointestinal bleeding. Am J Surg 2000; 180(3):181–4.
11. Pohl J, Delvaux M, Ell C, et al. ESGE Clinical Guidelines Committee. European Society of Gastrointestinal Endoscopy (ESGE) Guidelines: flexible enteroscopy for diagnosis and treatment of small-bowel diseases. Endoscopy 2008;40(7): 609–18.
12. Lepère C, Cuillerier E, Van Gossum A, et al. Predictive factors of positive findings in patients explored by push enteroscopy for unexplained GI bleeding. Gastrointest Endosc 2005;61(6):709–14.

13. Sidhu R, McAlindon ME, Kapur K, et al. Push enteroscopy in the era of capsule endoscopy. J Clin Gastroenterol 2008;42(1):54–8.
14. Pennazio M, Arrigoni A, Risio M, et al. Clinical evaluation of push-type enteroscopy. Endoscopy 1995;27(2):164–70.
15. Hayat M, Axon TR, O'Mahony S. Diagnostic yield and effect on clinical outcomes of push enteroscopy in suspected small-bowel bleeding. Endoscopy 2000; 32(5):369–72.
16. Nguyen NQ, Rayner CK, Schoeman MN. Push enteroscopy alters management in a majority of patients with obscure gastrointestinal bleeding. J Gastroenterol Hepatol 2005;20(5):716–21.
17. Bezet A, Cuillerier E, Landi B, et al. Clinical impact of push enteroscopy in patients with gastrointestinal bleeding of unknown origin. Clin Gastroenterol Hepatol 2004;2(10):921–7.
18. Landi B, Cellier C, Gaudric M, et al. Long-term outcome of patients with gastrointestinal bleeding of obscure origin explored by push enteroscopy. Endoscopy 2002;34(5):355–9.
19. Vakil N, Huilgol V, Khan I. Effect of push enteroscopy on transfusion requirements and quality of life in patients with unexplained gastrointestinal bleeding. Am J Gastroenterol 1997;9(3):425–8.
20. Askin MP, Lewis BS. Push enteroscopic cauterization: long-term follow-up of 83 patients with bleeding small intestinal angiodysplasia. Gastrointest Endosc 1996;43(6):580–3.
21. Morris AJ, Mokhashi M, Straiton M, et al. Push enteroscopy and heater probe therapy for small bowel bleeding. Gastrointest Endosc 1996;44(4):394–7.
22. Schmit A, Gay F, Adler M, et al. Diagnostic efficacy of push-enteroscopy and long-term follow-up of patients with small bowel angiodysplasias. Dig Dis Sci 1996;41(12):2348–52.
23. Barkin JS, Ross BS. Medical therapy for chronic gastrointestinal bleeding of obscure origin. Am J Gastroenterol 1998;93(8):1250–4.
24. Pennazio M, Santucci R, Rondonotti E, et al. Outcome of patients with obscure gastrointestinal bleeding after capsule endoscopy: report of 100 consecutive cases. Gastroenterology 2004;126(3):643–53.
25. Bresci G, Parisi G, Bertoni M, et al. The role of video capsule endoscopy for evaluating obscure gastrointestinal bleeding: usefulness of early use. J Gastroenterol 2005;40(3):256–9.
26. Carey EJ, Leighton JA, Heigh RI, et al. A single-center experience of 260 consecutive patients undergoing capsule endoscopy for obscure gastrointestinal bleeding. Am J Gastroenterol 2007;102(1):89–95.
27. Ge ZZ, Chen HY, Gao YJ, et al. Best candidates for capsule endoscopy for obscure gastrointestinal bleeding. J Gastroenterol Hepatol 2007;22(12):2076–80.
28. Apostolopoulos P, Liatsos C, Gralnek IM, et al. Evaluation of capsule endoscopy in active, mild-to-moderate, overt, obscure GI bleeding. Gastrointest Endosc 2007;66(6):1174–81.
29. May A, Wardak A, Nachbar L, et al. Influence of patient selection on the outcome of capsule endoscopy in patients with chronic gastrointestinal bleeding. J Clin Gastroenterol 2005;39(8):684–8.
30. Estévez E, González-Conde B, Vázquez-Iglesias JL, et al. Diagnostic yield and clinical outcomes after capsule endoscopy in 100 consecutive patients with obscure gastrointestinal bleeding. Eur J Gastroenterol Hepatol 2006;18(8): 881–8.

31. Hartmann D, Schmidt H, Bolz G, et al. A prospective two-center study comparing wireless capsule endoscopy with intraoperative enteroscopy in patients with obscure GI bleeding. Gastrointest Endosc 2005;61(7):826–32.
32. Delvaux M, Fassler I, Gay G. Clinical usefulness of the endoscopic video capsule as the initial intestinal investigation in patients with obscure digestive bleeding: validation of a diagnostic strategy based on the patient outcome after 12 months. Endoscopy 2004;36(12):1067–73.
33. Saurin JC, Delvaux M, Vahedi K, et al. Clinical impact of capsule endoscopy compared to push enteroscopy: 1-year follow-up study. Endoscopy 2005; 37(4):318–23.
34. de Leusse A, Vahedi K, Edery J, et al. Capsule endoscopy or push enteroscopy for first-line exploration of obscure gastrointestinal bleeding? Gastroenterology 2007;132(3):855–62.
35. Triester SL, Leighton JA, Leontiadis GI, et al. A meta-analysis of the yield of capsule endoscopy compared to other diagnostic modalities in patients with obscure gastrointestinal bleeding. Am J Gastroenterol 2005;100(11):2407–18.
36. Marmo R, Rotondano G, Piscopo R, et al. Meta-analysis: capsule enteroscopy vs. conventional modalities in diagnosis of small bowel diseases. Aliment Pharmacol Ther 2005;22(7):595–604.
37. Saperas E, Dot J, Videla S, et al. Capsule endoscopy versus computed tomographic or standard angiography for the diagnosis of obscure gastrointestinal bleeding. Am J Gastroenterol 2007;102(4):731–7.
38. Rondonotti E, Herrerias JM, Pennazio M, et al. Complications, limitations, and failures of capsule endoscopy: a review of 733 cases. Gastrointest Endosc 2005;62(5):712–6.
39. Cave D, Legnani P, de Franchis R, et al. ICCE consensus for capsule retention. Endoscopy 2005;37(10):1065–7.
40. Pennazio M. Capsule endoscopy: where are we after 6 years of clinical use? Dig Liver Dis 2006;38(12):867–78.
41. Herrerias JM, Leighton JA, Costamagna G, et al. Agile patency system eliminates risk of capsule retention in patients with known intestinal strictures who undergo capsule endoscopy. Gastrointest Endosc 2008;67(6):902–9.
42. Lee BI, Choi H, Choi KY, et al. Retrieval of a retained capsule endoscope by double- balloon enteroscopy. Gastrointest Endosc 2005;62(3):463–5.
43. Neu B, Ell C, May A, et al. Capsule endoscopy versus standard tests in influencing management of obscure digestive bleeding: results from a German multicenter trial. Am J Gastroenterol 2005;100(8):1736–42.
44. Lai LH, Wong GL, Chow DK, et al. Long-term follow-up of patients with obscure gastrointestinal bleeding after negative capsule endoscopy. Am J Gastroenterol 2006;101(6):1224–8.
45. Macdonald J, Porter V, McNamara D. Negative capsule endoscopy in patients with obscure GI bleeding predicts low rebleeding rates. Gastrointest Endosc 2008;68(6):1122–7.
46. Mergener K, Ponchon T, Gralnek I, et al. Literature review and recommendations for clinical application of small-bowel capsule endoscopy, based on a panel discussion by international experts. Consensus statements for small-bowel capsule endoscopy, 2006/2007. Endoscopy 2007;39(10):895–909.
47. Jones BH, Fleischer DE, Sharma VK, et al. Yield of repeat wireless video capsule endoscopy in patients with obscure gastrointestinal bleeding. Am J Gastroenterol 2005;100(5):1058–64.

48. Bar-Meir S, Eliakim R, Nadler M, et al. Second capsule endoscopy for patients with severe iron deficiency anemia. Gastrointest Endosc 2004;60(5):711–3.
49. Viazis N, Papaxoinis K, Vlachogiannakos J, et al. Is there a role for second-look capsule endoscopy in patients with obscure GI bleeding after a nondiagnostic first test? Gastrointest Endosc 2009;69(4):850–6.
50. Lewis BS, Eisen GM, Friedman S. A pooled analysis to evaluate results of capsule endoscopy trials. Endoscopy 2005;37(10):960–5.
51. Chong AK, Chin BW, Meredith CG. Clinically significant small-bowel pathology identified by double-balloon enteroscopy but missed by capsule endoscopy. Gastrointest Endosc 2006;64(3):445–9.
52. Ross A, Mehdizadeh S, Tokar J, et al. Double balloon enteroscopy detects small bowel mass lesions missed by capsule endoscopy. Dig Dis Sci 2008;53(8): 2140–3.
53. Baichi MM, Arifuddin RM, Mantry PS. Small-bowel masses found and missed on capsule endoscopy for obscure bleeding. Scand J Gastroenterol 2007;42(9): 1127–32.
54. Postgate A, Despott E, Burling D, et al. Significant small-bowel lesions detected by alternative diagnostic modalities after negative capsule endoscopy. Gastrointest Endosc 2008;68(6):1209–14.
55. Madisch A, Schimming W, Kinzel F, et al. Locally advanced small-bowel adenocarcinoma missed primarily by capsule endoscopy but diagnosed by push enteroscopy. Endoscopy 2003;35(10):861–4.
56. Fukumoto A, Tanaka S, Shishido T, et al. Comparison of detectability of small-bowel lesions between capsule endoscopy and double-balloon endoscopy for patients with suspected small-bowel disease. Gastrointest Endosc 2009;69(4): 857–65.
57. Yamamoto H, Kita H, Sunada K, et al. Clinical outcomes of double-balloon endoscopy for the diagnosis and treatment of small-intestinal diseases. Clin Gastroenterol Hepatol 2004;2(11):1010–6.
58. Heine GD, Hadithi M, Groenen MJ, et al. Double-balloon enteroscopy: indications, diagnostic yield, and complications in a series of 275 patients with suspected small-bowel disease. Endoscopy 2006;38(1):42–8.
59. Mönkemüller K, Fry LC, Neumann H, et al. Diagnostic and therapeutic utility of double balloon endoscopy: experience with 225 procedures. Acta Gastroenterol Latinoam 2007;37(4):216–23.
60. May A, Nachbar L, Schneider M, et al. Prospective comparison of push enteroscopy and push-and-pull enteroscopy in patients with suspected small-bowel bleeding. Am J Gastroenterol 2006;101(9):2016–24.
61. Kaffes AJ, Siah C, Koo JH. Clinical outcomes after double-balloon enteroscopy in patients with obscure GI bleeding and a positive capsule endoscopy. Gastrointest Endosc 2007;66(2):304–9.
62. Sun B, Rajan E, Cheng S, et al. Diagnostic yield and therapeutic impact of double-balloon enteroscopy in a large cohort of patients with obscure gastrointestinal bleeding. Am J Gastroenterol 2006;101(9):2011–5.
63. Mehdizadeh S, Ross A, Gerson L, et al. What is the learning curve associated with double-balloon enteroscopy? Technical details and early experience in 6 U.S. tertiary care centers. Gastrointest Endosc 2006;64(5):740–50.
64. Ohmiya N, Yano T, Yamamoto H, et al. Diagnosis and treatment of obscure GI bleeding at double balloon endoscopy. Gastrointest Endosc 2007;66(Suppl 3):S72–7.

65. Madisch A, Schmolders J, Brückner S, et al. Less favorable clinical outcome after diagnostic and interventional double balloon enteroscopy in patients with suspected small-bowel bleeding? Endoscopy 2008;40(9):731–4.
66. Tanaka S, Mitsui K, Yamada Y, et al. Diagnostic yield of double-balloon endoscopy in patients with obscure GI bleeding. Gastrointest Endosc 2008;68(4): 683–91.
67. Byeon JS, Chung JW, Choi KD, et al. Clinical features predicting the detection of abnormalities by double balloon endoscopy in patients with suspected small bowel bleeding. J Gastroenterol Hepatol 2008;23(7 Pt 1):1051–5.
68. Adler SN, Bjarnason I, Metzger YC. New balloon-guided technique for deep small-intestine endoscopy using standard endoscopes. Endoscopy 2008; 40(6):502–5.
69. Akerman PA, Agrawal D, Cantero D, et al. Spiral enteroscopy with the new DSB overtube: a novel technique for deep peroral small-bowel intubation. Endoscopy 2008;40(12):974–8.
70. May A, Nachbar L, Ell C. Double-balloon enteroscopy (push-and-pull enteroscopy) of the small bowel: feasibility and diagnostic and therapeutic yield in patients with suspected small bowel disease. Gastrointest Endosc 2005;62(1): 62–70.
71. Hadithi M, Heine GD, Jacobs MA, et al. A prospective study comparing video capsule endoscopy with double-balloon enteroscopy in patients with obscure gastrointestinal bleeding. Am J Gastroenterol 2006;101(1):52–7.
72. Nakamura M, Niwa Y, Ohmiya N, et al. Preliminary comparison of capsule endoscopy and double-balloon enteroscopy in patients with suspected small-bowel bleeding. Endoscopy 2006;38(1):59–66.
73. Matsumoto T, Esaki M, Moriyama T, et al. Comparison of capsule endoscopy and enteroscopy with the double-balloon method in patients with obscure bleeding and polyposis. Endoscopy 2005;37(9):827–32.
74. Kameda N, Higuchi K, Shiba M, et al. A prospective, single-blind trial comparing wireless capsule endoscopy and double-balloon enteroscopy in patients with obscure gastrointestinal bleeding. J Gastroenterol 2008;43(6):434–40.
75. Arakawa D, Ohmiya N, Nakamura M, et al. Outcome after enteroscopy for patients with obscure GI bleeding: diagnostic comparison between double-balloon endoscopy and videocapsule endoscopy. Gastrointest Endosc 2009; 69(4):866–74.
76. Pasha SF, Leighton JA, Das A, et al. Double-balloon enteroscopy and capsule endoscopy have comparable diagnostic yield in small-bowel disease: a meta-analysis. Clin Gastroenterol Hepatol 2008;6(6):671–6.
77. Gross SA, Stark ME. Initial experience with double-balloon enteroscopy at a U.S. center. Gastrointest Endosc 2008;67(6):890–7.
78. Mehdizadeh S, Han NJ, Cheng DW, et al. Success rate of retrograde double-balloon enteroscopy. Gastrointest Endosc 2007;65(4):633–9.
79. Pennazio M. Diagnostic and therapeutic utility of double-balloon endoscopy in small-bowel bleeding. Tech Gastrointest Endosc 2008;10:77–82.
80. Gay G, Delvaux M, Fassler I. Outcome of capsule endoscopy in determining indication and route for push-and-pull enteroscopy. Endoscopy 2006;38(1): 49–58.
81. Hendel JW, Vilmann P, Jensen T. Double-balloon endoscopy: who needs it? Scand J Gastroenterol 2008;43(3):363–7.
82. Mensink PB, Haringsma J, Kucharzik T, et al. Complications of double balloon enteroscopy: a multicenter survey. Endoscopy 2007;39(7):613–5.

83. May A, Nachbar L, Pohl J, et al. Endoscopic interventions in the small bowel using double balloon enteroscopy: feasibility and limitations. Am J Gastroenterol 2007;102(3):527–35.
84. Gerson L, Chiorean M, Tokar J, et al. Complications associated with double balloon enteroscopy: the US experience. Am J Gastroenterol 2008;103: S109–10.
85. Albert JG, Schülbe R, Hahn L, et al. Impact of capsule endoscopy on outcome in mid-intestinal bleeding: a multicentre cohort study in 285 patients. Eur J Gastroenterol Hepatol 2008;20(10):971–7.
86. Ahmad NA, Iqbal N, Joyce A. Clinical impact of capsule endoscopy on management of gastrointestinal disorders. Clin Gastroenterol Hepatol 2008;6(4):433–7.
87. Toy E, Rojany M, Sheikh R, et al. Capsule endoscopy's impact on clinical management and outcomes: a single-center experience with 145 patients. Am J Gastroenterol 2008;103(12):3022–8.
88. Sidhu R, Sanders DS, Kapur K, et al. Capsule endoscopy changes patient management in routine clinical practice. Dig Dis Sci 2007;52(5):1382–6.
89. García-Compean D, Armenta JA, Marrufo C, et al. Impact of therapeutic interventions induced by capsule endoscopy on long term outcome in chronic obscure GI bleeding. Gastroenterol Clin Biol 2007;31(10):806–11.
90. Redondo-Cerezo E, Pérez-Vigara G, Pérez-Sola A, et al. Diagnostic yield and impact of capsule endoscopy on management of patients with gastrointestinal bleeding of obscure origin. Dig Dis Sci 2007;52(5):1376–81.
91. Baichi MM, Arifuddin RM, Mantry PS. Capsule endoscopy for obscure GI bleeding: therapeutic yield of follow-up procedures. Dig Dis Sci 2007;52(5): 1370–5.
92. Rastogi A, Schoen RE, Slivka A. Diagnostic yield and clinical outcomes of capsule endoscopy. Gastrointest Endosc 2004;60(6):959–64.
93. van Tuyl SA, van Noorden JT, Stolk MF, et al. Clinical consequences of videocapsule endoscopy in GI bleeding and Crohn's disease. Gastrointest Endosc 2007; 66(6):1164–70.
94. Hindryckx P, Botelberge T, De Vos M, et al. Clinical impact of capsule endoscopy on further strategy and long-term clinical outcome in patients with obscure bleeding. Gastrointest Endosc 2008;68(1):98–104.
95. Hartmann D, Schmidt H, Schilling D, et al. Follow-up of patients with obscure gastrointestinal bleeding after capsule endoscopy and intraoperative enteroscopy. Hepatogastroenterology 2007;54(75):780–3.
96. Endo H, Matsuhashi N, Inamori M, et al. Rebleeding rate after interventional therapy directed by capsule endoscopy in patients with obscure gastrointestinal bleeding. BMC Gastroenterol 2008;8:12.
97. Gubler C, Fox M, Hengstler P, et al. Capsule endoscopy: impact on clinical decision making in patients with suspected small bowel bleeding. Endoscopy 2007; 39(12):1031–6.
98. de Graaf AP, Westerhof J, Weersma RK, et al. Correlation between predicted and actual consequences of capsule endoscopy on patient management. Dig Liver Dis 2008;40(9):761–6.
99. Pasha SF, Leighton J, Das A, et al. Diagnostic yield and therapeutic utility of double-balloon enteroscopy (DBE) in patients with obscure gastrointestinal bleeding (OGIB): a systematic review [abstract]. Gastrointest Endosc 2007; 65(5):366.
100. Manabe N, Tanaka S, Fukumoto A, et al. Double-balloon enteroscopy in patients with GI bleeding of obscure origin. Gastrointest Endosc 2006;64(1):135–40.

101. Fujimori S, Seo T, Gudis K, et al. Diagnosis and treatment of obscure gastrointestinal bleeding using combined capsule endoscopy and double balloon endoscopy: 1-year follow-up study. Endoscopy 2007;39(12):1053–8.
102. Lewis BS, Salomon P, Rivera-MacMurray S, et al. Does hormonal therapy have any benefit for bleeding angiodysplasia? J Clin Gastroenterol 1992;15(2): 99–103.
103. Rossini FP, Pennazio M. Small-bowel endoscopy. Endoscopy 2000;32(2): 138–45.
104. Pennazio M, Eisen G, Goldfarb N. ICCE consensus for obscure gastrointestinal bleeding. Endoscopy 2005;37(10):1046–50.
105. Descamps C, Schmit A, Van Gossum A. "Missed" upper gastrointestinal tract lesions may explain "occult" bleeding. Endoscopy 1999;31(6):452–5.
106. Kitiyakara T, Selby W. Non-small-bowel lesions detected by capsule endoscopy in patients with obscure GI bleeding. Gastrointest Endosc 2005;62(2):234–8.
107. Fry LC, Bellutti M, Neumann H, et al. Incidence of bleeding lesions within reach of conventional upper and lower endoscopes in patients undergoing double-balloon enteroscopy for obscure gastrointestinal bleeding. Aliment Pharmacol Ther 2009;29(3):342–9.
108. Das A, Leighton JA. Is double balloon enteroscopy the best initial imaging method for obscure gastrointestinal bleeding? Nat Clin Pract Gastroenterol Hepatol 2007;4(3):120–1.
109. Rey JF, Ladas S, Alhassani A, et al. ESGE Guidelines Committee. European Society of Gastrointestinal Endoscopy (ESGE). Video capsule endoscopy: update to guidelines (May 2006). Endoscopy 2006;38(10):1047–53.
110. Mishkin DS, Chuttani R, Croffie J, et al. Technology Assessment Committee, American Society for Gastrointestinal Endoscopy. ASGE Technology Status Evaluation Report: wireless capsule endoscopy. Gastrointest Endosc 2006; 63(4):539–45.
111. Sidhu R, Sanders DS, Morris AJ, et al. Guidelines on small bowel enteroscopy and capsule endoscopy in adults. Gut 2008;57(1):125–36.
112. Huprich JE, Fletcher JG, Alexander JA, et al. Obscure gastrointestinal bleeding: evaluation with 64-section multiphase CT enterography -initial experience. Radiology 2008;246(2):562–71.
113. Hogan RB III, Pareek N, Phillips P, et al. Video capsule endoscopy in life-threatening GI hemorrhage after negative primary endoscopy (with video). Gastrointest Endosc 2009;69(2):366–71.

Enteroscopy in the Diagnosis and Management of Crohn Disease

Shabana F. Pasha, MD[a,b], Jonathan A. Leighton, MD[a,b,*]

KEYWORDS

- Crohn disease • Strictures • Push enteroscopy
- Capsule endoscopy • Video capsule endoscopy
- Balloon-assisted enteroscopy • Double-balloon enteroscopy

Crohn disease (CD) is a chronic disorder that can affect any part of the gastrointestinal tract, and is characterized by mucosal and transmural inflammation of the bowel wall. The disease most commonly involves the small bowel in approximately 70% of patients. Up to 30% of these patients have disease confined only to the small bowel, usually the distal ileum. Evaluation of patients with suspected CD has traditionally involved the use of ileocolonoscopy. However, ileoscopy can investigate only the distal few centimeters of the ileum. Push enteroscopy is another conventional endoscopic technique that permits limited examination of the proximal small bowel. Hence, a large proportion of patients with mild small bowel disease or involvement of the mid-small bowel can potentially be missed if only these tests are used.

Barium small bowel radiography has also traditionally been used in suspected CD, but recent studies suggest a low sensitivity for mild mucosal disease. Because of its low sensitivity, barium small bowel radiography is gradually being replaced by CT and magnetic resonance (MR) enterography, which seem to be more sensitive and can better evaluate transmural disease and extraintestinal findings. However, even these studies are limited by the inability to perform biopsies and therapeutic interventions.

Conflicts of interest: Shabana F. Pasha, Given Imaging, Olympus and Fujinon: research and Jonathan A. Leighton, Given Imaging-research and consulting, Olympus-research, Fujinon-research, Intramedic-consulting.

[a] Division of Gastroenterology and Hepatology, Department of Internal Medicine, Mayo Clinic, 13400 E. Shea Boulevard, Scottsdale, AZ 85259, USA

[b] Inflammatory Bowel Disease Clinic, Division of Gastroenterology and Hepatology, Department of Internal Medicine, Mayo Clinic, 13400 E. Shea Boulevard, Scottsdale, AZ 85259, USA

* Corresponding author. Division of Gastroenterology and Hepatology, Department of Internal Medicine, Mayo Clinic, Scottsdale, AZ, USA.

E-mail address: leighton.jonathan@mayo.edu (J.A. Leighton).

Gastrointest Endoscopy Clin N Am 19 (2009) 427–444
doi:10.1016/j.giec.2009.04.004 giendo.theclinics.com
1052-5157/09/$ – see front matter © 2009 Published by Elsevier Inc.

Enteroscopy is defined as direct visualization of the small bowel using a fiber optic or wireless endoscope. Conventional modes of enteroscopy include ileocolonoscopy (IC), push enteroscopy (PE), sonde enteroscopy (SE) and intraoperative enteroscopy (IOE); new technologies include video capsule endoscopy (CE), balloon-assisted enteroscopy (BAE) (double-balloon enteroscopy [DBE] and single-balloon enteroscopy [SBE]) and spiral-assisted enteroscopy. Following recent advances in technology, enteroscopy currently plays a pivotal role not only in the diagnosis of small bowel CD but also in the management of its complications, such as bleeding and strictures. Enteroscopy may have additional roles in the future, including the objective assessment of mucosal response to therapy, and surveillance for SB malignancy. This article focuses on the usefulness of enteroscopy, and its advantages and limitations in the evaluation and long-term management of CD.

ILEOCOLONOSCOPY

Ileocolonoscopy is usually the initial procedure of choice in the evaluation of patients with suspected CD. Studies have reported successful intubation of the terminal ileum in 80% to 97% of patients when colonoscopy is performed by experienced endoscopists.[1,2] Ileocolonoscopy has a positive predictive value of 96% for the diagnosis of CD in patients who have an abnormal small bowel radiograph.[3] The test also serves to accurately differentiate CD from ulcerative colitis in more than 85% of patients with inflammatory bowel disease.[4] The main advantage of this procedure over radiologic studies is its ability to allow direct visualization of the terminal ileal mucosa, and the capacity to obtain biopsies. It thereby enables the diagnosis of CD, and also the differentiation between CD and other causes of ileitis, such as infection, ischemia, radiation- or drug-induced ileitis.[5]

In addition to diagnosing ileocolonic CD, ileocolonoscopy is also of value in the detection of postoperative recurrence of disease. Clinical recurrence of CD after surgery occurs in approximately 20% to 35% of patients, whereas endoscopic recurrence is much more common, in up to 90% of patients, usually within a year after surgery. In patients who have undergone terminal ileal resection, the most common location of postoperative recurrence is at the ileocolonic anastomosis.[6,7] Hence, colonoscopy with neoterminal ileal intubation has been recommended 6 to 12 months after surgery for identification of those patients with recurrence of CD who would benefit from initiation of maintenance therapy, if they are not already on prophylaxis.[5]

Endoscopic balloon dilation of distal ileal and colonic strictures, anastomotic strictures, and ileocecal valve stenoses have been successfully performed using the standard colonoscope. The technical success rate of endoscopic dilation is reported to be as high as 90%, with long-term symptomatic relief in 41% to 62% of patients.[8,9] However, strictures that are angulated, have a narrow lumen, or are longer than 4 cm, are probably not conducive to endoscopic dilation. Moreover, the risk of perforation with balloon dilation of complicated strictures is reported to range from 1.6% to 11%.[8,10]

The estimated distance of ileal intubation with ileoscopy is approximately 20 cm, and may be limited by poor patient tolerance, looping, or compromised preparation.[11,12] Another major limitation of the procedure is failure to achieve ileal intubation, especially in the presence of a stricture or ileocecal valve stenosis.

PUSH ENTEROSCOPY

The push enteroscope has a working length of 220 to 250 cm and an external diameter of 11.5 cm. Push enteroscopy enables visualization of the small bowel up to 70 cm distal to the ligament of Treitz. Deeper intubation, up to 140 cm, is feasible when the enteroscope is used in conjunction with an overtube. The technique of push enteroscopy is useful in the diagnosis of CD involving the duodenum or proximal jejunum. Taylor et al[13] evaluated the diagnostic and therapeutic impact of push enteroscopy in 77 patients referred for various indications, including abdominal pain and anemia. PE detected duodenal and jejunal ulcerations in 4 patients with known CD, in whom SB barium X ray was normal. In a study of eight patients with suspected CD, the diagnosis was established with push enteroscopy in 50% of patients. Histology was consistent with CD on biopsies in three patients, even in the absence of endoscopic evidence of inflammation. The investigators suggested that random biopsies be obtained if there is high clinical suspicion for CD, even in the absence of gross inflammation.[14] The same investigators have also reported on the usefulness of PE for balloon dilation of multiple jejunal strictures in a patient with CD.[15]

The main shortcomings of PE include limited depth of insertion due to looping and patient discomfort. Following the introduction of CE and BAE, the role of PE is restricted to evaluation and therapeutics of proximal small bowel lesions detected on radiologic studies or CE.[16]

INTRAOPERATIVE ENTEROSCOPY

Intraoperative enteroscopy (IOE) refers to laparoscopic-assisted endoscopic evaluation of the entire small bowel, and can be performed orally, rectally, or by an enterotomy. This technique has been used in the past for accurately assessing the extent of small bowel involvement in CD, and for the exclusion of small bowel inflammation in patients with indeterminate colitis before colectomy.[5] IOE has also been reported as useful in influencing surgical decisions in patients with CD. According to a study of 33 patients with CD, surgical options, including the decision to perform small bowel resection and the length of planned resections, were affected by findings at IOE in 66% of patients.[17] A similar study evaluated 20 patients with IOE before definitive surgery for CD. Thirty-five percent of patients were found to have small bowel lesions, which were not detected on prior evaluations. Surgical decisions were altered in 10% of patients based on new findings at IOE.[18]

However, IOE is not only a time consuming procedure but also has a high morbidity and mortality rate of up to 17%, with major complications of serosal tears, prolonged ileus, and avulsion of the mesenteric vessels.[19] Hence, following improvements in our ability to examine the small bowel and perform endoscopic interventions with newer modalities, the use of IOE in CD has declined significantly.

VIDEO CAPSULE ENDOSCOPY

Video capsule endoscopy (CE) is a noninvasive method of visualizing the small bowel with the use of a wireless capsule endoscope, which may be swallowed by the patient, or delivered into the small bowel with endoscopic assistance. The capsule measures 26 × 11 mm, and is propelled through the small bowel by peristalsis. It has the capacity to take images at the rate of two frames per second over an 8-hour period. The images are transmitted by radiofrequency to a sensor array strapped to the patient's waist. At the end of the study, the images are downloaded to a workstation and viewed by a gastroenterologist.

Pillcam SB (Given Imaging, Yoqneam, Israel) was the first video capsule endoscope to be introduced in 2001, followed by the Endo Capsule (Olympus Medical Systems Corporation, Tokyo, Japan), which was approved by the US Food and Drug Administration (FDA) in 2007. Preliminary studies in patients with obscure gastrointestinal bleeding have reported comparable functionality and safety profiles with both capsules.[20] CE is currently approved by the FDA for use in adult and pediatric patients over the age of 10 years, for the evaluation of obscure gastrointestinal bleeding, Crohn disease, celiac disease, polyposis syndromes, small bowel abnormalities detected on imaging studies, and symptom evaluation. It has been reported to allow visualization of the entire small bowel in 79% to 90% of patients (**Fig. 1**).[21]

Fireman and colleagues[22] first reported on the effectiveness of CE for the diagnosis of Crohn disease. The study found a diagnostic yield of 71% with CE in patients with high clinical suspicion for CD, but negative ileocolonoscopy and barium small bowel radiography. Since then, the usefulness of CE has been established for the evaluation of suspected and established CD. Based on results from multiple studies, the yield of CE for CD has been reported to range from 43% to 71% (**Fig. 2**).[23–25]

CE has a superior yield compared with other modalities in the evaluation of patients with nonstricturing CD. Several retrospective and prospective studies have compared the yield of CE with other endoscopic and radiologic modalities in patients with suspected CD. Capsule endoscopy has been reported to have a higher yield compared with barium small bowel radiography (9%–77% compared with 0%–23%),[26–31] push enteroscopy (9%–28% compared with 0%–10%),[29,30] ileocolonoscopy (28%–58% compared with 21%–53%),[26,27,29,31] and CT enterography (37.5%–77% compared with 20%–25%).[26,28] A meta-analysis of 11 prospective studies with 223 patients compared CE to ileoscopy, push enteroscopy, barium small bowel radiography and CT enterography in patients with suspected or established CD. CE was found to have an incremental yield (IY_W) of 40% (63% versus 23%) compared with small bowel radiography; IY_W of 15% compared with ileoscopy (61% versus 46%); IY_W of 38% compared with PE (46% versus 8%) and IY_W of 38% compared with CT enterography (69% versus 30%). Subanalysis of the data showed a significantly higher yield with CE for established, but not suspected CD, which may have been related to the sample

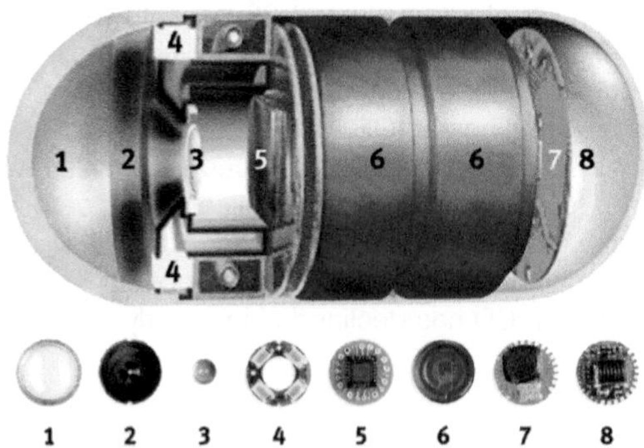

INSIDE THE PillCam

1. Optical dome
2. Lens holder
3. Lens
4. Illuminating LEDs (Light Emitting Diode)
5. CMOS (Complementary Metal Oxide Semiconductor) imager
6. Battery
7. ASIC (Application Specific Integrated Circuit) transmitter
8. Antenna

Fig. 1. Components of the Pillcam capsule. (*Courtesy of* Given Imaging, Inc., Duluth, GA; with permission.)

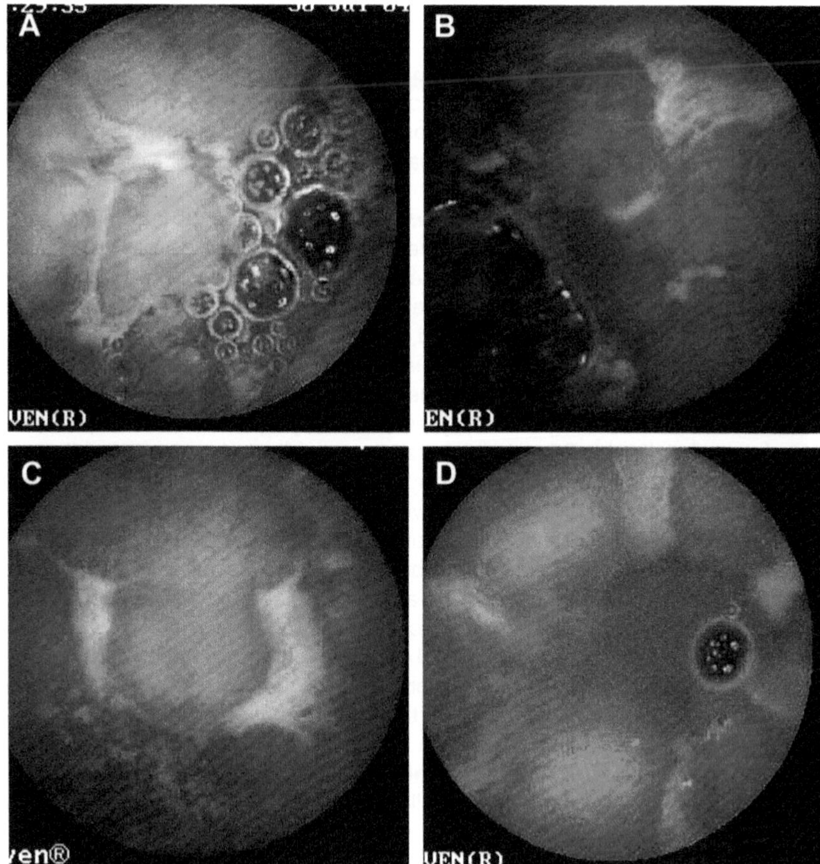

Fig. 2. Findings of Crohn disease seen on video capsule endoscopy. (*A, B, C*) Deep ulcerations in the small bowel consistent with Crohn disease. (*D*) A circumferential ulcerated stricture.

size of the study.[32] An updated analysis performed by the same investigators suggested that CE has a higher yield than barium small bowel radiography even in patients with suspected CD.[33]

Another meta-analysis of 17 studies that included 526 patients showed that the pooled difference in the rate of positive findings for CD between CE and other techniques was 45%.[34] In addition to facilitating the diagnosis of CD, CE allows an accurate assessment of the severity and extent of small bowel inflammation. Based on a study by Mow and colleagues[24] CE detected more extensive small bowel disease than was suspected on initial evaluation in 40% of patients with CD.

A prospective, blinded, four-way comparison trial was conducted by Solem and colleagues[35] to assess the sensitivity and specificity of CE, CT enterography, small bowel radiography, and ileocolonoscopy for the diagnosis of Crohn disease. Based on their results, the sensitivity of CE (83%) was found to be comparable to CT enterography (83%), ileocolonoscopy (74%), and small bowel radiography (65%). In comparison, the specificity of CE (53%) was significantly lower than all the other tests (100%). The investigators suggested that the combination of ileocolonoscopy and CT enterography should be the first-line investigation for suspected CD, with CE reserved for patients with a high clinical suspicion but negative evaluation with these tests.

The high negative predictive value of CE is an important advantage of using this test in the evaluation of patients with suspected CD. A pooled analysis of the results of 24 capsule endoscopy trials, which included 530 patients, found that CE had a low miss rate of 0.5% for small bowel ulcerations, compared with 78.7% with other modalities (small bowel radiography, PE or Ileocolonoscopy).[36] Hence, the diagnosis of CD can be excluded with a negative CE in most patients referred for symptom evaluation of chronic abdominal pain or diarrhea.

It is often challenging to differentiate between CD and other causes of inflammation. There has been a dearth of standardized criteria for measurement of small bowel inflammation in patients with CD. Two scoring indexes have been proposed.[37,38] The integration of these indexes into clinical practice may serve as an effective means to objectively classify severity of inflammation in CD, and, exclude other causes.

Findings at CE have been reported to influence medical management of patients with CD. In a study by Voderholzer and colleagues,[39] medical therapy was modified in 24% of patients based on CE findings. Similarly, another study reported clinical improvement in 70% of patients following CE-guided alterations in medical management.[24] The International Conference on Capsule Endoscopy (ICCE) Consensus Committee has stated that CE influence management in patients with established CD, and may have a potential role in patients with clinical suspicion for CD, but negative endoscopic and radiologic tests.[40] With the increasing focus on the importance of mucosal healing in inflammatory bowel disease, CE may have an additional role in the future for objective and noninvasive assessment of endoscopic response to therapy.

In patients who have undergone surgical management, early detection of recurrent CD is crucial for initiation of postoperative prophylactic therapy to prevent progression of the disease. CE may be a useful tool for the diagnosis of postoperative recurrence. A study by Bourreille and colleagues[41] that compared the yield of CE and ileocolonoscopy found that ileoscopy (90%) had a higher sensitivity than CE (62%) for detection of recurrence in the small bowel, but CE allowed detection of small bowel inflammation in 67% of patients in proximal locations of the small bowel inaccessible to ileoscopy.

Usefulness of CE in Classification of Indeterminate Colitis

Indeterminate colitis (IC) constitutes 5% to 15% of patients with inflammatory bowel disease, and can pose a challenge to gastroenterologists, especially for decisions regarding surgery.[42] Several studies have reported on the usefulness of CE for the appropriate classification of IC. A study by Maunoury and colleagues[43] evaluated 30 patients with IC, who underwent CE. CE was diagnostic for small bowel CD in 17% of patients, with 100% interobserver agreement. Similarly, Mow and colleagues[24] showed that CE facilitated a diagnosis of CD in 22% patients with IC, with small bowel findings suspicious for CD in an additional 7% of patients. Viazis and Karamanolis[44] reported a diagnosis of small bowel CD in 38% (5/13) of patients with indeterminate colitis, who underwent CE. A prospective study evaluated 8 patients with IC, of whom 75% were found to have small bowel lesions detected on CE. Fifty percent of these patients were diagnosed with CD at the end of a 1-year follow-up period.[45]

LIMITATIONS AND COMPLICATIONS OF CE IN CROHN DISEASE

Despite the high sensitivity of CE for small bowel CD, its usefulness is limited by its low specificity, and hence inability to accurately differentiate CD from other causes of inflammation.[46] Causes of small bowel inflammation seen on CE include CD, celiac disease, infection, ischemia, immunodeficiency, radiation- and drug-induced enteropathy. Up to 13% of patients on nonsteroidal antiinflammatory medications (NSAIDs) have erosions or ulcerations detected on CE. Hence NSAIDS should ideally be avoided for at least a month before performance of CE in patients with suspected CD.[47]

CE may also be limited by compromised visibility in the distal small bowel, and more importantly, failure to reach the cecum in up to 25% of patients.[35,48] Due to the potential for missed lesions in the distal ileum, CE should be used in conjunction with ileocolonoscopy in the evaluation of patients with suspected CD.

The overall incidence of capsule retention is less than 1%. However, the risk increases to 6.7% to 13% in patients with advanced CD and known strictures.[49–51] As significant strictures can sometimes be missed even with radiologic studies, barium small bowel radiography and CT enterography may be inadequate as screening tests before CE.[52,53] The use of a patency capsule (described below) before CE in patients with suspected obstruction has led to a significant reduction in the incidence of capsule retention.[54] Other rare complications of CE include impaction at the cricopharyngeus due to inability to swallow the capsule,[55] aspiration into the trachea,[56] impaction in small bowel diverticula,[57] and disintegration of the capsule.[58]

AGILE PATENCY CAPSULE

The Agile Patency Capsule (Given Imaging Inc) has been approved by the FDA for use in patients with suspected small bowel strictures or obstruction, to facilitate selection of patients who can safely undergo CE.[59] The system is comprised of a patency capsule, scanner and Testag. The patency or sham capsule is 26 × 11 mm in size, and contains a radiofrequency identification (RFID) tag covered with lactose and barium, with a timer plug on both sides (**Fig. 3**). The sham capsule is designed to dissolve in gastrointestinal secretions 30 hours after ingestion. It is hence a useful test to diagnose small bowel obstruction. Significant obstruction can be excluded by witnessed passage of the patency capsule or failure to detect the RFID tag at or before 30 hours after ingestion. Fluoroscopy may be used instead of the RFID scanner for accurate localization of the tag in the small bowel and in patients who have pacemakers.

In a study by Herrerias and colleagues, 106 patients with suspected small bowel obstruction ingested the patency capsule. The capsule was excreted intact in 56% of

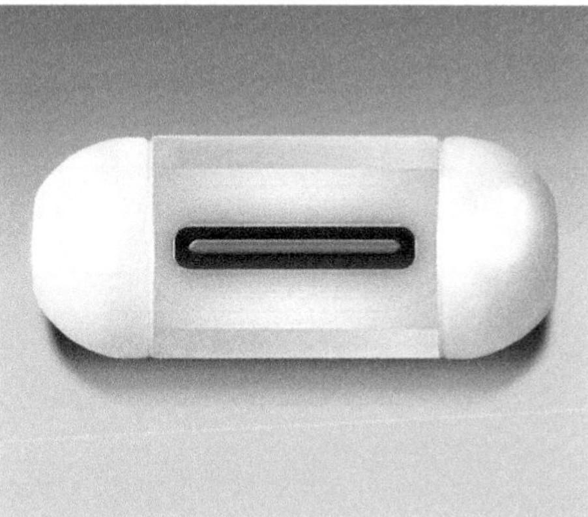

Fig. 3. The components of the patency capsule include a body, which comprises of a radiofrequency identification (RFID) covered with lactose and barium, and a timer plug on either side. (*Courtesy of* Given Imaging, Inc., Duluth, GA; with permission.)

patients, who subsequently underwent CE without retention. Forty percent of these patients had positive findings on CE.[60] A similar study by Spada and colleagues showed that the patency capsule was excreted intact after a mean transit time of 25.6 hours in 65.3% of patients with known or suspected intestinal strictures. CE was performed in all of these patients without any cases of retention.[61] Signorelli and colleagues evaluated 32 patients, of whom 18 had CD. Twenty-four patients excreted the patency capsule intact within 72 hours of ingestion. Of the remaining eight patients, four excreted the capsule between 72 and 96 hours. Of all the patients who excreted the capsule intact, the 25 who agreed to undergo CE did not experience any capsule-related complications.[54] The results of these studies confirm the usefulness of the patency capsule as a screening tool before CE to eliminate the risk of capsule retention.

BALLOON-ASSISTED ENTEROSCOPY

Balloon-assisted enteroscopy or push-and-pull enteroscopy allows deeper intubation of the small bowel, compared with push enteroscopy and ileoscopy. There are two balloon-assisted enteroscopes (BAE) currently available (the double-balloon enteroscope from Fujinon Inc, Japan, and the single-balloon enteroscope from Olympus Optical Company Ltd, Tokyo, Japan). Studies using BAE in the evaluation and management of Crohn disease have thus far been performed using the double-balloon enteroscope (DBE), which was the first balloon-assisted enteroscope to be introduced in 2003 (**Figs. 4–6**).

DBE allows real time evaluation of the entire small bowel, either with a single or combined (antegrade and retrograde) approach. The DBE system includes an enteroscope with a working length of 2 m and an overtube that is 1.4 m long. The working channel of the therapeutic DBE scope is 2.8 mm in diameter. The scope and overtube have a latex balloon attached at their distal end.

The procedure entails a series of steps called advancement cycles, performed using a push-and-pull technique. The enteroscope and overtube are inserted into the small

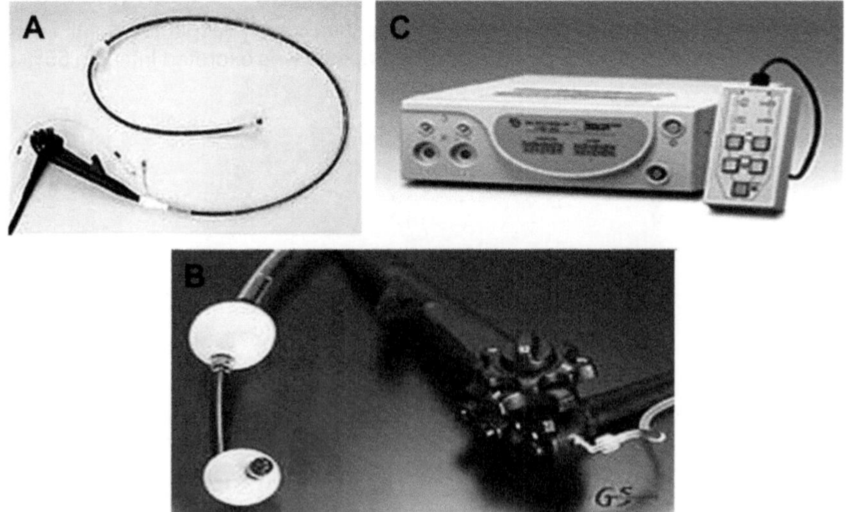

Fig. 4. Components of the double-balloon enteroscopy system. (*A*) The double-balloon enteroscope. (*B*) Inflated balloons at the distal end of the enteroscope and overtube. (*C*) The balloon controller pump system. (*Courtesy of* Fujinon, Inc., Wayne, NJ; with permission.)

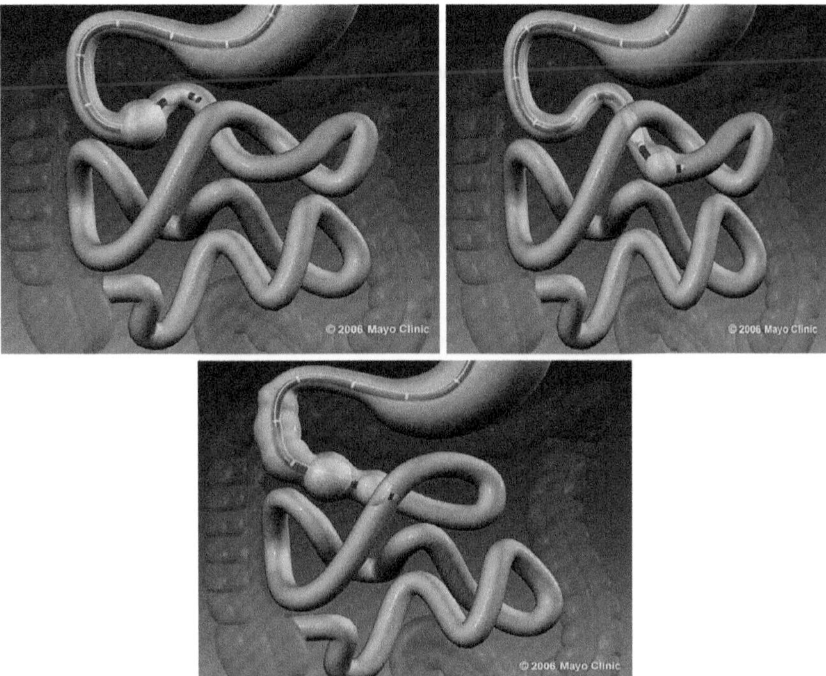

Fig. 5. Technique of antegrade double-balloon enteroscopy. Step 1: enteroscope and overtube are advanced into the small intestine and the balloon on the overtube is inflated. Step 2: the enteroscope is further advanced into the small intestine and the balloon on the enteroscope is inflated. Step 3: the overtube with the balloon deflated is advanced over the endoscope. Step 4: with both balloons inflated, the system is withdrawn which allows telescoping of the small intestine (*Courtesy of* Mayo Clinic, copyright 2008, with permission.).

bowel and advanced together as far as possible before the formation of a loop. The balloon on the overtube is then inflated, and the enteroscope is advanced beyond the overtube. The balloon on the enteroscope is then inflated to anchor it in the small bowel. With its balloon now deflated, the overtube is advanced over the enteroscope. After advancement, the balloon on the overtube is inflated. In this fixed position with

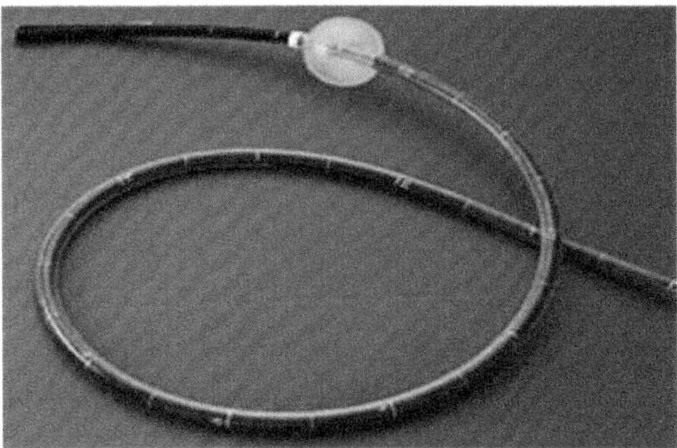

Fig. 6. The single-balloon enteroscope. The system has a balloon only at the distal end of the overtube.

both balloons inflated, the enteroscope and overtube are gently withdrawn to facilitate pleating of the small bowel over the enteroscope. DBE allows significantly deeper intubation of the small bowel (240–360 cm with the antegrade approach and 102–140 cm with the retrograde approach), compared with push enteroscopy (90–150 cm) and ileoscopy (50–80 cm).[62,63] The success rate of total enteroscopy with DBE has been reported to range from 16% to 86%.[64,65] The major advantage of DBE over CE is its capacity to allow diagnostic and therapeutic interventions, including biopsies, tattoo, hemostasis, polypectomy, dilation, foreign body removal (including retained capsules), and chromoendoscopy.[66–68]

Evaluation of Crohn Disease

The yield of CD in patients who undergo DBE for suspected small bowel disorders, predominantly obscure gastrointestinal bleeding, has been reported as 5% to 13%.[62,69] In comparison, the yield for small bowel CD with DBE has been reported to be significantly higher in patients with known inflammatory bowel disease. A study that evaluated 22 patients with inflammatory bowel disease using DBE found that 96% of patients had small bowel involvement confirmed with DBE.[70] Another study evaluated 35 patients with inflammatory bowel disease (17 with known CD) using DBE. The diagnosis of small bowel CD was established in 74% of patients, and impacted medical management in 63%. The procedure was unsuccessful in 26% of patients due to a presumed fixed small bowel.[71]

A recent study compared the yield of DBE and barium small bowel radiography in 40 patients with suspected small bowel CD. Sixty percent of patients were found to have small bowel involvement in locations proximal to the distal 20 cm of the ileum and hence not accessible to detection by ileoscopy. DBE detected subtle findings of mucosal erosions and ulcerations in 22% (4/18) of patients that were not detected on barium small bowel radiography. In comparison, small bowel radiography detected a larger number of ileal strictures compared with DBE (9 versus 6). Both tests had a comparable yield for detection of deep and longitudinal ulcerations.[72]

DBE was compared with magnetic resonance enteroclysis (MRE) in a pilot study of 10 patients with suspected small bowel CD. DBE confirmed a diagnosis of CD in four patients, and facilitated the diagnosis of a malignant lymphoma in one patient, thereby resulting in a change in management in 50% of the patients. In comparison, MRE detected superficial lesions in three patients that were not detected on DBE. There were no abnormalities detected on either test in two patients.[73]

CE and DBE appear to have an equivalent yield for diagnosis of small bowel CD. A meta-analysis of 11 studies that compared CE and DBE in 375 patients with suspected small bowel diseases, found that the pooled overall yield for small bowel findings was similar with both tests (60% with DBE and 57% with CE; IY_W 3%). Subanalysis of the data also showed a comparable yield for detection of small bowel inflammation (pooled yield 18% with DBE and 16% with CE; IY_W 0%). Hence, CE may be the preferred initial test of choice in the evaluation of small bowel CD, due to its relative noninvasiveness and higher success rate for achieving total enteroscopy. DBE is useful for tissue diagnosis in patients with positive findings on CE, in patients with suspected or known small bowel strictures in whom CE is contraindicated, and also in those patients with a negative CE, but a high clinical suspicion for CD.[74]

A study evaluated 52 patients with CD using DBE, and 26 patients with CE. The rate of total enteroscopy with CE was 77.8% and there were four cases of retention. The distribution of CD was the distal ileum in 86%, proximal ileum and distal jejunum in 71%, and proximal jejunum in 64% of patients. The investigators reported progressive worsening of inflammation from the jejunum to the ileum. DBE was successful in 11%

of patients in obtaining biopsies and performing therapeutics, but was unsuccessful in 87% due to the presence of adhesions or severe inflammation. DBE also facilitated the retrieval of a retained capsule. There was one reported case of perforation related to DBE. The study showed that CE and DBE have a complementary role in the evaluation and management of small bowel CD.[75]

Therapeutics in Crohn Disease

The management of strictures related to CD continues to pose a significant challenge, with surgery being the mainstay of treatment. Up to 30% of patients with CD are prone to develop strictures, with significant narrowing necessitating stricturoplasty or a segmental small bowel resection in 78% of patients.[76,77] Despite resection or stricturoplasty, strictures can commonly recur, often leading to multiple surgeries and risk for short bowel syndrome (**Figs. 7** and **8**).[78]

DBE appears to be useful in facilitating endoscopic dilation of small bowel strictures, thereby decreasing the need for surgery. One study reported successful dilation of strictures in four patients, of whom two had CD, resulting in symptomatic improvement in all the patients. DBE also facilitated diagnosis of three patients with malignant strictures.[79]

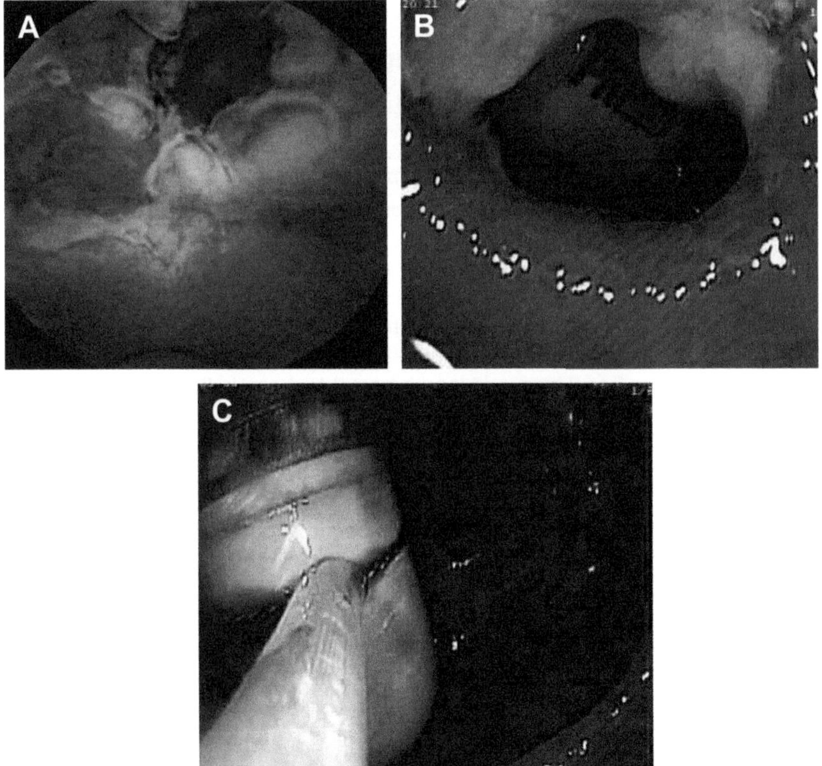

Fig. 7. (*A*) Inflammatory Crohn's stricture in the distal ileum seen on video capsule endoscopy, resulting in retention of the capsule. (*B*) The same stricture with proximal retention of CE, seen on retrograde double-balloon enteroscopy. (*C*) Successful retrieval of CE using a snare.

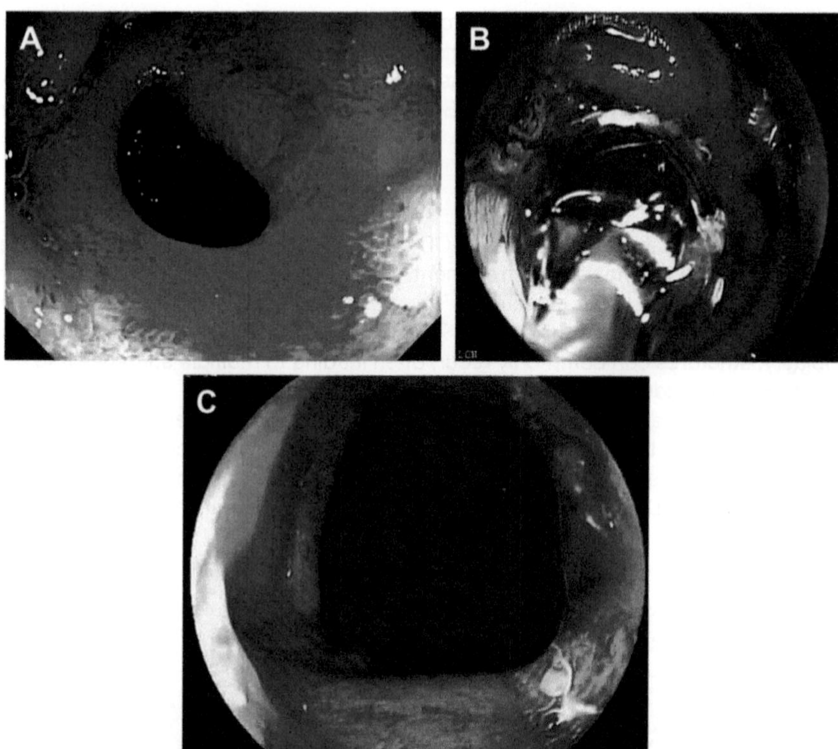

Fig. 8. (*A*) Crohn's stricture in the distal ileum. (*B*) Sequential balloon dilation (10, 13.5 and 15 mm) performed at retrograde double-balloon enteroscopy. (*C*) Image of stricture after dilation.

Another study evaluated the role of DBE in 19 patients with symptomatic small bowel strictures secondary to CD. DBE detected 28 strictures, of which 75% (21/28) were primary, and 25% (7/28) were anastomotic. The predilation diameter of the strictures ranged from 5 to 8 mm, and length from 1 to 4 cm. In 32% (6/19) of patients, dilation was deferred and medical therapy was intensified due to detection of significant inflammation. Of the remaining 13 patients, three had long (>5 cm) and angulated strictures that were not amenable to dilation. Ten patients with 13 strictures ranging from 1 to 4 cm (mean 3 cm) underwent 15 endoscopic balloon dilations (median diameter 17 mm; range 12–20 cm) with DBE. Therapeutic success was achieved in eight patients. In the remaining two patients, endoscopic dilation failed due to failure to achieve stability of the overtube. The investigators reported that there were no procedure-related complications.[80]

In addition to endoscopic management of strictures, DBE also facilitates endoscopic treatment of actively bleeding small bowel ulcers with the use of epinephrine, electrocautery, and placement of hemoclips. It has an additional role in retrieval of retained capsules, thereby avoiding the need for surgery.[81]

Future Roles of DBE in the Management of Crohn Disease

The end points of endoscopic and histologic remission are of increasing importance in the objective assessment of effectiveness of therapy with immunomodulators and biologic agents.[82,83] DBE is a useful tool for monitoring mucosal response to medical therapy. This technique can be used in patients with stricturing CD in whom CE is contraindicated, and to obtain biopsies to document histologic remission.

Patients with small bowel CD are at increased risk for developing adenocarcinoma, with a 17- to 67-fold higher risk compared with the general population.[84–86] Small bowel strictures, which can form during the process of mucosal healing and remodeling, are more prone to develop malignant changes.[87] DBE may have a role in surveillance due to its ability to evaluate strictures and obtain biopsies in these patients. Furthermore, the concomitant use of chromoendoscopy with DBE, may potentially allow for enhanced detection of flat dysplastic lesions in the small bowel.[88]

SUMMARY

The diagnosis and management of small bowel CD has represented a major challenge due to the lack of a gold standard test and general inaccessibility of the small bowel. The introduction of new endoscopic technologies, such as video capsule endoscopy and double-balloon enteroscopy have led to a significant improvement in our ability to diagnose small bowel CD, objectively evaluate the extent and severity of disease, and accurately differentiate the disease from other small bowel inflammatory entities. The most important advantage of small bowel enteroscopy, however, is the ability to perform endoscopic therapeutics, thereby obviating the need for invasive surgical procedures and small bowel resections. Small bowel enteroscopy is evolving rapidly with the introduction of newer modalities like single-balloon enteroscopy and spiral-assisted enteroscopy, which have not yet been formally studied in CD. This increasing range of enteroscopies offers the major advantage of individualized use in selected patients, and the benefit of using their complementary roles in the evaluation and management of small bowel CD.

REFERENCES

1. Nagasako K, Yazawa C, Takemoto T. Biopsy of the terminal ileum. Gastrointest Endosc 1972;19(1):7–10.
2. Gaisford WD. Fiberendoscopy of the cecum and terminal ileum. Gastrointest Endosc 1974;21(1):13–8.
3. Coremans G, Rutgeerts P, Geboes K, et al. The value of ileoscopy with biopsy in the diagnosis of intestinal Crohn's disease. Gastrointest Endosc 1984;30(3):167–72.
4. Chutkan RK, Scherl E, Waye JD. Colonoscopy in inflammatory bowel disease. Gastrointest Endosc Clin N Am 2002;12(3):463–83, viii.
5. Leighton JA, Shen B, Baron TH, et al. ASGE guideline: endoscopy in the diagnosis and treatment of inflammatory bowel disease. Gastrointest Endosc 2006;63(4):558–65.
6. Rutgeerts P, Geboes K, Vantrappen G, et al. Predictability of the postoperative course of Crohn's disease. Gastroenterology 1990;99(4):956–63.
7. Rutgeerts P, Geboes K, Vantrappen G, et al. Natural history of recurrent Crohn's disease at the ileocolonic anastomosis after curative surgery. Gut 1984;25(6):665–72.
8. Couckuyt H, Gevers AM, Coremans G, et al. Efficacy and safety of hydrostatic balloon dilatation of ileocolonic Crohn's strictures: a prospective longterm analysis. Gut 1995;36(4):577–80.

9. Thomas-Gibson S, Brooker JC, Hayward CM, et al. Colonoscopic balloon dilation of Crohn's strictures: a review of long-term outcomes. Eur J Gastroenterol Hepatol 2003;15(5):485–8.
10. Breysem Y, Janssens JF, Coremans G, et al. Endoscopic balloon dilation of colonic and ileo-colonic Crohn's strictures: long-term results. Gastrointest Endosc 1992;38(2):142–7.
11. Harewood GC, Mattek NC, Holub JL, et al. Variation in practice of ileal intubation among diverse endoscopy settings: results from a national endoscopic database. Aliment Pharmacol Ther 2005;22(6):571–8.
12. Bernstein C, Thorn M, Monsees K, et al. A prospective study of factors that determine cecal intubation time at colonoscopy. Gastrointest Endosc 2005; 61(1):72–5.
13. Taylor AC, Buttigieg RJ, McDonald IG, et al. Prospective Assessment of the Diagnostic and Therapeutic Impact of Small-Bowel Push Enteroscopy. Endoscopy 2003;35:951–6.
14. Perez-Cuadrado E, Macenlle R, Iglesias J, et al. Usefulness of oral video push enteroscopy in Crohn's disease. Endoscopy 1997;29(8):745–7.
15. Perez-Cuadrado E, Molina Perez E. Multiple strictures in jejunal Crohn's disease: push enteroscopy dilation. Endoscopy 2001;33(2):194.
16. Sidhu R, McAlindon ME, Kapur K, et al. Push enteroscopy in the era of capsule endoscopy. J Clin Gastroenterol 2008;42(1):54–8.
17. Smedh K, Olaison G, Nystrom PO, et al. Intraoperative enteroscopy in Crohn's disease. Br J Surg 1993;80(7):897–900.
18. Lescut D, Vanco D, Bonniere P, et al. Perioperative endoscopy of the whole small bowel in Crohn's disease. Gut 1993;34(5):647–9.
19. Ress AM, Benacci JC, Sarr MG. Efficacy of intraoperative enteroscopy in diagnosis and prevention of recurrent, occult gastrointestinal bleeding. Am J Surg 1992;163(1):94–8 [discussion: 98–9].
20. Cave D, Fleischer D, Heigh R, et al. First study involving simultaneous ingestion of two video capsules (VCs): a comparison of Olympus VC and Given Imaging VC in the detection of obscure GI bleeding (OGIB). [abstract]. Gastrointest Endosc 2006;63:171.
21. Rondonotti E, Villa F, Mulder CJ, et al. Small bowel capsule endoscopy in 2007: indications, risks and limitations. World J Gastroenterol 2007;13(46):6140–9.
22. Fireman Z, Mahajna E, Broide E, et al. Diagnosing small bowel Crohn's disease with wireless capsule endoscopy. Gut 2003;52(3):390–2.
23. Herrerias JM, Caunedo A, Rodriguez-Tellez M, et al. Capsule endoscopy in patients with suspected Crohn's disease and negative endoscopy. Endoscopy 2003;35(7):564–8.
24. Mow WS, Lo SK, Targan SR, et al. Initial experience with wireless capsule enteroscopy in the diagnosis and management of inflammatory bowel disease. Clin Gastroenterol Hepatol 2004;2(1):31–40.
25. Marmo R, Rotondano G, Piscopo R, et al. Capsule endoscopy versus enteroclysis in the detection of small-bowel involvement in Crohn's disease: a prospective trial. Clin Gastroenterol Hepatol 2005;3(8):772–6.
26. Hara AK, Leighton JA, Heigh RI, et al. Crohn disease of the small bowel: preliminary comparison among CT enterography, capsule endoscopy, small-bowel follow-through, and ileoscopy. Radiology 2006;238(1):128–34.
27. Dubcenco E, Jeejeebhoy KN, Petroniene R, et al. Diagnosing Crohn's disease (CD) of the small bowel (SB): should capsule endoscopy (CE) be used? CE vs other diagnostic modalities [abstract]. Gastrointest Endosc 2004;59:174.

28. Eliakim R, Suissa A, Yassin K, et al. Wireless capsule video endoscopy compared to barium follow-through and computerised tomography in patients with suspected Crohn's disease – final report. Dig Liver Dis 2004;36(8):519–22.
29. Toth E, Fork FT, Almqvist P, et al. Wireless capsule enteroscopy: a comparison with enterography, push enteroscopy and ileocolonoscopy in the diagnosis of small bowel Crohn's disease [abstract]. Gastrointest Endosc 2004;59:173.
30. Chong AK, Taylor A, Miller A, et al. Capsule endoscopy vs. push enteroscopy and enteroclysis in suspected small-bowel Crohn's disease. Gastrointest Endosc 2005;61(2):255–61.
31. Bloom P, Rosenberg M, Klein S, et al. Wireless capsule endoscopy (CE) is more informative than ileoscopy and SBFT for the evaluation of the small intestine (SI) in patients with known or suspected Crohn's disease (CD). Paper presented at: International Conference on Capsule Endoscopy (ICCE); March 23–25, 2003; Berlin, Germany.
32. Triester SL, Leighton JA, Leontiadis GI, et al. A meta-analysis of the yield of capsule endoscopy compared to other diagnostic modalities in patients with non-stricturing small bowel Crohn's disease. Am J Gastroenterol 2006;101(5):954–64.
33. Dionisio PM, Leighton JA, Leontiadis GI, et al. Capsule endoscopy (CE) has a significantly higher yield in patients with suspected and established non-stricturing Crohn disease (NSCD): a meta-analysis [abstract]. Gastrointest Endosc 2007;65:369.
34. Marmo R, Rotondano G, Piscopo R, et al. Meta-analysis: capsule enteroscopy vs. conventional modalities in diagnosis of small bowel diseases. Aliment Pharmacol Ther 2005;22(7):595–604.
35. Solem CA, Loftus EV Jr, Fletcher JG, et al. Small-bowel imaging in Crohn's disease: a prospective, blinded, 4-way comparison trial. Gastrointest Endosc 2008;68(2):255–66.
36. Lewis BS, Eisen GM, Friedman S. A pooled analysis to evaluate results of capsule endoscopy trials. Endoscopy 2005;37(10):960–5.
37. Gal E, Geller A, Fraser G, et al. Assessment and validation of the new capsule endoscopy Crohn's disease activity index (CECDAI). Dig Dis Sci 2008;53(7):1933–7.
38. Gralnek IM, Defranchis R, Seidman E, et al. Development of a capsule endoscopy scoring index for small bowel mucosal inflammatory change. Aliment Pharmacol Ther 2008;27(2):146–54.
39. Voderholzer WA, Beinhoelzl J, Rogalla P, et al. Small bowel involvement in Crohn's disease: a prospective comparison of wireless capsule endoscopy and computed tomography enteroclysis. Gut 2005;54(3):369–73.
40. Kornbluth A, Colombel JF, Leighton JA, et al. ICCE consensus for inflammatory bowel disease. Endoscopy 2005;37(10):1051–4.
41. Bourreille A, Jarry M, D'Halluin PN, et al. Wireless capsule endoscopy versus ileocolonoscopy for the diagnosis of postoperative recurrence of Crohn's disease: a prospective study. Gut 2006;55(7):978–83.
42. Stewenius J, Adnerhill I, Ekelund G, et al. Ulcerative colitis and indeterminate colitis in the city of Malmo, Sweden. A 25-year incidence study. Scand J Gastroenterol 1995;30(1):38–43.
43. Maunoury V, Savoye G, Bourreille A, et al. Value of wireless capsule endoscopy in patients with indeterminate colitis (inflammatory bowel disease type unclassified). Inflamm Bowel Dis 2007;13(2):152–5.
44. Viazis N, Karamanolis DG. Indeterminate colitis – the role of wireless capsule endoscopy. Aliment Pharmacol Ther 2007;25(7):859 [author reply 860].

45. Llach J, Mata A, Pellise M, et al. The role of capsule endoscopy in patients with indeterminate colitis: preliminary results of a prospective trial. Paper presented at: 5th International Conference on Capsule Endoscopy; Paris, France; June 9–10, 2006.
46. Goldstein JL, Eisen GM, Lewis B, et al. Video capsule endoscopy to prospectively assess small bowel injury with celecoxib, naproxen plus omeprazole, and placebo. Clin Gastroenterol Hepatol 2005;3(2):133–41.
47. Graham DY, Opekun AR, Willingham FF, et al. Visible small-intestinal mucosal injury in chronic NSAID users. Clin Gastroenterol Hepatol 2005;3(1):55–9.
48. Toy E, Rojany M, Sheikh R, et al. Capsule endoscopy's impact on clinical management and outcomes: a single-center experience with 145 patients. Am J Gastroenterol 2008;103(12):3022–8.
49. Barkin JS, Friedman S. Wireless capsule endoscopy requiring surgical intervention: the world's experience. Am J Gastroenterol 2002;97:S298.
50. Cave D, Legnani P, de Franchis R, et al. ICCE consensus for capsule retention. Endoscopy 2005;37(10):1065–7.
51. Sears DM, Avots-Avotins A, Culp K, et al. Frequency and clinical outcome of capsule retention during capsule endoscopy for GI bleeding of obscure origin. Gastrointest Endosc 2004;60(5):822–7.
52. Delvaux MM, Laurent V, Regent D. Should an entero-CT scanner (CT) necessarily precede capsule endoscopy (CE) recording when exploring patients with suspected small intestinal disease (SID) [abstract]. Gastrointest Endosc 2004;59: 175.
53. Fernandez-Diez S, Asteinza M, Gonzales F, et al. Capsule retention in small bowel strictures: a retrospective study. Paper presented at: International Conference on Capsule Endoscopy (ICCE); Florida: March 7–8, 2005.
54. Signorelli C, Rondonotti E, Villa F, et al. Use of the Given Patency System for the screening of patients at high risk for capsule retention. Dig Liver Dis 2006;38(5): 326–30.
55. Fleischer DE, Heigh RI, Nguyen CC, et al. Videocapsule impaction at the cricopharyngeus: a first report of this complication and its successful resolution. Gastrointest Endosc 2003;57(3):427–8.
56. Tabib S, Fuller C, Daniels J, et al. Asymptomatic aspiration of a capsule endoscope. Gastrointest Endosc 2004;60(5):845–8.
57. Giday SA, Pickett-Blakely OE, Buscaglia JM, et al. Capsule retention in a patient with small-bowel diverticulosis. Gastrointest Endosc 2009;69(2):384–6.
58. Fry LC, De Petris G, Swain JM, et al. Impaction and fracture of a video capsule in the small bowel requiring laparotomy for removal of the capsule fragments. Endoscopy 2005;37(7):674–6.
59. Delvaux M, Ben Soussan E, Laurent V, et al. Clinical evaluation of the use of the M2A patency capsule system before a capsule endoscopy procedure, in patients with known or suspected intestinal stenosis. Endoscopy 2005;37(9): 801–7.
60. Herrerias JM, Leighton JA, Costamagna G, et al. Agile patency system eliminates risk of capsule retention in patients with known intestinal strictures who undergo capsule endoscopy. Gastrointest Endosc 2008;67(6):902–9.
61. Spada C, Shah SK, Riccioni ME, et al. Video capsule endoscopy in patients with known or suspected small bowel stricture previously tested with the dissolving patency capsule. J Clin Gastroenterol 2007;41(6):576–82.
62. May A, Nachbar L, Ell C. Double-balloon enteroscopy (push-and-pull enteroscopy) of the small bowel: feasibility and diagnostic and therapeutic yield in

patients with suspected small bowel disease. Gastrointest Endosc 2005;62(1):62–70.
63. Mehdizadeh S, Ross A, Gerson L, et al. What is the learning curve associated with double-balloon enteroscopy? Technical details and early experience in 6 U.S. tertiary care centers. Gastrointest Endosc 2006;64(5):740–50.
64. Ell C, May A. Mid-gastrointestinal bleeding: capsule endoscopy and push-and-pull enteroscopy give rise to a new medical term. Endoscopy 2006;38(1):73–5.
65. Yamamoto H, Sekine Y, Sato Y, et al. Total enteroscopy with a nonsurgical steerable double-balloon method. Gastrointest Endosc 2001;53(2):216–20.
66. Nakamura M, Niwa Y, Ohmiya N, et al. Preliminary comparison of capsule endoscopy and double-balloon enteroscopy in patients with suspected small-bowel bleeding. Endoscopy 2006;38(1):59–66.
67. Heine GD, Hadithi M, Groenen MJ, et al. Double-balloon enteroscopy: indications, diagnostic yield, and complications in a series of 275 patients with suspected small-bowel disease. Endoscopy 2006;38(1):42–8.
68. May A, Ell C. Push-and-pull enteroscopy using the double-balloon technique/double-balloon enteroscopy. Dig Liver Dis 2006;38(12):932–8.
69. Yamamoto H, Kita H, Sunada K, et al. Clinical outcomes of double-balloon endoscopy for the diagnosis and treatment of small-intestinal diseases. Clin Gastroenterol Hepatol 2004;2(11):1010–6.
70. Numata M, Kodama M, Sasaki F, et al. Usefulness of double-balloon enteroscopy as a diagnostic and therapeutic method for small intestinal involvement in patients with inflammatory bowel disease [abstract]. Gastrointest Endosc 2007;65:188.
71. Ross AS, Leighton JA, Schembre D, et al. Double-balloon enteroscopy in Crohn's disease: findings and impact. Gastroenterology 2007;132:A654.
72. Oshitani N, Yukawa T, Yamagami H, et al. Evaluation of deep small bowel involvement by double-balloon enteroscopy in Crohn's disease. Am J Gastroenterol 2006;101(7):1484–9.
73. Seiderer J, Herrmann K, Diepolder H, et al. Double-balloon enteroscopy versus magnetic resonance enteroclysis in diagnosing suspected small-bowel Crohn's disease: results of a pilot study. Scand J Gastroenterol 2007;42(11):1376–85.
74. Pasha SF, Leighton JA, Das A, et al. Double-balloon enteroscopy and capsule endoscopy have comparable diagnostic yield in small-bowel disease: a meta-analysis. Clin Gastroenterol Hepatol 2008;6(6):671–6.
75. Kenji W, Hosomi S, Hirata N, et al. Useful diagnostic strategy in combination capsule endoscopy with double-balloon endoscopy for Crohn's disease. Paper presented at: 5th International Conference on Capsule Endoscopy, 2006; Paris, France.
76. Cosnes J, Cattan S, Blain A, et al. Long-term evolution of disease behavior of Crohn's disease. Inflamm Bowel Dis 2002;8(4):244–50.
77. Mekhjian HS, Switz DM, Watts HD, et al. National Cooperative Crohn's Disease Study: factors determining recurrence of Crohn's disease after surgery. Gastroenterology 1979;77(4 Pt 2):907–13.
78. Stebbing JF, Jewell DP, Kettlewell MG, et al. Recurrence and reoperation after strictureplasty for obstructive Crohn's disease: long-term results [corrected]. Br J Surg 1995;82(11):1471–4.
79. Sunada K, Yamamoto H, Kita H, et al. Clinical outcomes of enteroscopy using the double-balloon method for strictures of the small intestine. World J Gastroenterol 2005;11(7):1087–9.

80. Pohl J, May A, Nachbar L, et al. Diagnostic and therapeutic yield of push-and-pull enteroscopy for symptomatic small bowel Crohn's disease strictures. Eur J Gastroenterol Hepatol 2007;19(7):529–34.
81. Lee BI, Choi H, Choi KY, et al. Retrieval of a retained capsule endoscope by double-balloon enteroscopy. Gastrointest Endosc 2005;62(3):463–5.
82. D'Haens G, Geboes K, Rutgeerts P. Endoscopic and histologic healing of Crohn's (ileo-) colitis with azathioprine. Gastrointest Endosc 1999;50(5):667–71.
83. D'Haens G, Van Deventer S, Van Hogezand R, et al. Endoscopic and histological healing with infliximab anti-tumor necrosis factor antibodies in Crohn's disease: a European multicenter trial. Gastroenterology 1999;116(5):1029–34.
84. Persson PG, Karlen P, Bernell O, et al. Crohn's disease and cancer: a population-based cohort study. Gastroenterology 1994;107(6):1675–9.
85. Jess T, Winther KV, Munkholm P, et al. Intestinal and extra-intestinal cancer in Crohn's disease: follow-up of a population-based cohort in Copenhagen County, Denmark. Aliment Pharmacol Ther 2004;19(3):287–93.
86. Jess T, Loftus EV Jr, Velayos FS, et al. Risk of intestinal cancer in inflammatory bowel disease: a population-based study from Olmsted County, Minnesota. Gastroenterology 2006;130(4):1039–46.
87. Partridge SK, Hodin RA. Small bowel adenocarcinoma at a strictureplasty site in a patient with Crohn's disease: report of a case. Dis Colon Rectum 2004;47(5):778–81.
88. Monkemuller K, Fry LC, Ebert M, et al. Feasibility of double-balloon enteroscopy-assisted chromoendoscopy of the small bowel in patients with familial adenomatous polyposis. Endoscopy 2007;39(1):52–7.

Enteroscopy in the Diagnosis and Management of Celiac Disease

Emanuele Rondonotti, MD, PhD*, Federica Villa, MD, Valeria Saladino, MD, Roberto de Franchis, MD

KEYWORDS

• Celiac disease • Enteroscopy • Capsule endoscopy
• Double balloon enteroscopy • Duodenal biopsy

Celiac disease (CD) is a chronic systemic autoimmune disorder induced in genetically susceptible individuals by gluten fractions present in wheat, barley, and rye.[1] In the lamina propria of predisposed subjects, an immune reaction, triggered when gliadin binds to either DQ2 or DQ8 molecules, leads to an inflammatory reaction resulting in intraepithelial lymphocytosis and villous injury.[2–4]

Several sero-epidemiologic studies have shown that, in Europe and the United States, 1% to 3% of the general population develop celiac disease at some point in life,[5] whereas population-based studies have estimated that the biopsy-confirmed incidence of celiac disease in adults varies from 2 to 13 per 100,000 per year.[1,6,7] The prevalence of celiac disease is significantly increased in patients with autoimmune disorders (particularly in patients with diabetes mellitus type 1 or thyroid disorders) or with extraintestinal signs or symptoms such as anemia, fatigue, hypertransaminasemia, and osteoporosis.[8–11]

Although in the past, celiac disease was deemed to be primarily a disease of infancy, recent studies clearly demonstrated that this disease can become symptomatic at any age of life. Nowadays the diagnosis is typically made in adults[12,13] and even in older subjects.[14,15] Adults account for more than 60% of newly diagnosed cases of celiac disease,[16] and recent studies underlined that there are several differences between children and adults.[17] In children, diarrhea, vomiting, and failure to thrive are the leading symptoms, whereas adults often present with mild or vague gastrointestinal

Conflict of interest: Roberto de Franchis is a member of the speakers board of Given Imaging Inc. (Yoqneam, Israel).

Department of Medical Sciences, Gastroenterology 3 Unit, University of Milan, IRCCS Policlinico, Mangiagalli, Regina Elena Foundation, Via F. Sforza 35 (pad. Beretta Est, 1° piano). 20122 Milan, Italy
* Corresponding author.
E-mail address: emanuele.rondonotti@unimi.it (E. Rondonotti).

Gastrointest Endoscopy Clin N Am 19 (2009) 445–460
doi:10.1016/j.giec.2009.04.006 **giendo.theclinics.com**
1052-5157/09/$ – see front matter © 2009 Elsevier Inc. All rights reserved.

complaints, such as abdominal pain, occasional diarrhea, irritable bowel syndrome, dyspeptic symptoms, or isolated, subclinical malabsorption.[9,14,17,18]

Regardless of the age, an early and effective diagnosis warrants a complete and life-long withdrawal of the gluten from the diet. A gluten-free diet leads to the restoration of the small-bowel mucosa architecture,[19] the resolution of gastrointestinal[20] and extra-intestinal symptoms,[20–22] and the normalization of standardized mortality ratio,[23,24] and it significantly improves the patient's quality of life.[25,26] In addition, a possible correlation between the duration of gluten exposure and the risk of complications related to celiac disease has been hypothesized.[24,27] Some authors not only confirmed an increased risk of autoimmune disorders in patients with celiac disease,[28–31] but also showed a possible protective effect of a gluten-free diet,[22] highlighting the need of a diagnosis early in life.

Despite recent advances, the accurate diagnosis of celiac disease often remains a challenge for gastroenterologists. For each diagnosed case, there may be three to seven cases that remain undiagnosed;[1] several studies have shown that patients with celiac disease experience a long duration of symptoms before diagnosis,[8,32–34] and this diagnostic delay has also been noted for children, in whom the duration of symptoms before diagnosis can reach half of their life.[35]

Even when a definitive diagnosis is reached and a gluten-free diet is started, the patients must be carefully followed to verify the clinical response to the diet and mucosal recovery.

DIAGNOSING CELIAC DISEASE

Antibodies and Duodenal Histology

When the suspicion of celiac disease exists, the first recommended step is testing for specific antibodies. The most sensitive tests are based on the use of IgA isotypes. The available tests include antigliadin, antiendomysial, and anti-tissue transglutaminase antibodies. The use of anti-gliadin antibodies[36,37] for the diagnosis of celiac disease has been called into question because of their low sensitivity (55%–100%).[5] However,[38,39] the new gliadin peptide (deamidated gliadin) antibody tests have been shown to be highly accurate in the diagnostic work-up and follow-up of celiac disease.[40]

In everyday clinical practice, the IgA anti-endomysial and anti-tissue transglutaminase tests, which are both highly sensitive and specific (with values for both parameters exceeding 95% in most studies),[37] are used to identify both symptomatic and asymptomatic individuals at risk. Antibody-positive subjects require an intestinal biopsy to confirm the diagnosis. Despite the impressive performances of the serologic tests mentioned earlier, it has been clear for a long time[41] that the diagnosis of celiac disease requires the histologic demonstration of compatible small-bowel abnormalities.

The spectrum of pathologic changes in celiac disease ranges from near-normal villous architecture with a prominent intraepithelial lymphocytosis to various degrees of villous atrophy:[4] Marsh type 0 lesion indicates normal histology; Marsh type I is characterized by an increased number of intraepithelial lymphocytes in an architecturally normal small-bowel mucosa; Marsh type II presents crypt hyperplasia but normal villi; and Marsh type III is characterized by increasing degrees of villous atrophy.

Although jejunal biopsies, obtained by means of unguided suction devices (such as the Crosby capsule), are of better quality than those obtained by endoscopy (because they show less fragmentation and fewer crush artifacts), several studies have shown that, for diagnostic purposes, the biopsies obtained during esophagogastroduodenoscopy (EGD) are equivalent to jejunal suction biopsies.[2,42,43] Several studies have also been aimed at defining the site and the number of biopsies needed to optimize the diagnosis of celiac disease because of the possible patchy distribution of atrophic areas. Although this issue is still under discussion, it appears that at least three biopsies randomly taken from the descending duodenum (plus one to two biopsies taken from the duodenal bulb) can detect 95% to 100% of patients with celiac disease.[44–46] On the other hand, in everyday clinical practice, small-bowel biopsies taken during EGD can be[47] affected by some pitfalls (such as poor orientation or presence of artifacts) that can hamper or prevent the final diagnosis.

For all the reasons mentioned earlier, several efforts have been made to find new tools to improve the sampling methods (ie, jumbo forceps[48]), to better identify the areas of atrophic small-bowel mucosa on which to target biopsies (ie, chromoendoscopy, immersion and/or magnification techniques;[49] **Fig. 1**A, **Fig. 2**) or to completely avoid small-bowel biopsies (ie, capsule endoscopy).

Endoscopy

EGD

Characteristic endoscopic findings have been described by conventional endoscopy in the duodenum and jejunum in patients with celiac disease. These findings include reduction in number or scalloping of duodenal folds, mucosal fissures or grooves, mosaic pattern, visible mucosal vessels, or micronodules in the duodenal bulb (**Fig. 3**).[2] Although these endoscopic markers have shown good specificity (about 95%–100%) for the diagnosis of celiac disease, they are lacking in sensitivity. The sensitivity of these endoscopic markers, when detected by standard endoscopes, is so low (50%–80%) that in case of serologic suspicion of celiac disease 4 to 6 duodenal biopsies are warranted, regardless of the appearance of the duodenal mucosa at endoscopy.[2]

Capsule endoscopy

Capsule endoscopy cannot take biopsies, and therefore the diagnosis of celiac disease by this device is based on the recognition of those relatively “insensitive” markers. However, capsule endoscopy differs from regular endoscopy in several technical aspects, which can increase its capability in recognizing these endoscopic

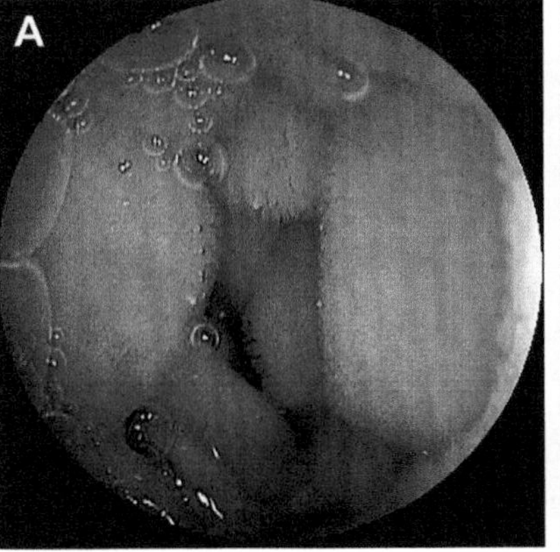

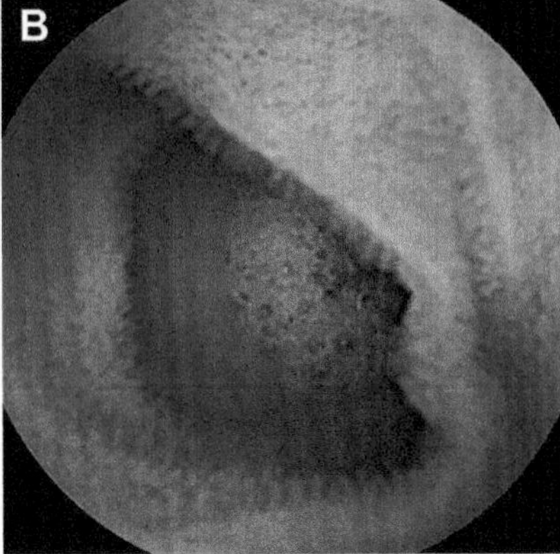

Fig. 1. Normal small bowel seen at EGD by immersion technique (*A*) and by capsule endoscopy (*B*).

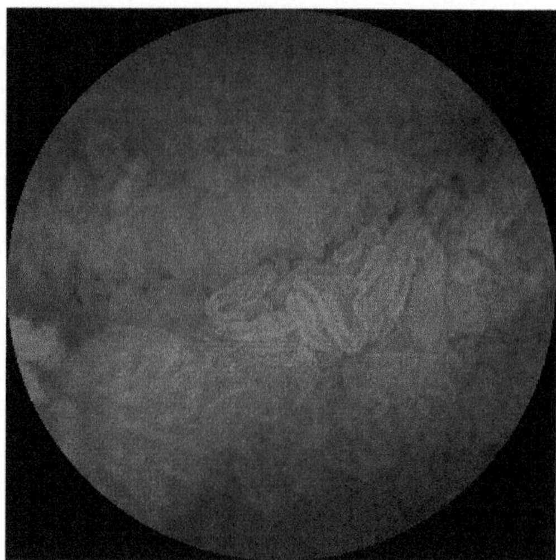

Fig. 2. Normal small-bowel mucosa seen with immersion technique—closer look.

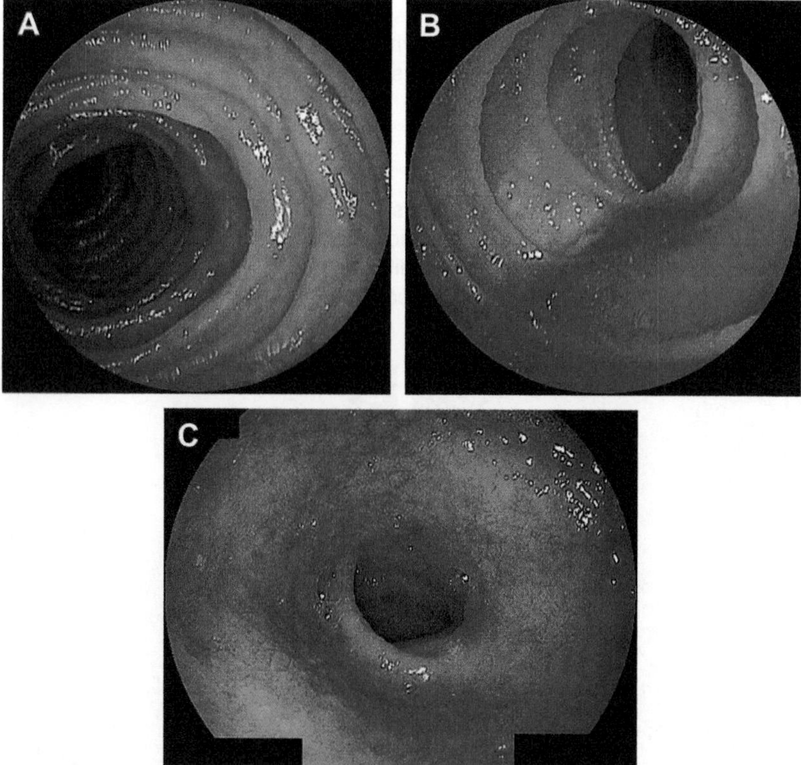

Fig. 3. Endoscopic markers compatible with celiac disease seen at EGD. (*A*) Normal small bowel; (*B*) scalloping of duodenal folds; (*C*) loss of duodenal folds.

markers. Capsule endoscopy, by navigating through the small bowel without air insufflation, inspects the small-bowel mucosa in a similar way as in the immersion technique (**Fig. 1**B) (which has been proved to be highly sensitive and specific in recognizing atrophic areas[49]) (**Fig. 4**). In addition, capsule endoscopy, with an eight-fold magnification, provides high-quality images of the entire small bowel, potentially overcoming the patchiness of mucosal lesions described in patients with celiac disease. When capsule endoscopy was first tested in patients with RCD, it was able to show not only possible complications in the distal small bowel, but also the presence of typical endoscopic markers, supporting the diagnosis of celiac disease.[50]

Only a few papers that aimed at evaluating the possible role of capsule endoscopy in establishing the diagnosis of celiac disease have been published so far. In the first one, Petroniene and colleagues[51] examined 10 patients with histologically proven villous atrophy (Marsh III lesions) with capsule endoscopy and found that the overall sensitivity, specificity, and positive and negative predictive values of this technique, when compared with histology, were excellent (70%, 100%, 100%, and 77% respectively). The authors underlined that, in recognizing mucosal lesions compatible with celiac disease, capsule endoscopy appears to be superior to conventional endoscopy, but at the same time, they highlighted some possible limitations (ie, capsule endoscopy may not be able to identify infiltrative or hyperplastic

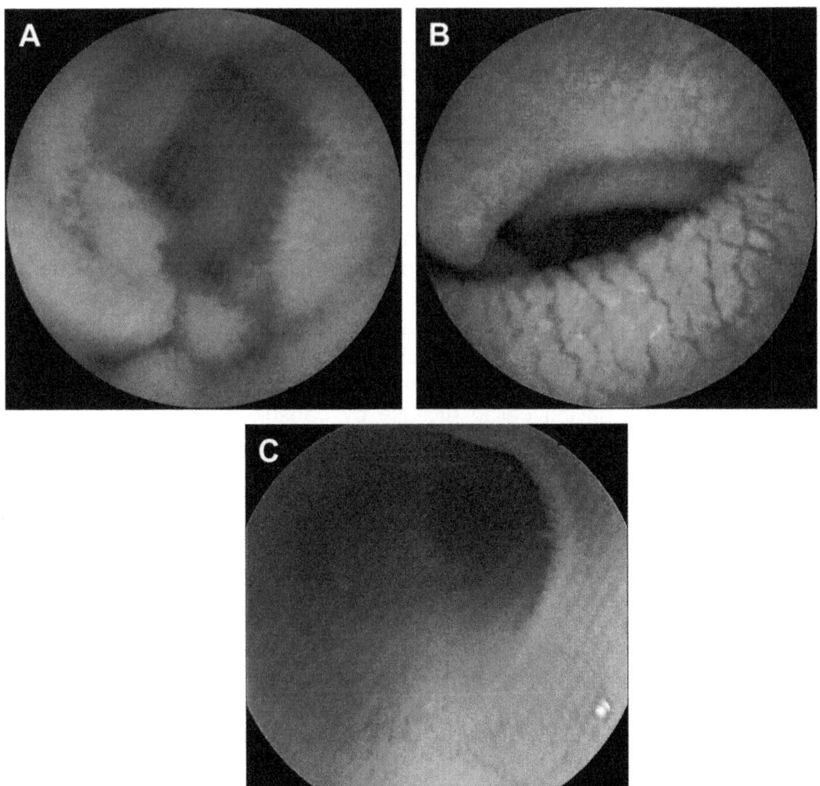

Fig. 4. Endoscopic markers compatible with celiac disease seen at capsule endoscopy. (*A*) Normal small bowel; (*B*) scalloping of duodenal folds; (*C*) loss of duodenal folds.

mucosal changes–Marsh I or II) that may prevent the use of this tool as a new gold standard.

This point has also been addressed in the study by Hopper and colleagues,[52] which included 1 patient with Marsh I lesion, and in a multicenter international study published in 2007,[53] where three patients with Marsh type II and one patient with Marsh type I lesion were included. Capsule endoscopy was unable to identify the two patients with Marsh I lesions as persons with celiac disease (in whom the indication to start a gluten-free diet was still under discussion). However, the capsule correctly identified all three patients with Marsh II lesions. A possible explanation of this phenomenon is related to the sampling error of small-bowel biopsies because biopsies are normally taken randomly, whereas capsule endoscopy, enabling to inspect the entire surface of the proximal small bowel, can overcome this problem. The two studies also confirmed the good accuracy (sensitivity 85%–87.5%, specificity 90.9%–100%) of capsule endoscopy in diagnosing celiac disease in patients with clinical suspicion and positive serology.

However, despite the demonstration that capsule endoscopy has high sensitivity and specificity and is potentially able to overcome the issue of the patchiness of mucosal atrophy, its performance in diagnosing celiac disease is not close enough to that of duodenal biopsies. In most of these studies, capsule endoscopy videos have been reviewed by endoscopists with a large experience in capsule endoscopy. Even in this setting, the interobserver agreement was only fair (K values range between 0.49 and 0.50),[54] and when videos were evaluated by reviewers with limited experience,[51] the accuracy parameters decreased further. Concerning the diagnostic work-up of celiac disease, EGD with biopsies is easily available worldwide and appears to be cheaper in comparison with capsule endoscopy, although no specific cost-effectiveness studies have yet been performed.

At the time of introduction of capsule endoscopy in clinical practice, it was hoped that this device, owing to its ability to explore the entire small bowel, would also provide significant information about the medium-distal small bowel at the time of diagnosis (ie, explaining reasons for different clinical presentations of celiac disease).

A study on this topic,which included 10 patients with positive serology and symptoms suggesting celiac disease, has been published by Ersoy and colleagues.[55] In this study, all patients had celiac disease with Marsh type III lesions, and the authors underlined that all patients had mucosal changes in the proximal small bowel and none showed patchy mucosal lesions. Therefore, although all patients had been correctly identified as having celiac disease by capsule endoscopy, the authors concluded that capsule endoscopy does not add any clinically relevant information in the diagnosis of patients with suspected celiac disease.

As far as the extent of mucosal atrophy in newly diagnosed celiac patients is concerned, beside the demonstration that in about two-thirds of patients the mucosal changes tend to extend distally involving the jejunum (and even reaching the terminal ileum in 10% of cases),[53] two studies confirmed that there is no significant correlation between the extent of enteropathy and clinical manifestations.[53,56] The authors found that patients with antiendomysial antibodies tend to have a more extensive involvement of the small bowel, but the clinical relevance of this relationship remains to be established.

For all these reasons, EGD with four to six biopsies in the descending duodenum remains the gold standard for the diagnosis of celiac disease, and an extensive evaluation of the small bowel at the time of diagnosis does not appear to be necessary. However, capsule endoscopy can be considered as a valid alternative in patients unable or unwilling to undergo EGD with biopsies.

PATIENTS WITH POSITIVE ANTIBODIES AND NEGATIVE HISTOLOGY

Capsule Endoscopy

Capsule endoscopy has also been proposed in selected cases with strong suspicion of celiac disease, positive antibody tests, and negative histology. In these difficult patients, when other rare diseases causing the patient's complaints have been excluded, repeat small-bowel tissue sampling (eventually by push enteroscopy) or starting gluten withdrawal may be indicated. As far as the symptomatic response to gluten withdrawal is concerned, this is not a strong indicator of celiac disease[57,58] (the positive predictive value for clinical improvement after gluten withdrawal was 36%).[57]

Push Enteroscopy

The repetition of small-bowel biopsies may be as inconclusive as the first attempt. A few reports[59,60] exist on the use of push enteroscopy in difficult cases. These studies include a small number of celiac disease patients with positive serology and negative duodenal biopsies diagnosed only on the basis of jejunal biopsies. However, because Cellier and colleagues[61] showed that, for diagnostic purposes, push enteroscopy does not add significant data to EGD in patients with different stages of celiac disease, this technique has been progressively abandoned. In addition, Sidhu and colleagues[62] showed that, if an evaluation of the small bowel is needed, the diagnostic yields of push enteroscopy and capsule endoscopy appear to be comparable.

Double Balloon Enteroscopy

Some authors[63] suggested the superiority of double balloon enteroscopy (DBE) when compared with push enteroscopy. However, a meta-analysis by Pasha and colleagues,[64] of studies directly comparing capsule endoscopy with DBE, even if not focused on celiac disease, clearly demonstrated that these two techniques have comparable diagnostic yields.

Based on these data, the evaluation of the small bowel in these difficult patients, when needed, should be better performed by means of capsule endoscopy (which is superior to push enteroscopy in identifying other possible small-bowel diseases and is less invasive than push- and DBE).

FOLLOW-UP OF PATIENTS WITH KNOWN CELIAC DISEASE

Patients Clinically Improving on a Gluten-Free Diet

Small-bowel histology

The mucosal changes described in patients with celiac disease, although non–disease-specific,[42] permit a presumptive diagnosis of celiac disease and eventually the initiation of a gluten-free diet.[20] Histologic recovery after gluten withdrawal, requiring months or even years, especially in adults, remains the final confirmation of the diagnosis.[20] Confirmation of the diagnosis, based only on resolution of symptoms after gluten exclusion, may be misleading. This point can be exemplified by patients with irritable bowel syndrome, who despite a normal duodenal biopsy may benefit from a gluten-free diet.[65] For this reason, in adult patients with clinical improvement following a strict gluten-free diet, a second EGD with biopsies,1.5 to 2 years after the diagnosis, is generally recommended to verify mucosal recovery and dietary compliance.[19,25–27,66]

Capsule endoscopy

To explore the possible role of capsule endoscopy in the follow-up of celiac disease patients clinically responding to a gluten-free diet, Murray and colleagues[56] repeated capsule endoscopy in 37 histologically proven celiac disease patients after 6 months of a gluten-free diet. In these patients, the mucosal improvement was readily apparent with a reduction in the frequency and distribution of features of atrophy in both the duodenum and jejunum. The authors highlighted that biopsy specimens of the proximal small bowel alone may not reflect the healing that has occurred more distally in response to a gluten-free diet. However, in this study, capsule endoscopy was performed quite early after gluten withdrawal, probably leading to an overestimation of the significance of the distal healing and, by consequence, of the possible role of capsule endoscopy in this setting.

The study by Biagi and colleagues[54] clearly demonstrated that capsule endoscopy provides only partial indications on the degree of mucosal intestinal atrophy; it seems to be able to discriminate between atrophic and normal mucosa, but it does not allow a correct evaluation of the degree of mucosal atrophy. Consequently, the estimation of the histologic recovery by means of capsule endoscopy can be extremely difficult.

For all these reasons, capsule endoscopy cannot substitute EGD with biopsies in the follow-up of patients with clinical improvement after gluten withdrawal.

Refractory Celiac Disease

In about 30% of patients diagnosed with celiac disease, symptoms persist despite a gluten-free diet, or relapse after an initial response.[67] The major cause of failure is the continued inadvertent ingestion of gluten. A minimal, but continuous, intake of gluten can prevent mucosal recovery.[68] However, when the dietary compliance is established by a dietician, and the patient still does not respond, the initial diagnosis of celiac disease must be reassessed, and other reasons for persisting symptoms (ie, pancreatic insufficiency, irritable bowel syndrome, bacterial overgrowth, inflammatory bowel disease, microscopic colitis, tropical sprue) must be ruled out.[69] When clinical symptoms and histologic abnormalities persist or recur despite a strict adherence to the diet for more than 12 months, patients are defined as suffering from RCD.[16,70–72] They represent a small minority of patients with celiac disease (about 1%–2%) but are more prone to have aberrant clonal intraepithelial T-cell population and finally to develop ulcerative jejunitis and T-cell lymphoma.[73]

EGD plus duodenal biopsy

In this subset of patients, EGD plus biopsy has a key role in discriminating between two different types of RCD (type I: normal and polyclonal intraepithelial lymphocytes, and type II: abnormal and monoclonal, intraepithelial lymphocytes), which considerably differ in prognosis and response to medical therapies.[74] There are several studies aimed at understanding the pathogenesis of possible complications of celiac disease, in particular whether the progression from RCD type I to type II truly exists.

Nevertheless, conventional EGD allows limited examination of the extent of the small bowel, whereas mucosal lesions consistent with ulcerative jejunitis and/or T-cell lymphoma may be located in the mid or distal small bowel. For this reason, deep endoscopic techniques, such as intraoperative enteroscopy, push enteroscopy, capsule endoscopy, and balloon-assisted enteroscopy, have been tested in this subgroup of patients.

Enteroscopy

There is limited experience about the role of intraoperative enteroscopy[75,76] in refractory-unresponsive celiac disease. Only isolated cases have been reported so far, mainly because of the invasiveness of this technique.

As far as push enteroscopy is concerned, Cellier and colleagues[61] clearly demonstrated that lesions compatible with RCD are often located beyond the reach of conventional endoscopes. In their study of 8 patients, of whom only one had duodenal lesions, push enteroscopy detected jejunal ulcerations in five, leading to a change in the management. However, despite being better than EGD, push enteroscopy can evaluate only about 100 to 150 cm beyond the ligament of Treitz, whereas the majority of the small bowel remains unexplored.[77]

Device-assisted enteroscopes allow the direct inspection of most of the small-bowel mucosa, with the possibility of taking targeted biopsies. After their introduction in clinical practice, these tools, particularly the double balloon enteroscope, have been used to evaluate the small bowel in many different conditions.[78,79] However, to the best of our knowledge, although there are only a few case series in which individual cases of RCD undergoing DBE have been described, there is only one peer-reviewed paper specifically devoted to this topic.[80]

Hadithi and colleagues[80] performed 24 DBE procedures in 21 RCD patients without complications. The authors were able not only to discover two cases of ulcerative jejunitis (**Fig. 5**) and five lymphomas, but also to rule out T-cell lymphomas in four patients with strong suspicion based on radiologic findings. Despite the significant diagnostic yield of the DBE in this series, the authors missed the opportunity to perform a formal comparison between DBE results and CT findings (CT was performed only in a minority of patients), and none of the included patients underwent capsule endoscopy. In addition, DBE is an invasive, time consuming, and potentially risky technique, particularly in these frail patients. Therefore, based on this study, it cannot be judged whether DBE is mandatory in every patient suffering from RCD or if this procedure should be reserved to a particular subgroup of patients (ie, patients with positive imaging).

It should be emphasized that, in patients with RCD, examination of the entire small bowel is mandatory. Unfortunately, even in experienced hands in the Western world, complete enteroscopy is possible with DBE (combining oral and anal approach) in only 30% to 60% of patients.[81,82] This goal can be easily achieved with less invasive techniques such as imaging techniques or capsule endoscopy.

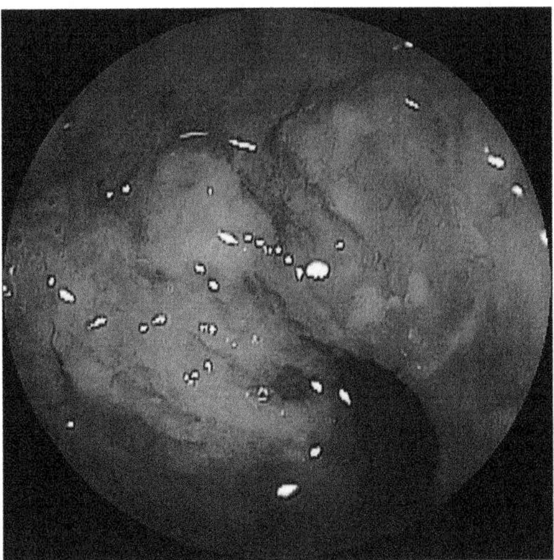

Fig. 5. Ulcerated stenosis identified by DBE in a patient with RCD.

Maiden and colleagues[83] performed EGD with biopsies and capsule endoscopy in 19 patients who had been on a gluten-free diet for at least 12 months with continuing gastrointestinal symptoms. Comparing capsule endoscopy findings (**Fig. 6**) and histology (obtained during EGD), the authors found a complete concordance in 78% of cases (k statistic 0.65, 95% confidence interval, 0.36–0.95) and showed that the accuracy parameters of capsule endoscopy were similar to those reported in the case of new diagnosis of celiac disease. The authors confirmed that even in this case, capsule endoscopy cannot substitute the histologic evaluation of the small-bowel mucosa, but they pointed out that the capsule was able to detect two cases of ulcerative jejunitis missed by EGD.

In another study performed by Daum and colleagues,[84] the authors tried to identify those nonresponsive celiac disease patients who would benefit from capsule endoscopy. These authors performed capsule endoscopy in seven patients with type I and seven patients with type II RCD and found that capsule endoscopy detects additional cases with ulcerative jejunitis among RCD type II patients, whereas the diagnostic yield of this technique remains low in patients with RCD type I.

In agreement with the above study, Culliford and colleagues[50] showed that the diagnostic yield of capsule endoscopy in diagnosing complications of the disease significantly increases when celiac disease patients with high risk of harboring a malignancy (ie, those with iron deficiency anemia and positive fecal occult blood test or previous history of small-bowel carcinoma) are evaluated. In these highly selected patients, capsule endoscopy frequently revealed ulcerations or cancers (45% and 2.1% of cases respectively) and directly influenced further management. The authors also reported that in these patients a comparison between capsule endoscopy and standard radiologic techniques was not systematically done, but in those in which the comparison was done, the radiologic techniques appeared not to be sensitive enough.

Imaging techniques

Some studies explored the possible role of imaging techniques (such as CT scan, CT enteroclysis, MRI enteroclysis, positron emission tomography [PET] scan) in evaluating the small bowel and in excluding small-bowel neoplasms. Van Weyenberg and colleagues[85] tested a four-point MRI-enteroclysis score able to discriminate RCD patients with low or high chance to develop enteropathy-associated T-cell lymphoma,

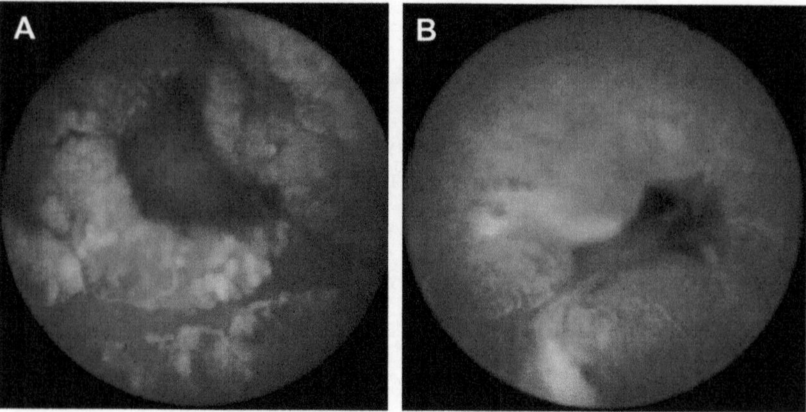

Fig. 6. Endoscopic findings identified by capsule endoscopy in a patient with RCD. (*A*) Linear ulcer; (*B*) ulcerated stenosis.

whereas Hadithi and colleagues,[86] in a cohort of 30 patients with RCD, showed that 18-fluorodeoxyglucose PET scan is superior to CT scan, in visualizing sites affected by lymphomas.[87]

The exact diagnostic algorithm in RCD patients remains uncertain, because a prospective comparison between different diagnostic tools in these patients is lacking. The new imaging techniques mentioned earlier and capsule endoscopy appear to be complementary. The latter is capable of inspecting the entire small bowel and is able to identify even subtle premalignant superficial changes, whereas the former techniques have the indubitable advantage of providing information about intestinal wall thickness and extraluminal abnormalities, thus providing complete preoperative staging if a lymphoma is present.

SUMMARY

Several studies have demonstrated that biopsies taken from the descending duodenum are comparable, for diagnostic purposes, with those taken in the jejunum. EGD has become the technique of choice for taking tissue samples, completely replacing jejunal biopsy for the diagnosis of celiac disease.The demonstration of histologic changes in the small-bowel mucosa by EGD remains the gold standard. Because of its technical characteristics and its minimal invasiveness, capsule endoscopy has been tested as a possible substitute for EGD with biopsies in this setting. Although capsule endoscopy has been found to be highly sensitive and specific for this purpose, its performance is still considered insufficient to replace EGD. Capsule endoscopy can only be considered as a valid alternative in patients unable or unwilling to undergo EGD with biopsies. It might also be proposed in selected cases with a strong suspicion of celiac disease and negative first-line tests. Capsule endoscopy has so far failed to demonstrate any correlation between the length of small-bowel involvement and clinical presentation. For the same reasons, the use of other endoscopic tools to evaluate the entire small bowel at the time of initial diagnosis does not seem to be justified.

Conversely, enteroscopy can play a key role in the case of unresponsive celiac disease or RCD. In this particular subset of patients, EGD may have a role as an easy way to take biopsies aimed at distinguishing between RCD type I and type II. However, the exploration of the entire small bowel is mandatory. Complications such as ulcerative jejunitis or enteropathy-associated T-cell lymphoma can be located at any point along the small bowel. Push enteroscopy has been shown to be superior to EGD in detecting lesions in the proximal small bowel, but it can only inspect 100 to 150 cm of this organ. Therefore, both capsule endoscopy and DBE have been found, for different reasons, to be helpful in patients with RCD (particularly in case of RCD type II). There are only few studies on this topic at the present time, which include a small number of patients, and a comparison between different diagnostic tools (including imaging techniques) is also lacking. In addition, whether the progression from type I to type II RCD truly exists is still under discussion. It is also important to clarify whether enteroscopy (capsule endoscopy and/or DBE) should be performed in all patients with RCD or only in RCD type II or in case of alarm symptoms.

Although technical and clinical advances in the field of small-bowel endoscopy have been numerous, there is still much room for further technical improvement (ie, new capsules with a wider angle of view, improved optical systems, therapeutic capsule devices driven from outside the body, or newly designed overtubes and enteroscopes). It can reasonably be assumed that the present scenario may change substantially in the not too distant future.

REFERENCES

1. Rewers M. Epidemiology of celiac disease: what are the prevalence, incidence and progression of celiac disease. Gastroenterology 2005;128:S47–51.
2. Lee SK, Green PHR. Endoscopy in celiac disease. Curr Opin Gastroenterol 2005; 21:589–94.
3. Shan L, Molberg O, Parrot I, et al. Structural basis for gluten intolerance in celiac sprue. Science 2002;297:2275–9.
4. Marsh MN. Gluten, major histocompatibility complex and the small intestine: a molecular and immunologic approach to the spectrum of gluten sensitivity ('celiac sprue'). Gastroenterology 1992;102:330–54.
5. James SP. National Institute of Health consensus development conference statement on celiac disease, June 28–30, 2004. Gastroenterology 2005;128:S1–9.
6. Murray JA, Van Dyke C, Plevak MF, et al. Trends in the identification and clinical features of celiac disease in North American community, 1950–2001. Clin Gastroenterol Hepatol 2003;1:19–27.
7. Cook B, Oxner R, Chapman B, et al. A thirty-year (1970–1999) study of celiac disease in the Canterbury region of New Zealand. N Z Med J 2004;117:U772.
8. Lo W, Sano K, Lebwohl B, et al. Changing presentation of adult celiac disease. Dig Dis Sci 2003;48:395–8.
9. Catassi C, Kryszak, Jacques OL, et al. Detection of celiac disease in primary care: a multicenter case-finding study in North America. Am J Gastroenterol 2007;102:1454–60.
10. Rubio-Tapia A, Murray JM. Celiac disease beyond the gut. Clin Gastroenterol Hepatol 2008;6:722–3.
11. Cosnes J, Cellier C, Viola S, et al. Incidence of autoimmune diseases in celiac disease: protective effect of the gluten free diet. Clin Gastroenterol Hepatol 2008;6:753–8.
12. Fasano A, Catassi C. Current approaches to diagnosis and treatment of celiac disease: an evolving spectrum. Gastroenterology 2001;120:636–51.
13. Mulder CJ, Cellier C. Coeliac disease: changing views. Best Pract Res Clin Gastroenterol 2005;19:313–21.
14. Vippula A, Collin P, Maki M, et al. Undetected celiac disease in the elderly. A biopsy-proven population-based study. Dig Liver Dis 2008;40:809–13.
15. Muhammad A, Pitchumoni CS. Newly detected celiac disease by wireless capsule endoscopy in older adults with iron deficiency anemia. J Clin Gastroenterol 2008;42:980–3.
16. United European Gastroenterolgy. When is a coeliac a coeliac. Report of a working group of the United European Gastroenterology Week in Amsterdam 2001. Eur J Gastroenterol Hepatol 2001;13:1123–8.
17. Vivas S, Ruiz de Morales JM, Fernandez M, et al. Age-related clinical, serological and histopathological features of celiac disease. Am J Gastroenterol 2008;103: 2360–5.
18. Green PH, Cellier C. Celiac disease. N Engl J Med 2007;357:1731–43.
19. Tursi A, Brandimarte G, Giorgetti GM, et al. Endoscopic and histological findings in the duodenum of adults with celiac disease before and after changing to a gluten-free diet: a 2-year prospective study. Endoscopy 2006;38:702–7.
20. Dewar DH, Ciclitira PJ. Clinical features and diagnosis of celiac disease. Gastroenterology 2005;128:S19–24.
21. Tau C, Mautalen C, De Rosa S, et al. Bone mineral density in children with celiac disease: effect of a gluten free diet. Eur J Clin Nutr 2006;60:358–63.

22. Annibale B, Severi C, Chistolini A, et al. Efficacy of gluten-free diet alone on recovery from iron deficiency anemia in adult celiac patients. Am J Gastroenterol 2001;96:132–7.
23. Corrao G, Corazza GR, Bagnardi V, et al. Mortality in patients with celiac disease and their relatives: a cohort study. Lancet 2001;358:356–61.
24. West J, Logan RF, Smith CJ, et al. Malignancy and mortality in people with celiac disease: population-based cohort study. Br Med J 2004;329:716–9.
25. Nachman F, Mauriño E, Vázquez H, et al. Quality of life in celiac disease patients: prospective analysis on the importance of clinical severity at diagnosis and the impact of treatment. Dig Liver Dis 2009;41:15–25.
26. Casellas F, Rodrigo L, Vivancos JL, et al. Factors that impact health-related quality of life in adults with celiac disease: a multicenter study. World J Gastroenterol 2008;14:46–52.
27. Green PH, Fleischauer AT, Bhagat G, et al. Risk of malignancy in patients with celiac disease. Am J Med 2003;115:191–5.
28. Cataldo F, Marino V. Increased prevalence of autoimmune diseases in first-degree relatives of patients with celiac disease. J Pediatr Gastroenterol Nutr 2003;36:470–3.
29. Ventura A, Magazzu G, Greco L. Duration of exposure to gluten and risk for autoimmune disorders in patients with celiac disease. Gastroenterology 1999;117: 297–303.
30. Viljamaa M, Kaukinen K, Huhtala H, et al. Coeliac disease, autoimmune diseases and gluten exposure. Scand J Gastroenterol 2005;40:437–43.
31. Sategna Guidetti C, Solerio E, Scaglione N, et al. Duration of gluten exposure in adult celiac disease does not correlate with the risk for autoimmune disorders. Gut 2001;49:502–5.
32. Green PHR, Stavropoulos SN, Panagi SG, et al. Characteristics of adult celiac disease in the USA: results of a national survey. Am J Gastroenterol 2001;96: 126–31.
33. Rampertab SD, Pooran N, Brar P, et al. Trends in the presentation of celiac disease. Am J Med 2006;119. 355.e9–14.
34. Green PHR. Where are all those patients with celiac disease? Am J Gastroenterol 2007;102:1461–3.
35. D'Amico MA, Holmes J, Stavropoulos N, et al. Presentation of pediatric celiac disease in the United States: prominent effect of breastfeeding. Clin Pediatr (Phila) 2005;44:249–58.
36. Green PHR, Rostami K, Marsh MN. Diagnosis of celiac disease. Best Pract Res Clin Gastroenterol 2005;19:389–400.
37. Hill ID. What are the sensitivity and the specificity of serologic tests for celiac disease? Do sensitivity and specificity vary in different populations? Gastroenterology 2005;128:S25–32.
38. Volta U, Granito A, Fiorini E, et al. Usefulness of antibodies to deaminated gliadin peptides in celiac disease diagnosis and follow up. Dig Dis Sci 2008; 53:1582–8.
39. Kaukinen K, Collin P, Laurila K, et al. Resurrection of gliadin antibodies in coeliac disease. Deamidated gliadin peptide antibody test provides additional diagnostic benefit. Scand J Gastroenterol 2007;42:1428–33.
40. Holdstock G, Eade OE, Isaacson P, et al. Endoscopic duodenal biopsies in celiac disease and duodenitis. Scand J Gastroenterol 1979;14:717–20.
41. Paulley JW, Fairweather FA, Leemin A. Postgastrectomy steatorrhoea and patchy jejunal atrophy. Lancet 1957;1:406–7.

42. Mee AS, Burke M, Valon AG, et al. Small bowel biopsies for malabsorption: comparison of the diagnostic adequacy of endocopi forceps and capsule biopsy specimens. Br Med J (Clin Res Ed) 1985;291:769–72.
43. Achkar E, Casey WD, Petras R, et al. Comparaison of suction capsule and endoscopic biopsy of small bowel mucosa. Gastrointest Endosc 1986;32:278–81.
44. Hopper AD, Cross SS, Sanders DS. Patchy villous atrophy in adult patients with suspected gluten-sensitive enteropathy: is a multiple duodenal biopsy strategy appropriate? Endoscopy 2007;39:219–24.
45. Green PHR. Celiac disease: how many biopsies for diagnosis? Gastrointest Endosc 2008;67:1088–90.
46. Pais WP, Duerksen DR, Pettigrew NM, et al. How many duodenal biopsy specimens are required to make a diagnosis of celiac disease? Gastrointest Endosc 2008;67:1082–7.
47. Collin P, Kaukinen K, Vogelsang H, et al. Antiendomysial and antihuman recombinant tissue transglutaminase antibodies in the diagnosis of coeliac disease: a biopsy-proven European multicentre study. Eur J Gastroenterol Hepatol 2005;17:85–91.
48. Dandalides SM, Carey WD, Petras R, et al. Endoscopic small bowel mucosal biopsy: a controlled trial evaluating forceps size and biopsy location in the diagnosis of normal and abnormal mucosal architecture. Gastrointest Endosc 1989; 35(3):197–200.
49. Cammarota G, Fedeli P, Gasbarrini A. Emerging technologies in upper gastrointestinal endoscopy and celiac disease. Nat Clin Pract Gastroenterol Hepatol 2009;6:47–56.
50. Culliford A, Daly J, Diamond B, et al. The value of wireless capsule endoscopy in patients with complicated celiac disease. Gastrointest Endosc 2005;62:55–61.
51. Petroniene R, Dubcenco E, Baker JP, et al. Given capsule endocopy in celiac disease: evaluation of diagnostic accuracy and interobserver agreement. Am J Gastroenterol 2005;100:685–94.
52. Hopper AD, Sidhu R, Hurlstone DP, et al. Capsule endoscopy: an alternative to duodenal biopsy for the recognition of villous atrophy in coelic disease? Dig Liver Dis 2007;39:140–5.
53. Rondonotti E, Spada C, Cave D, et al. Video capsule enteroscopy in the diagnosis of celiac disease: a multicenter study. Am J Gastroenterol 2007;102: 1624–31.
54. Biagi F, Rondonotti E, Campanella J, et al. Video capsule endoscopy and histology for small bowel mucosa evaluation: a comparison performed by blinded observers. Clin Gastroenterol Hepatol 2006;4:998–1003.
55. Ersoy O, Akin E, Ugras S, et al. Capsule endoscopy findings in celiac disease. Dig Dis Sci 2009;54(4):825–9.
56. Murray JA, Rubio-Tapia A, Van Dike C, et al. Mucosal atrophy in celiac disease: extent of involvement, correlation with clinical presentation and response to treatment. Clin Gastroenterol Hepatol 2008;6:186–93.
57. Campanella J, Biagi F, Bianchi PI, et al. Clinical response to gluten withdrawal is not an indicator of coeliac disease. Scand J Gastroenterol 2008;43:1311–4.
58. Wahab PJ, Crusius JB, Meijer JW, et al. Gluten challenge in borderline gluten-sensitive enteropathy. Am J Gastroenterol 2001;96:1464–9.
59. De Vitis I, Spada C, Pirozzi PA, et al. Role of enteroscopy in the diagnosis of celiac disease [abstract]. Gastrointest Endosc 2003;58:147.
60. Horoldt B, McAlindon ME, Sthenson TJ, et al. Making the diagnosis of celiac disease: is there a role for push enteroscopy? Eur J Gastroenterol Hepatol 2004;16:1143–6.

61. Cellier C, Cullerier E, Patey-Mariaud de Serre M, et al. Push enteroscopy in celiac sprue and refractory sprue. Gastrointest Endosc 1999;50:613–7.
62. Sidhu R, McAlindon M, Kapur K, et al. Push enteroscopy in the era of capsule endoscopy. J Clin Gastroenterol 2008;42:54–8.
63. Matsumoto T, Tomohiko M, Esaki M, et al. Performance of anterograde double-balloon enteroscopy: comparison with push enteroscopy. G Ital Endod 2005; 62:392–8.
64. Pasha SF, Leighton JA, Das A, et al. Double-balloon enteroscopy and capsule endoscopy have comparable diagnostic yield in small-bowel disease: a meta-analysis. Clin Gastroenterol Hepatol 2008;6:671–6.
65. Hopper AD, Hadjivassiliou, Butt S, et al. Adult celiac disease. Br Med J 2007;335: 558–62.
66. Ciacci C, Cirillo M, Cavallaro R, et al. Long term follow up of celiac adults on gluten-free diet: prevalence and correlates of intestinal damage. Digestion 2002;66:178–85.
67. Pink IJ, Creamer B. Response to a gluten-free diet of patients with the celiac syndrome. Lancet 1967;1:300–4.
68. Biagi F, Campanella J, Martucci S, et al. A milligram of gluten a day keeps the mucosal recovery away: a case report. Nutr Rev 2004;62:360–3.
69. Schuppan D, Kelly CP, Krauss N. Monitoring non-responsive patients with celiac disease. Gastrointest Endosc Clin N Am 2006;16:593–603.
70. Al-Toma A, Visser OJ, van Roessel HM, et al. Autologous hematopoietic stem cell transplantation in refractory celiac disease with aberrant T cells. Blood 2007;109: 2243–9.
71. Patey-Mariaud De SN, Cellier C, Jabri B, et al. Distinction between coeliac disease and refractory sprue: a simple immunohistochemical method. Histopathology 2000;37:70–7.
72. Cellier C, Patey N, Mauvieux L, et al. Abnormal intestinal intraepithelial lymphocytes in refractory sprue. Gastroenterology 1998;114:471–81.
73. Verbeek WHM, van de Water JMW, Al-toma A, et al. The incidence of entheropathy associated T-cell lymphoma: a nation-wide study of population based registry in the Netherlands. Scand J Gastroenterol 2008;11:1–7.
74. Rubio-Tapia A, Kelly DG, Lahr BD, et al. Clinical staging and survival in refractory celiac disease: a single center experience. Gastroenterology 2009;136: 99–107.
75. Mesnard B, Bonniere P, Colombel JF, et al. [Intestinal ulceration in celiac disease in the adult. Value of preoperative enteroscopy]. Presse Med 1989;18:847 [French].
76. Daum S, Collier C, Mulder CJ, et al. Refractory celiac disease. Best Pract Res Clin Gastroenterol 2005;19:413–24.
77. Taylor AC, Buttigieg RJ, Mc Donald IG, et al. Prospective assessement of the diagnostic and therapeutic impact of small bowel push and pull enteroscopy. Endoscopy 2003;35:951–6.
78. May A, Ell C. European experiences with push-and-pull enteroscopy in double-balloon technique (double-balloon enteroscopy). Gastrointest Endosc Clin N Am 2006;16:377–82.
79. Kita H, Yamamoto H, Yano T, et al. Double balloon endoscopy in two hundred fifty cases for the diagnosis and treatment of small intestinal disorders. Inflammopharmacology 2007;15(2):74–7.
80. Hadithi M, Al-toma A, Oudejans J, et al. The value of double balloon enteroscopy in patients with refractory celiac disease. Am J Gastroenterol 2007; 102:987–96.

81. May A, Nachbar L, Schneider M, et al. Prospective comparison of push enteroscopy and push-and-pull enteroscopy in patients with suspected small-bowel bleeding. Am J Gastroenterol 2006;101:2016–24.
82. Yamamoto H, Sekine Y, Sato Y, et al. Total enteroscopy with a nonsurgical steerable double-balloon method. Gastrointest Endosc 2001;53:216–20.
83. Maiden L, Elliott T, McLaughlin SD. A blinded pilot comparison of capsule endoscopy and small bowel histology in unresponsive celiac disease. Dig Dis Sci 2009; 54(6):1280–3.
84. Daum S, Wahnschaffe U, Glasenapp R, et al. Capsule endocopy in refractory celiac disease. Endoscopy 2007;39:455–8.
85. van Weyenberg SJB, Mallant M, Al-Toma A, et al. Magnetic resonance enteroclysis in adult coeliac disease: findings and comparisons between subtypes with different prognosis. OP-G-239. Gut 2007;56(Suppl 3):A56.
86. Hadithi M, Mallant M, Oudejans J, et al. ^{18}F-FDG PET versus CT for the detection of enteropathy-associated T-Cell lymphoma in refractory celiac disease. J Nucl Med 2006;47:1622–7.
87. Verbeek WHM, Schreurs MWJ, Visser OJ, et al. Novel approaches in the management of refractory coeliac disease. Exp Rev Clin Immunol 2008;4:205–19.

Small Bowel Tumors

Shirley C. Paski, MSc, MD, Carol E. Semrad, MD*

KEYWORDS

• Small bowel tumor • Enteroscopy • Capsule endoscopy

Small bowel tumors are rare, accounting for only 2% of all primary gastrointestinal tumors.[1] Several theories to account for the scarcity of small bowel tumors have been hypothesized, including rapid intestinal transit time, dilution of carcinogens in chyme, reduced bacterial load limiting conversion of bile acids to carcinogens, rapid turnover of the small intestinal epithelium, conversion of dietary benzpyrene by benzpyrene hydroxylase into less toxic moieties, and protection by high levels of secretory IgA.[1,2] Benign small bowel tumors are often asymptomatic and cured at the time of resection. In contrast, malignant primary small bowel tumors have a poor prognosis and have often metastasized by the time they are discovered.[3] Videocapsule endoscopy (VCE) and new radiologic imaging techniques have greatly facilitated detection of small bowel tumors. Double-balloon enteroscopy (DBE) and newer overtube-assisted enteroscopes can detect small bowel tumors missed at VCE and allow for tissue sampling, tumor marking, and endoscopic resection when possible.

This article describes the general features of small bowel tumors, clinical presentation, and diagnostic tests followed by a description of the more common tumor types and their management.

EPIDEMIOLOGY

Epidemiologic studies on small bowel tumors are limited, in part, due to their low incidence. Benign small bowel tumors are usually asymptomatic, which makes the precise incidence difficult to determine. Older studies including 22,810 and 2648 autopsies found 35 and 22 benign small bowel tumors, respectively, for an incidence of 0.15% to 0.83%.[4,5] Amongst patients with symptomatic benign small bowel tumors, the most common types are leiomyomas, lipomas, adenomas, and angiomas.[6] In autopsy series, benign tumors are far more common than malignant tumors, accounting for up to 75% of all small bowel tumors.[7] However, the latter are more commonly reported in the medical literature.

The global incidence of primary small bowel cancers is highly variable. Incidence rates are highest in North America and Western Europe, particularly amongst African American men. Incidence rates are lowest in Asia and the Middle East. In most

Section of Gastroenterology, Department of Internal Medicine, University of Chicago Medical Center, 5841 S Maryland Avenue, MC 4076, Chicago, IL 60637, USA
* Corresponding author.
E-mail address: csemrad@medicine.bsd.uchicago.edu (C.E. Semrad).

Gastrointest Endoscopy Clin N Am 19 (2009) 461–479
doi:10.1016/j.giec.2009.04.012 giendo.theclinics.com
1052-5157/09/$ – see front matter © 2009 Elsevier Inc. All rights reserved.

countries, men have a slightly higher incidence compared with women.[2] Incidence increases with age, the mid-60s being the median age of diagnosis. Carcinoids (44.3%) and adenocarcinoma (32.6%) are the most common primary cancers of the small bowel, followed by lymphomas (14.8%) and sarcomas (8.3%).[3] Adenocarcinomas most commonly occur in the duodenum or proximal jejunum, carcinoids and lymphomas in the ileum. Recent studies show that the incidence of small bowel cancer is increasing in the United States. Using the National Cancer Institute's Surveillance Epidemiology and End Results (SEER) 9 Incidence database, Bilimoria and colleagues[3] found that the average annual age-adjusted incidence of small bowel cancer nearly doubled from 11.8 cases per million in 1973 to 22.7 cases per million in 2004. The greatest increase was seen in carcinoids, followed by lymphomas and adenocarcinomas. Gastrointestinal stromal tumor incidence has remained steady. Despite these increases, primary small bowel malignancies remain rare with only 6110 new cases and 1110 deaths in the United States in 2008.[8]

Metastatic cancers to the small bowel are more common than primary cancers. They occur by direct invasion from adjacent organs or by distant metastasis.[9]

RISK FACTORS

Several medical and genetic conditions are associated with an increased risk for developing small bowel cancer, including celiac disease, Crohn disease, polyposis syndromes, and hereditary nonpolyposis colorectal cancer. Dietary factors have been associated with small bowel tumors, although study results are inconsistent.

Inflammatory diseases of the small bowel are associated with an increased risk of malignancy. Celiac disease is associated with increased risk for developing small bowel lymphoma and adenocarcinoma. The incidence of malignancy has been reported to be highest within the first 3 to 4 years of diagnosis and in those with poor adherence to a gluten-free diet.[10] Early diagnosis and strict adherence to a gluten-free diet may lessen the risk of small bowel malignancy in celiac disease.[11,12] Crohn disease is associated with an increased risk of developing adenocarcinoma and, to a lesser extent, lymphoma of the small bowel. Increased risk is associated with male gender, extended duration of disease, location in the small bowel, strictures, and fistulas.[13]

Polyposis syndromes and hereditary nonpolyposis colorectal cancer (HNPCC) have been associated with an increased risk for small bowel cancer. New enteroscopy technologies that allow examination of the entire small bowel and therapeutics have the potential for improved surveillance and therapy.[14,15]

Studies exploring the relationship between diet and environmental factors and small bowel cancer have yielded mixed results. Several case-control studies have found a positive association between the development of small bowel cancer and increased consumption of red and processed meat,[16,17] sugar intake,[16] smoking, and alcohol.[16] Others found no relationship between smoking and alcohol consumption.[17,18] Prospective cohort studies found no relationship between red or processed meat and small bowel tumors, but did find a positive correlation between saturated fat and carcinoid,[19] and a negative correlation between whole grain fiber and small bowel cancer.[20] Further studies are needed to clarify the role of diet, if any, in small bowel cancer.

SYMPTOMS AND SIGNS

The diagnosis of small bowel tumors is often delayed because most are asymptomatic or have nonspecific symptoms during the early stages of development. Clinical symptoms reflect the tumor location and pathology. The most common clinical symptoms associated with small bowel tumors are related to obstruction and bleeding. Obstruction usually manifests as recurrent crampy abdominal pain. The pain is usually periumbilical or epigastric and occurs following meals. Some may experience associated bloating, nausea, or vomiting,[5,6,21] symptoms often noted in the much more common functional bowel disorders thereby causing diagnostic delay. Intussusception in adults is rare and most often occurs with lipomas and Peutz-Jeghers polyps.[22] Cases of volvulus have also been reported.[23]

Chronic occult bleeding is also a common clinical presentation of small bowel tumors. Severe bleeding is less common and typically involves tumors with a rich blood supply, such as leiomyomas, angiomas, and sarcomas. Weight loss, anorexia, and perforation are other presenting symptoms. Periampullary lesions may cause jaundice. Tumor spread to the retroperitoneum may manifest as back pain.[5,21]

Most patients have an unrevealing physical examination. A palpable mass may be present in the case of a large tumor. Cachexia, hepatomegaly, or ascites may be present in advanced metastatic disease. Physical findings occasionally suggest a specific tumor type, such as: buccal hyperpigmentation in Peutz-Jeghers syndrome; buccal and skin lesions in blue rubber bleb nevus syndrome; flushing, diarrhea, or a pulmonic stenosis murmur in carcinoid syndrome; or cutaneous angiomata in Rendu-Osler-Weber syndrome.[5,21,24]

Because small bowel tumors are rare and the sensitivity of clinical signs is low, astute clinicians must maintain a high index of suspicion and low threshold to order further investigations if presented with a patient who has a suggestive history.

DIAGNOSIS

The nonspecific symptoms of small bowel tumors often result in a long delay in diagnosis. A mean delay of up to 3 years from first symptoms to diagnosis of benign tumors and 18 months for malignant tumors has been reported.[9,25] Diagnosis is often made using a combination of laboratory, radiologic, and endoscopic techniques. Recent advances in radiologic and endoscopic imaging technologies now enable clinicians to visualize the entire small bowel (mucosa and wall). Using these new imaging modalities under the correct clinical circumstances has the potential to expedite the diagnosis of small bowel tumors using nonoperative techniques.

RADIOLOGIC IMAGING

Small Bowel Series (SBS)

In some centers with experienced GI radiologists, small bowel series continues to be used in the diagnosis of small bowel tumors. However, this imaging modality is falling out of favor as newer technologies are more sensitive at identifying small bowel tumors, allow simultaneous examination of abdominal organs, and are better tolerated.

Computed Tomographic Enterography and Enteroclysis

Computed tomographic (CT) enterography involves the rapid ingestion of diluted barium just before scanning. A major limitation is the inability of patients to consume a large amount of fluid in a short period of time. Delay in contrast ingestion or scan can result in incomplete bowel distention and limited study interpretation.[26] Enteroclysis overcomes this limitation by placing a nasojejunal catheter past the ligament of Treitz, which allows rapid filling of the intestine with contrast dye. Neutral enteral contrast is a sensitive method for detecting small bowel tumors as long as luminal distention is achieved.[27,28] False-positive readings usually result from incomplete distention, intestinal spasms, or functional invaginations.[29] Pilleul and colleagues[30] assessed 219 patients for possible small bowel tumors after negative findings on upper and lower endoscopy. Results were compared with intraoperative enteroscopy, surgery without resection, surgical or enteroscopic biopsy specimens, VCE, and clinical follow-up. CT enterography had an 84.7% sensitivity (95% CI, 75.5%, 93.9%) and 90.9% specificity (95% CI, 94.2%, 99.6%). Positive predictive value was 90.9% (95% CI, 83.3%, 98.5%) and negative predictive value 94.5% (95% CI, 91.1%, 97.9%). In addition, CT enterography/enteroclysis permits extraluminal visualization, which may provide valuable clues to the nature of the small bowel tumor, particularly in the case of suspected malignancy.

Magnetic Resonance Enterography and Enteroclysis

Magnetic resonance (MR) enterography and enteroclysis are similar to their CT counterparts, but avoid exposure to ionizing radiation. Adequate small bowel lumen distention is also essential. In some cases, it is possible to differentiate between different tumor types based on characteristics between the T1- and T2-weighted images.[31] Adenocarcinomas typically appear as a focal mass with an intra- and extraluminal growth or as a circumferential constricting lesion with luminal narrowing. Carcinoid tumors cause focal, nodular, asymmetric wall thickening or a smooth submucosal mass. Contrast markedly enhances primary carcinoid tumors. Gastrointestinal lymphomas can have a variety of appearances from polypoid lesions to large fungating masses to diffusely infiltrating, full thickness, mural thickening. Splenomegaly and mesenteric and retroperitoneal lymphadenopathy support the diagnosis.[32] In patients with celiac disease, a smooth marginal contour, diffuse segmental bowel loop aneurismal dilatation, and the absence of a distinct mesenteric or antimesenteric distribution are highly suggestive of the presence of enteropathy-associated T cell lymphoma.[33] Stromal tumors typically appear as a heterogeneously enhancing exophytic mass, often with regions of necrosis.

At present, the main limitations of MR enterography and enteroclysis are the lower resolution and greater motion artifact compared with CT. As MR technology improves, it will likely be preferred over CT imaging due to its lack of patient exposure to ionizing radiation.

Positron Emission Tomography

Positron emission tomography (PET) is a nuclear medicine technique using the tracer fluorine-18 fluorodeoxyglucose ([^{18}F]FDG) combined with CT or MR to identify anatomic areas of increased tissue metabolic activity. It is widely used for diagnosing and staging cancers and monitoring treatment. In a prospective study of patients with refractory celiac disease, [^{18}F]FDG PET was more sensitive than CT scan in detecting enteropathy = associated T cell lymphoma.[34] Isreal and colleagues[35] reported that [^{18}F]FDG PET identified foci of increased uptake in the small intestine that corresponded to metastasis of gastric and colon cancer. It is also useful for monitoring response to treatment of small bowel lymphoma[36] and gastrointestinal stromal tumor (GIST).[37,38] More studies are needed to determine the usefulness of PET in the clinical evaluation and staging of suspected small bowel tumors.

VIDEO CAPSULE ENDOSCOPY

The development of wireless VCE has enabled visualization of the entire small intestine in a noninvasive fashion that is well tolerated by patients. Several studies have assessed the diagnostic yield of capsule endoscopy (CE) compared with other small bowel imaging and endoscopic modalities. One meta-analysis found CE superior to push enteroscopy (63 versus 28%) and SBS (42 versus 6%) in detecting small bowel lesions in the setting of obscure GI bleeding.[39] In a review of 416 patients who underwent CE, in which 27 small bowel tumors were found, patients underwent an average of 4.6 negative investigations before VCE, including small bowel follow through or enteroclysis, push enteroscopy, or abdominal CT scan. The most common indication for a capsule study in these patients was obscure GI bleeding.[40]

CE has been shown to be useful in the diagnosis and surveillance of several specific small bowel tumors. In patients with gastrointestinal lymphoma, CE is useful to diagnose, determine the extent of small bowel disease, and assess efficacy of treatment.[41] Lymphomas or ulcerative jejunitis have been detected by CE in patients with type II refractory celiac disease.[42] Mata and colleagues[43] reported that CE was superior to SBS in the detection of Peutz-Jeghers and familial adenomatous polyps. The additional polyps found at CE contained low-grade dysplasia on resection by endoscopic polypectomy. In a similar study, Brown and colleagues[44] found that CE detected more clinically significant small bowel polyps (>1 cm) than SBS in patients with Peutz-Jeghers syndrome. Most patients preferred CE to SBS because of better comfort and convenience. Caspari and colleagues[45] compared the yield of CE to MR enterography in patients with either Peutz-Jeghers or familial adenomatous polyposis. The yield of detecting polyps >15 mm was similar with both modalities, whereas smaller polyps were seen more often with CE. Polyp location and size was more accurate by MR enterography.

Not all studies have found CE superior to other modalities at identifying small bowel tumors. CE is not superior to standard endoscopy in the detection of periampullary and duodenal polyps in familial adenomatous polyposis,[46] the most common site of malignancies in these patients. This finding may be due to rapid transit of the CE through the duodenal sweep.

Limitations of CE include capsule retention, poor localization of lesions, lack of tissue sampling, and missed small bowel lesions. The risk of capsule retention is increased in patients with small bowel tumors. Rondonotti and colleagues[47] found the rate of capsule retention to be 12/124 (9.8%). The polyp/mass or stenosis created by the small bowel tumor was the location of capsule retention in each of these cases. Removal was by push enteroscopy or surgery. No acute obstructions occurred. This retention rate is significantly greater than the 1.4% to 2.5% reported in other studies.[48,49] The use of a patency capsule in patients at higher risk for obstruction, such as suspected small bowel tumors, may lessen retention risk.[50]

CE used early in the diagnostic workup for symptoms that are suspicious for small bowel disease is noninvasive and has the potential to diagnose small bowel tumors earlier in their course. However, the highest miss rate of lesions using CE are solitary small bowel mass lesions (18.6% versus 10% overall).[51] If the clinical suspicion for a small bowel tumor is high, further evaluation with radiologic imaging, deep enteroscopy, or intraoperative enteroscopy must be pursued. Further studies are needed to determine whether the early use of CE leads to improved outcomes and to clarify its role in the surveillance of treated small bowel tumors.

ENTEROSCOPY

Push enteroscopy usually reaches the upper jejunum, to an average depth of 80 cm, and is useful for identification and sampling of tumors in the proximal jejunum.[52]

Double-balloon enteroscopy (DBE), also known as push-and-pull enteroscopy, is a new technique that allows visualization of the entire small bowel and therapeutics.[53] This is accomplished using a 2-m enteroscope inserted through an overtube, each with an inflatable balloon attached to its end. Sequential inflation and deflation of the balloons on the enteroscope and overtube allows advancement into new segments of small bowel and pleating of the bowel already examined on the back of the overtube. Depth of insertion into the small bowel from the oral route is significantly greater compared with push enteroscopy (230 cm versus 80 cm).[51]

In a meta-analysis study, the diagnostic yield for small bowel lesions was comparable using DBE and CE (57% [n = 360] and 60% [n = 397], respectively).[54] DBE has identified small bowel mass lesions that were missed on CE.[55] Missed lesions included adenocarcinomas, carcinoids, and stromal tumors. It is a valuable tool for obtaining a histologic diagnosis, marking lesions before surgery, and performing therapeutic interventions such as polyp resection, stenting, or hemostasis. Case studies have shown that biopsies obtained from DBE have been useful for diagnosing lymphangiectasia,[56] mantle cell lymphoma,[57] marginal cell lymphoma,[58] follicular cell lymphoma,[59] and carcinoid.[60] The diagnostic yield of DBE is highest in patients who have positive findings on previous radiologic studies, CE, or octreotide scan.[61] In one prospective study, DBE had a lower success rate in achieving total transit through the small bowel compared with CE (50% versus 73.3%, respectively).[62] Success rates for total enteroscopy using DBE vary and improvement requires a significant learning curve.[63] The main limitation of DBE is incomplete studies particularly in patients with previous abdominal surgery or large body habitus, invasiveness, and the long duration of the procedure (1–3 hours).

Since the development of DBE two other technologies for deep small bowel enteroscopy have emerged. Single-balloon enteroscopy (SBE) is similar to the double-balloon method with equivalent diagnostic yield reported in one study.[64] Spiral enteroscopy (SE) uses an overtube with spiral ridges. Clockwise spinning of the overtube allows faster visualization of the small bowel compared with DBE, on average 36 minutes in one small study.[65] In a larger study by Akerman and colleagues,[66] two patients had small bowel tumors. In both cases, endoscopic biopsies and tattooing of the tumor site were possible. Mucosal trauma with the passage of the spiral overtube is a potential concern if luminal projections such as small bowel mass lesions are present.[67] Spiral examination of the small bowel from the anal approach is not yet possible.

Diagnosis of small bowel tumors often requires multiple studies including radiologic imaging, CE, and balloon-assisted enteroscopy or SE. With these new technologies, the hope is that time from first symptom to diagnosis will decrease. A proposed approach for the diagnosis of small bowel tumors is presented in **Fig. 1**.

SMALL BOWEL TUMOR MORPHOLOGY, DIAGNOSIS, AND MANAGEMENT

Small bowel tumors are broadly classified as epithelial, mesenchymal, lymphoproliferative, or metastatic (**Table 1**). The more common tumors are described in the following sections.

Adenomas and Adenocarcinomas

Adenomas and adenocarcinomas arise from mucosal glands. Adenomas in the small intestine develop into adenocarcinoma in the same sequence as in the colon with mutations in k-ras, p53, and mismatch repair proteins. Approximately one third of solitary small bowel adenomas will transform into invasive carcinoma.[68] Small bowel

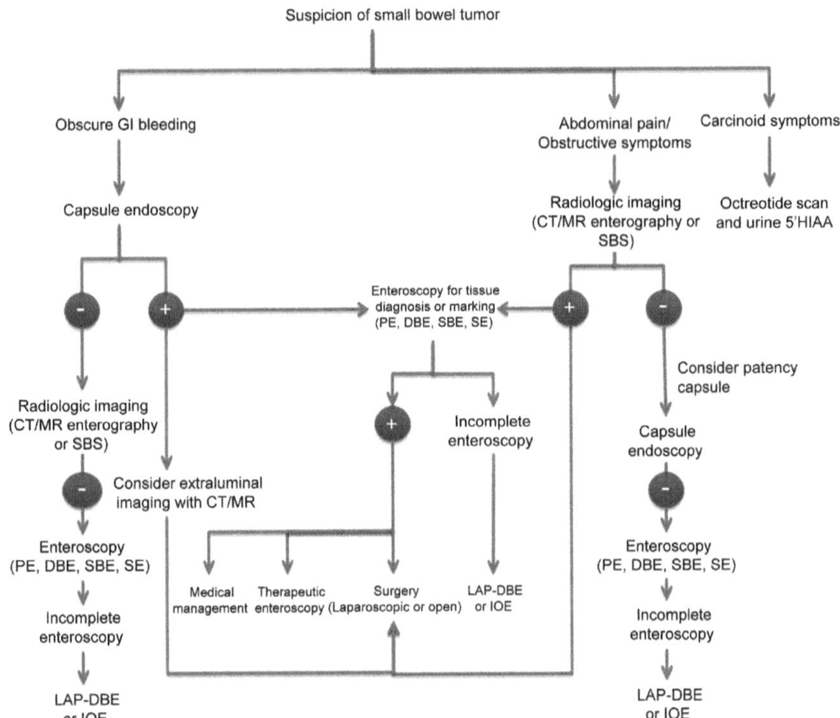

Fig. 1. Diagnostic approach to small bowel tumors.

adenocarcinoma is staged by the tumor-node-metastasis (TNM) method.[21] Most patients present with pain, obstruction, or bleeding, and 35% have metastatic disease at the time of diagnosis.[69] Proximal tumors are much more common with about 70% occurring in the duodenum and jejunum.[1] Surgical resection offers the only cure. Various adjuvant chemotherapy regimens have been attempted, most with 5-fluorouracil alone or in combination with other agents like doxorubicin, cisplatin, mitomycin C, cyclophosphamide, and oxaliplatin. One recent case report suggests bevicizumab may be promising.[70] In a retrospective study, 3-year survival and relapse-free survival rates after curative resection were 66.1% and 50.8%, respectively. Median survival of patients who received palliative chemotherapy was 8.0 months (95% CI, 3.5–12.4).[71] Overall median survival in a more recent retrospective study by Dabaja and colleagues[69] was 20 months and the 5-year overall survival rate was 25%. Cancer-directed surgery, presentation with early stage disease, and the absence of lymph node involvement were associated with improved overall survival.[69]

The detection of primary small bowel adenocarcinomas is usually by radiologic imaging or CE when presenting as obscure GI bleeding. However, even fungating

Table 1
Classification of small bowel tumors

	Cell Type	Benign	Malignant
Epithelial tumors	Glandular	Adenomas	Adenocarcinoma
	Neuroendocrine	Well-differentiated neuroendocrine tumor (carcinoid)	Well-differentiated neuroendocrine carcinoma (malignant carcinoid) Poorly differentiated neuroendocrine carcinoma
Mesenchymal tumors	Vasculature	Hemangioma Lymphangioma Angiomatoses	Angiosarcoma Kaposi sarcoma
	Adipocytes Spindle cells	Lipoma GIST Inflammatory myofibroblastic tumors Desmoid tumors	Liposarcoma GIST Inflammatory myofibroblastic tumors Desmoid tumors Malignant fibrous histiocytomas
	Smooth muscle cells	Leiomyoma Hamartoma	Leiomyosarcoma
	Nerve cells	Schwannoma Neurofibroma Perineuroma Peragangliomas	Schwannoma Malignant peripheral nerve sheath tumors Peragangliomas
Lymphoproliferative disorder	B cell	—	Diffuse large B cell lymphoma MALT lymphoma Mantle cell lymphoma Burkitt lymphoma Immunoproliferative small cell disease
	T cell	—	Enteropathy-associated T cell lymphoma
Metastatic	—	—	Direct invasion: ovarian, uterine, cervical, colon, gastric, pancreas, liver, kidney, adrenal
	—	—	Distant metastasis: melanoma, lung, breast, kidney, testes

Abbreviations: GIST, gastrointestinal stromal tumor; MALT, mucosa-associated lymphoid tissue.

intraluminal lesions may be missed by CE due to compression or cincturing of the bowel wall by tumor or intraluminal blood that obscures visualization. Push enteroscopy may fail to reach proximal lesions due to fixed bowel angulations at the tumor site. Therefore, balloon enteroscopy, with the overtube as a straightener, may be needed for detection of even proximal small bowel tumors. Tattoo at the tumor site may facilitate resection, particularly by the laparoscopic approach, although most tumors are visible serosally.

Carcinoid

Carcinoid tumors arise from argentaffin cells. They are most frequent in the gastrointestinal tract (67%), particularly the ileum.[3] Carcinoids often stimulate a fibrotic reaction in the surrounding tissue that can lead to functional obstruction or vascular compromise. They appear as submucosal mass lesions, sometimes with ulcerations (**Fig. 2**A). The most common presentation of small bowel carcinoid tumors is intermittent intestinal obstruction or vague abdominal pain.[72] Typical carcinoid syndrome is usually caused by metastatic midgut carcinoids that secrete high levels of serotonin. Serotonin release results in the symptoms of flushing, diarrhea, abdominal pain, and bronchospasm. Atypical carcinoid syndrome is usually associated with foregut tumors. The flushing tends to be patchier and associated with pruritus due to

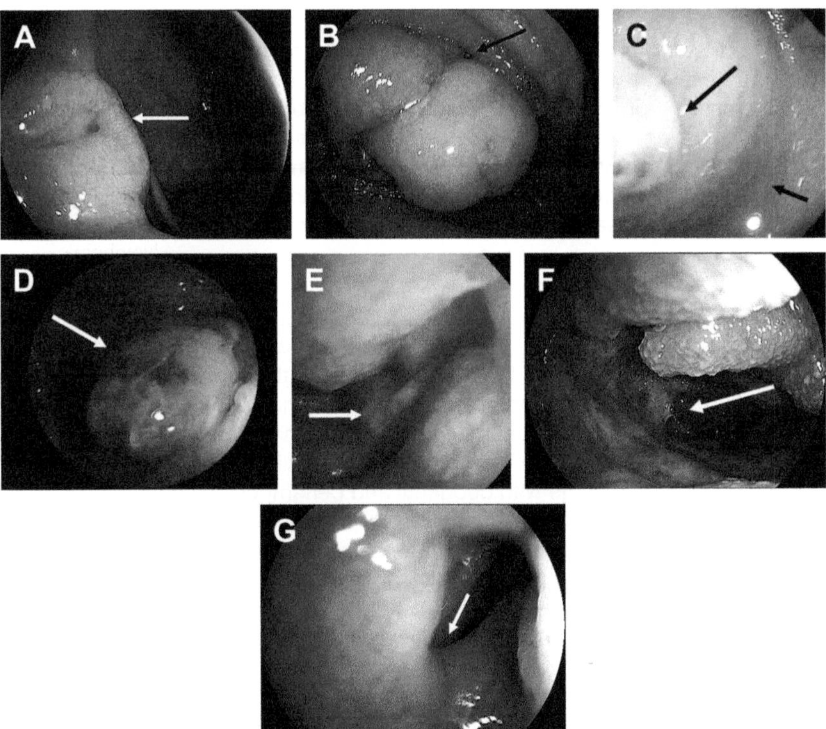

Fig. 2. Examples of small bowel tumors. (*A*) Ulcerating ileal carcinoid, (*B*) large intussuscepting Peutz-Jeghers polyp in jejunum, (*C*) endocentric ileal GIST with ulcerated tip and compressed surrounding mucosa, (*D*) mid-small bowel hemangioma with exudative-appearing surface, (*E*) ulcerating lymphoma in mid-ileum, (*F*) ulcerating jejunal adenocarcinoma metastatic from the lung, (*G*) jejunal metastatic melanoma.

histamine excess. Carcinoids may also secrete other bioactive amines, such as dopamine or norepinephrine or corticotropin, gastrin, vasopressin, and calcitonin, that dictate symptoms. Although 86% of small bowel carcinoids secrete seretonin, the presentation with typical carcinoid syndrome is rare. Seventy-five percent of primary small bowel carcinoids are <1.5 cm at the time of diagnosis and about 30% already have multifocal disease at the time of diagnosis.[73]

Diagnosis of carcinoid syndrome is made by a history of flushing, diarrhea, and measuring an elevated level of 5-hydroxyindoleacetic acid (5-HIAA) in 24-hour urine. Somatostatin analog scintigraphy (octreotide scan) is extremely useful for detecting primary and metastatic tumors as 80% to 90% of carcinoids express high levels of high-affinity receptors to somatostatin.[74]

Combined endoscopic and radiologic imaging techniques are usually needed to localize and stage the tumors. It is sometimes difficult to determine whether abdominal lesions are inside or outside the small bowel. CE is useful in detecting small bowel carcinoids.[75] However, it does not allow tissue sampling and is poor at localizing lesions particularly deep in the small bowel. Balloon-assisted enteroscopy of the entire small bowel may be necessary to detect, take a sample for biopsy, and tattoo multifocal lesions for surgical resection. Biopsies are not always diagnostic if tumors are deep in the submucosa. At present, endoscopic resection of carcinoid tumors in the small bowel is not recommended due to their submucosal location and risk of perforation. However, with the advancement of endoscopic small bowel therapeutics, endoscopic management of some lesions may be possible in the future.

Surgery is the only curative therapy for carcinoid tumors. Before surgical resection, somatostatin analog therapy should be administered to reduce the risk of carcinoid crisis that results from high levels of mediator under the stress of anesthesia or surgery.[76] If a patient is asymptomatic, it may be reasonable to undergo a period of observation. For those with symptoms, a somatostatin analog (octreotide or lantreotide) is effective in controlling flushing and diarrhea in most patients with carcinoid syndrome.[77,78] The 5-year survival rate for small bowel carcinoids is 55% to 60%.[73]

Polyposis Syndromes

Familial adenomatous polyposis (FAP) is an autosomal dominant condition due to a mutation in the APC gene and is characterized by the formation of hundreds of adenomas in the small bowel and colon. Within the small bowel, most polyps are in the duodenum and proximal jejunum.[79] The risk of small bowel adenocarcinoma is significantly increased,[80,81] particularly in the periampullary area of the duodenum.[82] Following colectomy, patients with duodenal and periampullary adenomas are prone to developing adenomas in the ileal pouch. Upper endoscopy with end- and side-viewing instruments is recommended for screening around the time of consideration for colectomy or early in the third decade of life.[83] CE has been reported to miss duodenal and periampullary lesions in patients with FAP. The role of CE for surveillance of the remaining small bowel is unknown. Capsule retention may occur in those with known mesenteric desmoids.

Peutz-Jeghers syndrome is an autosomal recessive condition characterized by benign hamartomatous polyps of the gastrointestinal tract and a characteristic buccal pigmentation. A recent meta-analysis found up to a 13% lifetime risk for the development of small intestinal cancer, which corresponds to a relative risk 520 times that of the general population.[14] Based on this finding, surveillance for small bowel polyps is recommended using either CE or MR/CT enterography at the time of diagnosis and, if positive, repeated every 2 years from the age of 8 years.[84] CE is better tolerated and avoids radiation exposure, but imaging studies are superior to estimate polyp size and location.

DBE has revolutionized the management of Peutz-Jeghers small bowel polyps. Endoscopic resection of large polyps (>1 cm) deep in the small bowel is now possible but requires significant technical skill. Positioning of polyps for resection can be difficult. The risk of bleeding is high (3.3%) for small bowel polypectomy using DBE, especially in polyps greater than 3 cm in size.[85] In patients with large polyps not reached because of fixed bowel due to previous resection and in those with multiple large polyps, laparoscopic-assisted DBE has been reported to be successful in removing all large polyps in 1 treatment session.[86] Surgical assistance helps with adhesiolysis, bowel pleating, positioning polyps for endoscopic resection, and immediate management of complications.

Hereditary nonpolyposis colorectal cancer (HNPCC) is characterized by mutations in genes HMLH1 and HMLH2 involved in DNA mismatch repair. The risk of small bowel adenocarcinoma is increased 25-fold in HNPCC.[15] However, there is no evidence to support screening at present.[83]

Gastrointestinal Stromal Tumor

GIST are rare tumors that originate from the interstitial cell of Cajal, an intestinal pacemaker cell in the normal myenteric plexus.[87] GISTs appear as submucosal masses that grow in an endocentric or exocentric pattern, and are sometimes ulcerated (**Fig. 2**C). Previously classified as leiomyomas, leiomyosarcomas, or schwannomas, GISTs are now recognized as a distinct group of mesenchymal tumors that are C-kit and CD34 positive. Mutations in the KIT gene (CD 117) lead to overexpression of the tyrosine kinase KIT protein, which seems to drive the neoplastic growth. GISTs can develop throughout the entire GI tract and are most common in the stomach (60%) followed by the jejunum and ileum (30%), duodenum (4%–5%), rectum (4%), colon and appendix (1%–2%), and esophagus (<1%).[88] Microscopic GISTs are also common in the general population and have been found in up to 23% of adults >50 years at autopsy.[89] Risk of an aggressive clinical course is based on tumor size and mitotic count: low for tumors less than 2 cm with a mitotic count less than 5 per 50 high power fields, and high for tumors greater than 10 cm with a mitotic count greater than 10 per 50 high power fields.[90] Coagulative necrosis, ulceration, diffuse nuclear atypia, and epithelioid cytology are also factors associated with unfavorable outcomes in patients with small intestine GISTs.[91]

GISTs in the small bowel can grow to a large size with no clinical symptoms. With large tumors, diagnosis is easily made on abdominal CT scan. In patients presenting with obscure GI bleeding, these tumors may be missed at CE due to incomplete studies or cincturing of the intestinal wall (**Fig. 3**). Reaching these lesions by balloon-assisted enteroscopy may also be difficult as the weight of the tumor may fix the bowel and limit endoscope advancement. Radiologic imaging remains an important modality for detection of small bowel GISTs, particularly in younger patients with obscure GI bleeding.

Surgical resection is the preferred treatment of GISTs if technically feasible.[92] Imatinib (Gleevec™) is a therapeutic agent that reduces C-kit tyrosine kinase activity and seems to be effective in the treatment of nonresectable or metastatic GIST and also in combination with surgery.[92–95] Sinitinib malate (Sutent) is a multitargeted tyrosine kinase inhibitor that has been used to control progressive disease in patients with imatinib-resistant GIST.[96]

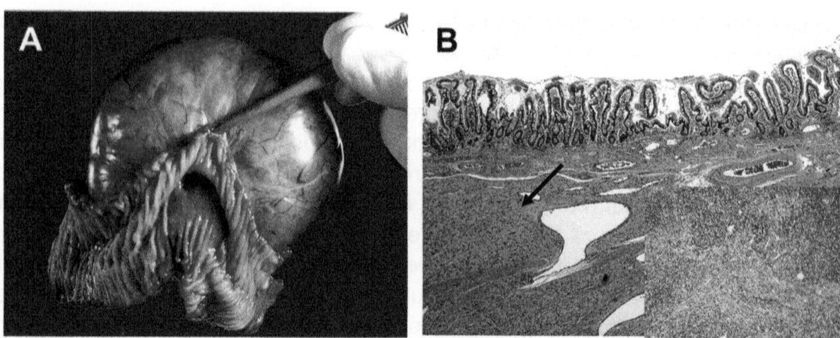

Fig. 3. (*A*) Large ileal GIST missed by CE and DBE. Mucosal ulceration site is recessed in the bowel walled cinctured by the tumor. (*B*) Stromal tumor cells nested beneath the epithelium. Inset shows cells that stained positive for C-kit, diagnostic of GIST.

Select Mesenchymal Tumors

Lipomas are benign tumors that arise from the submucosal adipose tissue and expand with compression of the lumen. Lipomas typically present in the ileum with symptoms of chronic intermittent obstruction or bleeding due to ulceration. Myxoid liposarcomas comprise about 30% to 35% of liposarcomas and are characterized by either t(12;16)(q13;p11) or t(12;22)(q13;q12) translocation. Fibromas and fibrosarcomas arise from fibroblasts.[6,21]

Vascular Tumors

Benign vascular tumors of the gastrointestinal tract are most commonly found in the small bowel. They present from infancy to elderly adult life. Hemangiomas and angiosarcomas arise from the vasculature and may be capillary, cavernous, or mixed. Hemangiomas appear as well circumscribed or encapsulated submucosal mass lesions, sometimes with an exudative surface (**Fig. 2**D). They can involve skin, subcutaneous tissue, and the GI tract as in the blue rubber bleb nevus syndrome. Bleeding is the most common presentation.

Detection of vascular tumors has improved since the introduction of CE and DBE. Balloon-assisted enteroscopy has the advantage of tattoo placement for laparoscopic or open surgical resection. There are two reports of successful endoscopic management of blue rubber bleb hemangiomas using snare polypectomy and argon plasma coagulation, one in the setting of intraoperative enteroscopy and the other using DBE.[97,98]

Lymphoproliferative Disorders

The gastrointestinal tract is the most common extranodal site of lymphoma with the small intestine accounting for approximately one third of these cases. Most gastrointestinal lymphomas are of B cell origin, including B cell lymphoma of mucosa-associated lymphoid tissue (MALT) type, diffuse large B cell lymphoma, mantle cell lymphoma, follicular lymphoma, Burkitt lymphoma, and immunoproliferative lymphoma. T cell lymphomas are less common and are usually associated with celiac disease.[99]

B cell lymphoproliferative disorders

B cell lymphoma of the MALT type is usually found in the stomach with only rare case reports of small bowel involvement in the medical literature. Similar to its gastric counterpart, MALT lymphoma of the small intestine may be associated with infection with *Helicobacter pylori* and there are reports of histologic remission after eradication of *H pylori* with antibiotics.[100] Diffuse large B cell lymphoma is the most common subtype of non-Hodgkin lymphoma. Stage at diagnosis is a key prognostic factor. Stage 1 disease is curable in 75% of cases with surgery and radiation of the abdomen. In more advanced disease, combination chemotherapy with cyclophosphamide, doxorubicin, vincristine, prednisone, rituximab (CHOP-R) is the standard regimen with or without radiation.[101] Post-transplant lymphoproliferative disorder (PTLD) is one of the complications of immunosuppression following solid organ or hematopoietic stem cell transplant. PTLD is usually associated with the Epstein Barr virus and most commonly occurs within 1 year of transplant.[102]

Follicular lymphoma is an indolent lymphoma characterized by t(14:18) translocation and rearrangement of the BCL2 gene in most cases. Primary follicular lymphoma of the small intestine is rare and accounts for only 1% to 3% of lymphomas in the GI tract. In one case series, the estimated 5-year disease-free survival rate was 62% and the median disease-free survival rate was 69 months.[103] Burkitt lymphoma is an extremely aggressive lymphoma characterized by translocation of the MYC gene and one of the three immunoglobulin genes. In the case of endemic Burkitt lymphoma, the Epstein Barr virus and malaria are associated with most cases. Burkitt lymphoma is also associated with HIV infection.[104]

Immunoproliferative lymphoma, also known as immunoproliferative small intestinal disease or alpha chain disease, is a MALT subtype characterized by plasma cell infiltration of the bowel wall, leading to malabsorption and protein-losing enteropathy. Immunoproliferative lymphoma occurs only in developing countries, accounting for one third of GI lymphoma in the Middle East. Infection with *Campylobacter jejuni* is associated with immunoproliferative lymphoma and early stage disease is often responsive to antibiotic treatment.[105]

CE has been reported to be useful in the diagnosis of small bowel lymphomas.[41] Their appearance at CE has been described as ulcerated, nodular, mucosal atrophy, or white plaques. DBE allows tissue sampling of lesions deep in the small bowel (**Fig. 2**E). One of the major reasons for a biopsy of ulcerating or nodular lesions in the small bowel remains assessment for lymphoma because this may change the management from surgical to medical. Taking multiple endoscopic biopsies provides sufficient material to diagnose lymphoma in nearly all cases.[99] There is increased risk for perforation in the setting of ulcerating lymphoma.

T cell lymphoproliferative disorders

Enteropathy-associated T cell lymphoma (EATL) are less common than B cell lymphomas and are typically associated with celiac disease. In a study of a Dutch population, the crude incidence was 0.1 per 100,000 and slightly higher in older individuals with the mean age of diagnosis of 64 years. Most EATLs were located in the proximal small intestine.[106] A small study of 32 patients with refractory celiac disease showed that 4/9 patients with type II refractory disease had EATL.[107] Refractory celiac disease type II is characterized by T cell antigen loss (CD8 or T cell receptor-[beta]), T cell clonality, or both abnormalities in biopsy specimens. The development of EATL in patients with refractory celiac disease type II is associated with high morbidity and mortality with an overall 5-year survival rate of only 8%.[108]

The diagnosis of small bowel lymphoma should be entertained in celiac patients who do not improve on a gluten-free diet or develop recurrent gastrointestinal symptoms, anemia, or weight loss. Evaluation for small bowel lymphoma should be part of the diagnostic workup for refractory celiac disease or to monitor EATL. CE and DBE are effective at detecting ulcerating jejunitis, lymphomas, and EATL;[109] DBE provides tissue diagnosis.

Metastatic Tumors

Secondary small bowel cancers occur either by direct invasion from adjacent organs or by distant metastasis. Direct invasion may occur from the stomach, pancreas, liver, kidneys, adrenal glands, uterus, ovaries, cervix, or mesentery. Distant metastasis spreads from melanoma, breast, lung, kidney, and testes. Melanoma is the most common tumor to metastasize to the small bowel.

Primary and metastatic tumors can be difficult to distinguish based on endoscopic appearance (**Fig. 2**F, G). Features suggestive of metastatic disease include evidence of cancer elsewhere by history or imaging, large lesions that protrude from the external surface, multiple lesions, or the presence of extensive lymphatic involvement.[110]

SUMMARY

Although rare, small bowel tumors may cause significant morbidity and mortality if left undetected. New endoscopic modalities allow full examination of the small bowel with improved diagnosis. However, isolated mass lesions may be missed by CE or incomplete balloon-assisted enteroscopy. Therefore the use of radiologic imaging and intraoperative enteroscopy for diagnosis should not be forgotten. Endoscopic resection of small bowel polyps and certain vascular tumors is possible but requires proper training. Advances in endoscopic tools are likely to broaden the endoscopic management of small bowel tumors.

REFERENCES

1. Schottenfeld D, Beebe-Dimmer JL, Vigneau FD. The epidemiology and pathogenesis of neoplasia in the small intestine. Ann Epidemiol 2009;19(1):58–69.
2. Haselkorn T, Whittemore A, Lilienfeld D. Incidence of small bowel cancer in the United States and worldwide: geographic, temporal, and racial differences. Cancer Causes Control 2005;16(7):781–7.
3. Bilimoria KY, Bentrem DJ, Wayne JD, et al. Small bowel cancer in the United States changes in epidemiology, treatment, and survival over the last 20 years. Ann Surg 2009;249(1):63–71.
4. Shandalow SL. Benign tumors of the small intestine. Arch Surg 1955;71(5):761–7.
5. Myhre J. Diagnosis of small-bowel tumors. Am J Dig Dis 1963;8(11):916–22.
6. Wilson J, Melvin D, Gray G, et al. Benign small bowel tumor. Ann Surg 1975;181(2):247–50.
7. O'Riordan B, Vilor M, Herrera L. Small bowel tumors: an overview. Dig Dis 1996;14(4):245–57.
8. American Cancer Society. Cancer facts & figures 2008. Atlanta (GA): American Cancer Society; 2008.
9. Gill SS, Heuman DM, Mihas AA. Small intestinal neoplasms. J Clin Gastroenterol 2001;33(4):267–82.
10. Corrao G, Corazza G, Bagnardi V, et al. Mortality in patients with coeliac disease and their relatives: a cohort study. Lancet 2001;358(9279):356–61.
11. Collin P, Reunala T, Pukkala E, et al. Coeliac disease – associated disorders and survival. Gut 1994;35(9):1215–8.
12. Logan R, Rifkind E, Turner I, et al. Mortality in celiac disease. Gastroenterology 1989;97(2):265–71.

13. Feldstein RC, Sood S, Katz S. Small bowel adenocarcinoma in Crohn's disease. Inflamm Bowel Dis 2008;14(8):1154–7.
14. Giardiello FM, Brensinger JD, Tersmette AC, et al. Very high risk of cancer in familial Peutz-Jeghers syndrome. Gastroenterology 2000;119(6):1447–53.
15. Watson P, Lynch H. Extracolonic cancer in hereditary nonpolyposis colorectal cancer. Cancer 1993;71(3):677–85.
16. Wu AH, Yu MC, Mack TM. Smoking, alcohol use, dietary factors and risk of small intestinal adenocarcinoma. Int J Cancer 1997;70(5):512–7.
17. Chow WH, Linet MS, McLaughlin JK, et al. Risk factors for small intestine cancer. Cancer Causes & Control 1993;4(2):163–9.
18. Negri E, Bosetti C, La Vecchia C, et al. Risk factors for adenocarcinoma of the small intestine. Int J Cancer 1999;82(2):171–4.
19. Cross AJ, Leitzmann MF, Subar AF, et al. A prospective study of meat and fat intake in relation to small intestinal cancer. Cancer Res 2008;68(22):9274–9.
20. Schatzkin A, Park Y, Leitzmann MF, et al. Prospective study of dietary fiber, whole grain foods, and small intestinal cancer. Gastroenterology 2008;135(4):1163–7.
21. Sleisenger MH, Feldman M, Friedman LS, et al. Sleisenger & Fordtran's gastrointestinal and liver disease: pathophysiology, diagnosis, management. 8th edition. Philadelphia: Saunders Elsevier; 2006.
22. Chiang J, Lin Y. Tumor spectrum of adult intussusception. J Surg Oncol 2008; 98(6):444–7.
23. Sheen A, Drake I, George P. A small bowel volvulus caused by a mesenteric lipoma: report of a case. Surg Today 2003;33(8):617–9.
24. Flutter L. Peutz-Jegher syndrome. Arch Dis Child 2008;93(2):163.
25. Gupta S. Primary tumors of the small bowel: a clinicopathological study of 58 cases. J Surg Oncol 1982;20(3):161–7.
26. Dave-Verma H, Moore S, Singh A, et al. Computed tomographic enterography and enteroclysis: pearls and pitfalls. Curr Probl Diagn Radiol 2008;37(6):279–87.
27. Orjollet-Lecoanet C, Menard Y, Martins A, et al. L'entéroscanner: une nouvelle méthode d'exploration du grêle. J Radiol 2000;81(6):618–27.
28. Romano S, De Lutio E, Rollandi G, et al. Multidetector computed tomography enteroclysis (MDCT-E) with neutral enteral and IV contrast enhancement in tumor detection. Eur Radiol 2005;15(6):1178–83.
29. Kermarrec E, Barbary C, Corby S, et al. [CT enteroclysis: a pictorial essay] [in French]. J Radiol 2007;88(2):235–50 [French].
30. Pilleul F, Penigaud M, Milot L, et al. Possible small-bowel neoplasms: contrast-enhanced and water-enhanced multidetector CT enteroclysis. Radiology 2006; 241(3):796–801.
31. Masselli G, Gualdi G. Evaluation of small bowel tumors: MR enteroclysis. Abdom Imaging 2008, in press.
32. Chou C, Chen L, Sheu R, et al. MRI manifestations of gastrointestinal lymphoma. Abdom Imaging 1994;19(6):495–500.
33. Lohan D, Alhajeri A, Cronin C, et al. MR enterography of small-bowel lymphoma: potential for suggestion of histologic subtype and the presence of underlying celiac disease. AJR Am J Roentgenol 2008;190(2):287–93.
34. Hadithi M, Mallant M, Oudejans J, et al. 18F-FDG PET versus CT for the detection of enteropathy-associated T-cell lymphoma in refractory celiac disease. J Nucl Med 2006;47(10):1622–7.
35. Israel O, Yefremov N, Bar-Shalom R, et al. PET/CT detection of unexpected gastrointestinal foci of 18F-FDG uptake: incidence, localization patterns, and clinical significance. J Nucl Med 2005;46(5):758–62.

36. Kumar R, Xiu Y, Potenta S, et al. 18F-FDG PET for evaluation of the treatment response in patients with gastrointestinal tract lymphomas. J Nucl Med 2004; 45(11):1796–803.
37. Gayed I, Vu T, Iyer R, et al. The role of 18F-FDG PET in staging and early prediction of response to therapy of recurrent gastrointestinal stromal tumors. J Nucl Med 2004;45(1):17–21.
38. Ertuk M, Van den Abbeele AD. Infrequent tumors of the gastrointestinal tract including gastrointestinal stromal tumor (GIST). PET Clin 2008;3:207–15.
39. Triester S, Leighton J, Leontiadis G, et al. A meta-analysis of the yield of capsule endoscopy compared to other diagnostic modalities in patients with obscure gastrointestinal bleeding. Am J Gastroenterol 2005;100(11):2407–18.
40. Bailey A, Debinski H, Appleyard M, et al. Diagnosis and outcome of small bowel tumors found by capsule endoscopy: a three-center Australian experience. Am J Gastroenterol 2006;101(10):2237–43.
41. Flieger D, Keller R, May A, et al. Capsule endoscopy in gastrointestinal lymphomas. Endoscopy 2005;37(12):1174–80.
42. Daum S, Wahnschaffe U, Glasenapp R, et al. Capsule endoscopy in refractory celiac disease. Endoscopy 2007;39(5):455–8.
43. Mata A, Llach J, Castells A, et al. A prospective trial comparing wireless capsule endoscopy and barium contrast series for small-bowel surveillance in hereditary GI polyposis syndromes. Gastrointest Endosc 2005;61(6):721–5.
44. Brown G, Fraser C, Schofield G, et al. Video capsule endoscopy in Peutz-Jeghers syndrome: a blinded comparison with barium follow-through for detection of small-bowel polyps. Endoscopy 2006;38(4):385–90.
45. Caspari R, von Falkenhausen M, Krautmacher C, et al. Comparison of capsule endoscopy and magnetic resonance imaging for the detection of polyps of the small intestine in patients with familial adenomatous polyposis or with Peutz-Jeghers' syndrome. Endoscopy 2004;36(12):1054–9.
46. Iaquinto G, Fornasarig M, Quaia M, et al. Capsule endoscopy is useful and safe for small-bowel surveillance in familial adenomatous polyposis. Gastrointest Endosc 2008;67(1):61–7.
47. Rondonotti E, Pennazio M, Toth E, et al. Small-bowel neoplasms in patients undergoing video capsule endoscopy: a multicenter European study. Endoscopy 2008;40(6):488–95.
48. Li F, Gurudu S, De Petris G, et al. Retention of the capsule endoscope: a single-center experience of 1000 capsule endoscopy procedures. Gastrointest Endosc 2008;68(1):174–80.
49. Cheon J, Kim Y, Lee I, et al. Can we predict spontaneous capsule passage after retention? A nationwide study to evaluate the incidence and clinical outcomes of capsule retention. Endoscopy 2007;39(12):1046–52.
50. Delvaux M, Ben Soussan E, Laurent V, et al. Clinical evaluation of the use of the M2A patency capsule system before a capsule endoscopy procedure, in patients with known or suspected intestinal stenosis. Endoscopy 2005;37(9): 801–7.
51. Lewis B, Eisen G, Friedman S. A pooled analysis to evaluate results of capsule endoscopy trials. Endoscopy 2005;37(10):960–5.
52. May A, Nachbar L, Schneider M, et al. Prospective comparison of push enteroscopy and push-and-pull enteroscopy in patients with suspected small-bowel bleeding. Am J Gastroenterol 2006;101(9):2016–24.
53. Yamamoto H, Sugano K. A new method of enteroscopy – the double-balloon method. Can J Gastroenterol 2003;17(4):273–4.

54. Pasha S, Leighton J, Das A, et al. Double-balloon enteroscopy and capsule endoscopy have comparable diagnostic yield in small-bowel disease: a meta-analysis. Clin Gastroenterol Hepatol 2008;6(6):671–6.
55. Ross A, Mehdizadeh S, Tokar J, et al. Double balloon enteroscopy detects small bowel mass lesions missed by capsule endoscopy. Dig Dis Sci 2008;53(8): 2140–3.
56. Safatle-Ribeiro A, Iriya K, Couto D, et al. Secondary lymphangiectasia of the small bowel: utility of double balloon enteroscopy for diagnosis and management. Dig Dis 2008;26(4):383–6.
57. Hotta K, Oyama T, Kitamura Y, et al. Mantle cell lymphoma presenting as multiple lymphomatous polyposis spreading widely to the small intestine and diagnosed by double-balloon endoscopy. Endoscopy 2007;39(Suppl 1):E347–8.
58. Giri K, Sudar C, Arya M, et al. Diagnosis of marginal cell lymphoma of small intestine by double balloon enteroscopy. South Med J 2008;101(5):561–4.
59. Higuchi K, Komatsu K, Wakamatsu H, et al. Small intestinal follicular lymphoma with multiple tumor formations diagnosed by double-balloon enteroscopy. Intern Med 2007;46(11):705–9.
60. Yamagishi H, Fukui H, Shirakawa K, et al. Early diagnosis and successful treatment of small-intestinal carcinoid tumor: useful combination of capsule endoscopy and double-balloon endoscopy. Endoscopy 2007;39(Suppl 1):E243–4.
61. Bellutti M, Fry L, Schmitt J, et al. Detection of neuroendocrine tumors of the small bowel by double balloon enteroscopy. Dig Dis Sci 2008;54:1050–8.
62. Kameda N, Higuchi K, Shiba M, et al. A prospective, single-blind trial comparing wireless capsule endoscopy and double-balloon enteroscopy in patients with obscure gastrointestinal bleeding. J Gastroenterol 2008;43(6):434–40.
63. Gross S, Stark M. Initial experience with double-balloon enteroscopy at a U.S. center. Gastrointest Endosc 2008;67(6):890–7.
64. Tsujikawa T, Saitoh Y, Andoh A, et al. Novel single-balloon enteroscopy for diagnosis and treatment of the small intestine: preliminary experiences. Endoscopy 2008;40(1):11–5.
65. Akerman P, Agrawal D, Chen W, et al. Spiral enteroscopy: a novel method of enteroscopy by using the Endo-Ease Discovery SB overtube and a pediatric colonoscope. Gastrointest Endosc 2009;69(2):327–32.
66. Akerman P, Agrawal D, Cantero D, et al. Spiral enteroscopy with the new DSB overtube: a novel technique for deep peroral small-bowel intubation. Endoscopy 2008;40(12):974–8.
67. Schembre D, Ross A. Spiral enteroscopy: a new twist on overtube-assisted endoscopy. Gastrointest Endosc 2009;69(2):333–6.
68. Sellner F. Investigations on the significance of the adenoma-carcinoma sequence in the small bowel. Cancer 1990;66(4):702–15.
69. Dabaja BS, Suki D, Pro B, et al. Adenocarcinoma of the small bowel: presentation, prognostic factors, and outcome of 217 patients. Cancer 2004;101(3): 518–26.
70. Tsang H, Yau T, Khong PL, et al. Bevacizumab-based therapy for advanced small bowel adenocarcinoma. Gut 2008;57(11):1631–2.
71. Hong SH, Koh YH, Rho SY, et al. Primary adenocarcinoma of the small intestine: presentation, prognostic factors and clinical outcome. Jpn J Clin Oncol 2009; 39(1):54–61.
72. Burke A, Thomas R, Elsayed A, et al. Carcinoids of the jejunum and ileum: an immunohistochemical and clinicopathologic study of 167 cases. Cancer 1997; 79(6):1086–93.

73. Modlin I, Lye K, Kidd M. A 5-decade analysis of 13,715 carcinoid tumors. Cancer 2003;97(4):934–59.
74. Anthony L, Martin W, Delbeke D, et al. Somatostatin receptor imaging: predictive and prognostic considerations. Digestion 1996;57(Suppl 1):50–3.
75. van Tuyl S, van Noorden J, Timmer R, et al. Detection of small-bowel neuroendocrine tumors by video capsule endoscopy. Gastrointest Endosc 2006;64(1): 66–72.
76. Vaughan D, Brunner M. Anesthesia for patients with carcinoid syndrome. Int Anesthesiol Clin 1997;35(4):129–42.
77. Harris A, Redfern J. Octreotide treatment of carcinoid syndrome: analysis of published dose-titration data. Aliment Pharmacol Ther 1995;9(4):387–94.
78. O'Toole D, Ducreux M, Bommelaer G, et al. Treatment of carcinoid syndrome: a prospective crossover evaluation of lanreotide versus octreotide in terms of efficacy, patient acceptability, and tolerance. Cancer 2000;88(4):770–6.
79. Matsumoto T, Esaki M, Yanaru-Fujisawa R, et al. Small-intestinal involvement in familial adenomatous polyposis: evaluation by double-balloon endoscopy and intraoperative enteroscopy. Gastrointest Endosc 2008;68(5):911–9.
80. Jagelman D, DeCosse J, Bussey H. Upper gastrointestinal cancer in familial adenomatous polyposis. Lancet 1988;1(8595):1149–51.
81. Nugent K, Spigelman A, Phillips R. Risk of extracolonic cancer in familial adenomatous polyposis. Br J Surg 1996;83(8):1121–2.
82. Offerhaus G, Giardiello F, Krush A, et al. The risk of upper gastrointestinal cancer in familial adenomatous polyposis. Gastroenterology 1992;102(6):1980–2.
83. Hirota WK, Zuckerman MJ, Adler DG, et al. ASGE guideline: the role of endoscopy in the surveillance of premalignant conditions of the upper GI tract. Gastrointest Endosc 2006;63(4):570–80.
84. Giardiello FM, Trimbath JD. Peutz-Jeghers syndrome and management recommendations. Clin Gastroenterol Hepatol 2006;4(4):408–15.
85. Mensink P, Haringsma J, Kucharzik T, et al. Complications of double balloon enteroscopy: a multicenter survey. Endoscopy 2007;39(7):613–5.
86. Ross A, Dye C, Prachand V. Laparoscopic-assisted double-balloon enteroscopy for small-bowel polyp surveillance and treatment in patients with Peutz-Jeghers syndrome. Gastrointest Endosc 2006;64(6):984–8.
87. Kindblom L, Remotti H, Aldenborg F, et al. Gastrointestinal pacemaker cell tumor (GIPACT): gastrointestinal stromal tumors show phenotypic characteristics of the interstitial cells of Cajal. Am J Pathol 1998;152(5):1259–69.
88. Miettinen M, Lasota J. Gastrointestinal stromal tumors: pathology and prognosis at different sites. Semin Diagn Pathol 2006;23(2):70–83.
89. Agaimy A, Wünsch P, Hofstaedter F, et al. Minute gastric sclerosing stromal tumors (GIST tumorlets) are common in adults and frequently show c-KIT mutations. Am J Surg Pathol 2007;31(1):113–20.
90. Fletcher C, Berman J, Corless C, et al. Diagnosis of gastrointestinal stromal tumors: a consensus approach. Hum Pathol 2002;33(5):459–65.
91. Miettinen M, Makhlouf H, Sobin L, et al. Gastrointestinal stromal tumors of the jejunum and ileum: a clinicopathologic, immunohistochemical, and molecular genetic study of 906 cases before imatinib with long-term follow-up. Am J Surg Pathol 2006;30(4):477–89.
92. Demetri G, Benjamin R, Blanke C, et al. NCCN Task Force report: management of patients with gastrointestinal stromal tumor (GIST) – update of the NCCN clinical practice guidelines. J Natl Compr Canc Netw 2007;5(Suppl 2):S1–29; quiz S30.

93. Gold J, Dematteo R. Combined surgical and molecular therapy: the gastrointestinal stromal tumor model. Ann Surg 2006;244(2):176–84.
94. Kobayashi M, Okamoto K, Nakatani H, et al. Complete remission of recurrent gastrointestinal stromal tumors after treatment with imatinib: report of a case. Surg Today 2006;36(8):727–32.
95. Schnadig I, Blanke C. Gastrointestinal stromal tumors: imatinib and beyond. Curr Treat Options Oncol 2006;7(6):427–37.
96. Demetri G, van Oosterom A, Garrett C, et al. Efficacy and safety of sunitinib in patients with advanced gastrointestinal stromal tumour after failure of imatinib: a randomised controlled trial. Lancet 2006;368(9544):1329–38 [German].
97. Fishman S, Smithers C, Folkman J, et al. Blue rubber bleb nevus syndrome: surgical eradication of gastrointestinal bleeding. Ann Surg 2005;241(3):523–8.
98. Anzinger M, Gospos J, Pitzl H, et al. [Blue rubber-bleb nevus syndrome and therapeutic double balloon enteroscopy] [in German]. Z Gastroenterol 2006; 44(11):1141–4.
99. Zucca E, Roggero E, Bertoni F, et al. Primary extranodal non-Hodgkin's lymphomas. Part 1: gastrointestinal, cutaneous and genitourinary lymphomas. Ann Oncol 1997;8(8):727–37.
100. Keung YK, Higgs V, Albertson DA, et al. Mucosa-associated lymhpoid tissue (MALT) lymphoma of the jejunum and *Helicobacter pylori* – chance association? Leuk Lymphoma 2003;44(8):1413–6.
101. Rawls R, Vega K, Trotman B. Small bowel lymphoma. Curr Treat Options Gastroenterol 2003;6(1):27–34.
102. Frey NV, Tsai DE. The management of posttransplant lymphoproliferative disorder. Med Oncol 2007;24(2):125–36.
103. Shia J, Teruya-Feldstein J, Pan D, et al. Primary follicular lymphoma of the gastrointestinal tract: a clinical and pathologic study of 26 cases. Am J Surg Pathol 2002;26(2):216–24.
104. Brady G, MacArthur GJ, Farrell PJ. Epstein-Barr virus and Burkitt lymphoma. Postgrad Med J 2008;84(993):372–7.
105. Lecuit M, Abachin E, Martin A, et al. Immunoproliferative small intestinal disease associated with *Campylobacter jejuni*. N Engl J Med 2004;350(3):239–48.
106. Verbeek WH, Van De Water JM, Al-Toma A, et al. Incidence of enteropathy-associated T-cell lymphoma: a nation-wide study of a population-based registry in The Netherlands. Scand J Gastroenterol 2008;43(11):1322–8.
107. Daum S, Ipczynski R, Schumann M, et al. High rates of complications and substantial mortality in both types of refractory sprue. Eur J Gastroenterol Hepatol 2009;21(1):66–70.
108. Al-toma A, Verbeek WHM, Hadithi M, et al. Survival in refractory coeliac disease and enteropathy-associated T-cell lymphoma: retrospective evaluation of single-centre experience. Gut 2007;56(10):1373–8.
109. Hadithi M, Al-toma A, Oudejans J, et al. The value of double-balloon enteroscopy in patients with refractory celiac disease. Am J Gastroenterol 2007; 102(5):987–96.
110. Fenoglio-Preiser CM. Gastrointestinal pathology: an atlas and text. 3rd edition. Philadelphia: Wolters Kluwer Health/Lippincott Williams & Wilkins; 2008.

Outcomes Associated with Deep Enteroscopy

Lauren B. Gerson, MD, MSc

KEYWORDS

- Obscure gastrointestinal hemorrhage • Deep enteroscopy
- Cost-effectiveness analysis • Endoscopic complications
- Outcomes assessment

In approximately 5% of patients with gastrointestinal hemorrhage, no source of bleeding is identified on conventional upper endoscopy or colonoscopy.[1] It has been estimated that in 75% of patients with obscure bleeding the source responsible will be in the small bowel.[2] The diagnosis of obscure GI bleeding (OGIB) has been associated with increased costs as a result of associated hospitalizations and diagnostic and therapeutic procedures[3,4] in addition to a significant impact on health-related quality of life.[5]

Outcome assessments for patients with obscure gastrointestinal bleeding are important to determine the impact of diagnostic and therapeutic interventions on the natural history of small bowel hemorrhage. Short-term outcome measurements can include the diagnostic or therapeutic yield associated with a diagnostic procedure, or immediate postprocedural complications. In the scenario of deep enteroscopy for patients with OGIB, these parameters also include cessation of bleeding or rate of total enteroscopy. Long-term outcome parameters require prospective or retrospective data collection and might include rates of bleeding cessation or bleeding recurrence months to years after an intervention, the need for subsequent or repeat therapeutic or diagnostic procedures, requirements for medical or surgical therapy or an ongoing transfusion requirement.

Long-term data collection is crucial to determine the impact that an intervention might have on the natural history of a disorder. Using the example of patients with OGIB from small bowel angiodysplastic lesions, the rate of spontaneous cessation of hemorrhage has been described to range between 40% and 50% per year.[6] It is important to determine whether patients undergoing endoscopic therapy for angiodysplastic lesions have a bleeding cessation rate greater than that observed with placebo therapy.

Conflicts of Interest: Dr. Gerson has received speaking honoraria from Given Imaging Inc. She has received grant support and speaking honoraria from Fujinon, Inc.
Division of Gastroenterology & Hepatology, Department of Medicine, Stanford University School of Medicine, Room A149, 300 Pasteur Drive, Stanford, CA 94305-5202, USA
E-mail address: lgerson@stanford.edu

Gastrointest Endoscopy Clin N Am 19 (2009) 481–496
doi:10.1016/j.giec.2009.04.007 **giendo.theclinics.com**
1052-5157/09/$ – see front matter © 2009 Published by Elsevier Inc.

The purpose of this article is to describe the available data regarding the short- and long-term outcomes associated with deep enteroscopy. Deep enteroscopy can be defined the use of an enteroscope to examine small bowel distal to the ligament of Treitz or proximal to the distal ileum. The term deep enteroscopy includes double-balloon (DBE), single-balloon (SBE), and spiral enteroscopy. Comparisons are made with push enteroscopy and intraoperative enteroscopy, the major therapeutic endoscopic options available to the gastroenterologist before the introduction of deep enteroscopy. The article concludes with a discussion on the cost-effectiveness of management strategies for obscure bleeding, and proposed changes to the current algorithm for management of OGIB.

SHORT-TERM OUTCOME ASSESSMENTS

Approximately 5% of patients presenting with gastrointestinal hemorrhage will have lesions located distal to the ligament of Treitz or proximal to the ileocecal valve.[7] Angiodysplastic lesions (AVMs) are the most common source of small bowel bleeding, found in approximately 30% to 40% of patients undergoing deep enteroscopy in the United States and Europe.[8,9] For reasons that remain unclear, ulcerative and neoplastic lesions are more commonly detected with deep enteroscopy performed in Asia.[10,11]

The remaining 25% of patients will have lesions located in the upper or lower gastrointestinal tracts not detected by initial upper endoscopy or colonoscopy. These lesions can include peptic ulcers, Cameron's ulcerations in a large herniasac, Dieulafoy's lesions or AVMs, gastric antral vascular ectasia (GAVE), or neoplasms. Studies on large series of patients undergoing DBE have confirmed that approximately 25% of patients will have sources of bleeding confirmed within reach of a traditional upper endoscopy or colonoscopy.[12]

Short-term outcomes associated with OGIB include diagnostic and therapeutic yields of the endoscopic procedures, complications, and bleeding cessation rates. The performance parameters of deep enteroscopy are compared with push enteroscopy and intraoperative enteroscopy (IOE). Capsule endoscopy (CE) has emerged as the major comparative technology to deep enteroscopy, but is not discussed in this article.

Push Enteroscopy

Push enteroscopy can be performed using a pediatric colonoscope or dedicated 220 to 250 cm push enteroscope to examine the proximal jejunum. There is evidence that utilization of an overtube during the examination may be associated with greater depth of insertion.[13] The expected depth of insertion with push enteroscopy ranges from 50 to 150 cm distal to the ligament of Treitz. Outcomes parameters associated with push enteroscopy from 22 published series are shown in **Table 1**. In 1389 patients, the diagnostic yield of push enteroscopy was 44%, with AVMs detected in 31% of examinations. Endoscopic therapy was performed in 12% to 100% of examinations. Bleeding cessation from AVMs was not measured in most of the studies, but ranged from 27% to 85% in series in which cessation rates were determined.

In a recent decision analysis, it was estimated that if small bowel AVMs were present in 40% of a cohort of patients with obscure bleeding, push enteroscopy would detect the lesions in approximately 18% of examinations with a sensitivity of 45%[34] based on the current published literature.

Intraoperative Enteroscopy

Although intraoperative enteroscopy (IOE) offers the ability to visualize the entire small bowel, the benefits of the procedure are offset by increased risks of morbidity and

Table 1
Push enteroscopy for obscure bleeding

Author, Year	No. of Patients and Type of Bleeding	Diagnostic Yield, n (%)	Examinations with AVMs (%)	Endoscopic Therapy (%)	Bleeding Cessation/Year AVM Cohort (%)[a]
Foutch, 1990[3]	20 overt 19 occult	15 (38)	31	92	44
Chong, 1994[14]	55 overt	35 (64)	4	N/A	N/A
Pennazio, 1995[2]	21 overt	9 (43)	38	12.5	N/A
Davies, 1995[15]	11 overt 7 occult	6 (33)	11	100	N/A
Schmit, 1996[16]	37 overt 46 occult	49 (59)	40	42	38
Adrain, 1998[17]	41 overt	32 (78)	49	N/A	27
Zaman, 1998[18]	75 overt 20 occult	39 (41)	46	61	60
Shackel, 1998[19]	23 overt 21 occult	23 (52)	65	73	40
Descamps, 1999[20]	110 overt 123 occult	125 (53)	63	N/A	N/A
Hayat, 2000[21]	50 occult 28 overt	43 (78)	26	100	70
Sharma, 2000[22]	21 overt 5 occult	9 (43)	4.7	N/A	N/A
Landi, 2002[23]	49 overt 56 occult	49 (47)	37	44	70
Lewis, 2002[24]	21 overt	6 (30)	30	100	N/A
Ell, 2002[25]	32 overt	9 (32)	22	14	N/A
Mylonaki, 2003[26]	50 overt	16 (32)	20	N/A	N/A
Saurin, 2003[27]	28 overt 32 occult	3 (3)	7	N/A	N/A
Keizman, 2003[28]	36 overt 57 occult	51 (40)	35	100	85
Romelaer, 2004[29]	66 overt 53 occult	50 (42)	66	76	76
Adler, 2004[30]	20 occult	5 (25)	10	100	60
Mata, 2004[31]	26 overt 16 occult	8 (19)	9.5	50	N/A
Pennazio, 2004[32]	34 overt 17 occult	15 (29)	N/A	N/A	N/A
Lara, 2005[33]	44 overt 19 occult	35 (56)	30	100	N/A
Totals and mean (±SD) values	1389 patients	611 (43 ± 0.2)	31 ± 0.2		

[a] Calculated from $P = 1 - e(-rt)$ where r is the rate and t is the time.

Data from Raju GS, Gerson L, Das A, et al. American Gastroenterological Association (AGA) Institute technical review on obscure gastrointestinal bleeding. Gastroenterology 2007;133:1697–717.

mortality. The diagnostic yield of IOE has been shown to be equivalent to capsule endoscopy[35] with a higher sensitivity than push enteroscopy. Published yields for intraoperative enteroscopy are presented in **Table 2**. In more than 300 patients with obscure bleeding, the diagnostic yield of IOE was 76 ± 9.7% with an associated mortality of 5 ± 6%. Bleeding was reported to recur within a year post-IOE in 12% to 60% of patients postoperatively. The major reasons for recurrent bleeding include missed lesions due to limited visibility, or the evanescent nature of ectasias. IOE should be reserved for patients failing other diagnostic modalities, or in patients in whom lysis of adhesions is required to perform deep enteroscopy.

Deep Enteroscopy: Double-Balloon Enteroscopy

DBE was first introduced by Yamamoto in 2001[43] and introduced into the United States in 2004. Single-balloon and spiral enteroscopy have been available in the United States since 2007.[44,45] Most of the outcome data regarding deep enteroscopy originate from the published DBE experience.

Short-term outcome data from published series of DBE, including more than 1370 patients and 2591 examinations, are shown in **Table 3**. The mean (±SD) diagnostic yield was 67 ± 14% (range 41%–81%) with a mean treatment success rate of 64 ± 13% (range 42%–84%). Total enteroscopy was performed in 86% of subjects in the original Yamamoto study; it was performed overall in 34% of patients. The low rate of total enteroscopy implies that either pathology was identified in most patients during an initial approach, thereby obviating the need for the complimentary procedure, or that it was not technically feasible due to the presence of adhesions or other limiting anatomic factors. Rebleeding rates were not measured in most of the studies.

Findings detected in patients with OGIB who have undergone deep enteroscopy are listed in **Table 4**. Of 980 patients and 1568 DBE examinations, the mean (±SD) diagnostic yield was 72 ± 50% (range 25%–92%) with ulcerations found in 15 ± 15% (range 2%–35%), tumors or polyps in 17 ± 26% (range 0%–59%) and vascular lesions in 24 ± 20% (range 5%–50%). As previously noted, it was more common to observe ulcerations and tumors in series of DBEs from Asia,[10,11,59] whereas AVMs were more commonly reported in patients from the United States or Europe.[48,50,53]

Table 2
Yield of intraoperative enteroscopy for obscure bleeding

Author, Year	No. of Patients with Bleeding	Diagnostic Yield (%)	Yearly Recurrence (%)[a]	Mortality (%)
Desa, 1991[36]	12	83	30	17
Ress, 1992[37]	44	70	60	11
Lopez, 1996[38]	16	88	12.5	0
Zaman, 1999[39]	14	58	43	0
Douard, 2000[40]	25	81	38	4
Kendrick, 2001[41]	70	74	48	6
Hartmann, 2005[35]	47	72	N/A	2
Jakobs, 2006[42]	81	84	N/A	0
Totals and mean (±SD) values	309	76 ± 9.7		5 ± 6

[a] Calculated from $P = 1 - e(-rt)$ where r is the rate and t is the time.

Data from Raju GS, Gerson L, Das A, et al. American Gastroenterological Association (AGA) Institute technical review on obscure gastrointestinal bleeding. Gastroenterology 2007;133:1697–717.

Table 3
Outcomes associated with double-balloon enteroscopy

Author, Year	Patients with Bleeding[a]/ DBE Exams (%)	Diagnostic Yield (%)	Diagnostic or Treatment Success (%)	Total DBE (%)[b]	Rebleed Rate (%)	Complications, n (%)
Yamamoto, 2004[10]	66/178 (37)	76	61	86	N/A	Perforation, 1 (0.6)
May, 2005[46]	90/248 (36)	80	76	45	N/A	None
Ell, 2005[47]	64/147 (44)	72	62	16	N/A	None
Di Caro, 2005[48]	33/89 (37)	80	42	44	N/A	None
Matsumoto, 2005[49]	13/22 (59)	46	N/A	14	N/A	None
Mehdizadeh, 2006[9]	130/237 (55)	43	60	0	N/A	Perforation, 1 (0.4)
Hadithi, 2006[50]	35/35 (100)	60	77	20	20	None
Heine, 2006[51]	168/275 (61)	73	55	42	N/A	Pancreatitis, 3 (1)
Kaffes, 2006[52]	32/40 (80)	48	75	0	N/A	Perforation, 1 (2.5)
Monkemuller, 2006[53]	29/70 (41)	67	57	30	0	Polypectomy bleed, 1 (1.4)
Nakamura, 2006[54]	32/28 (100)	41	43	62.5	6	Perforation, 1 (3.6)
Manabe, 2006[11]	31/31 (100)	74	74	29	91	None
Akahoshi, 2006[55]	20/103 (19)	43	43	40	N/A	None
Sun, 2006[56]	152/191 (80)	76	84	N/A	12 at 16 months	None
Barretto-Zuniga, 2007[57]	40/86 (47)	74	50	70	4 at 6 months	None
Cazzato, 2007[58]	71/100 (71)	69	65	N/A	N/A	None
Zhong, 2007[59]	191/378 (51)	65	84	56	7 at 6 months	Polypectomy bleed, 1 (0.5)
Zhi, 2007	92/155 (59)	81	61	N/A	N/A	Perforation, 1 (0.65)
Gross, 2008[60]	101/200 (50)	80	72	25	N/A	None
Totals and mean values (range)	1378 patients 2591 exams	67 ± 14 (41–81)	64 ± 13 (42–84)	34 ± 23 (0–86)		Perforation, 5 (0.2)

[a] Includes patients with obscure overt or obscure occult bleeding.
[b] Defined as initial DBE from 1 approach with tattoo at most distal insertion point followed by DBE from opposite direction with prior tattoo site identified.

Single-Balloon and Spiral Enteroscopy

Published data regarding the efficacy of SBE and spiral enteroscopy have been limited to date. Two series of SBE, including 78 and 37 examinations, reported diagnostic yields ranging between 30% and 55% with similar success rates for therapy. Total enteroscopy was reported in 6/24 (25%) of one series,[61] and in 1/10 (10%) of the second cohort.[62] Comparative studies between DBE and SBE have not been

Table 4
Findings on DBE in patients with obscure bleeding

Study	No. of Patients Bleeding	Yield, n (%)	Ulcers, n (%)	Tumor, n (%)	AVM, n (%)
Yamamoto	66	55 (83)	22 (33)	10 (15)	4 (6)
Di Caro	38	30 (79)	6 (16)	1 (3)	19 (50)
Mehdizadeh	130	66 (51)	13 (10)	11 (9)	47 (37)
Hadithi	35	21 (60)	2 (6)	1 (3)	16 (46)
Heine	168	123 (73)	4 (2)	8 (5)	60 (36)
Monkemuller	29	19 (66)	3 (10)	1 (3)	13 (45)
Manabe	31	23 (74)	11 (35)	9 (29)	2 (7)
Nakamura	28	12 (43)	3 (10)	0 (0)	2 (7)
Akahoshi	20	5 (25)	2 (11)	2 (10)	1 (5)
Zhong	191	154 (81)	48 (25)	37 (19)	32 (17)
Zhi	92	85 (93)	N/A	N/A	N/A
Sun	152	115 (76)	31 (20)	90 (59)	35 (23)
Mean values (range)	780	72 (25–93)	15 (2–35)	17 (0–59)	24 (5–50)

reported. In a preliminary report of 75 spiral enteroscopy examinations, the overall diagnostic yield and treatment success was 24%.[45] Spiral enteroscopy is not currently approved for retrograde examination.

Examination Duration

The time required to complete deep enteroscopy exceeds that of standard endoscopic procedures. For DBE, approximately 10 to 15 minutes is required to place the enteroscope balloon on the tip of the enteroscope before the start of the procedure. This step is not required for SBE or spiral enterscopy.

In the multicenter United States study,[9] the mean (±SD) examination time was 90 ± 37 minutes for the oral route with a mean depth of insertion of 360 ± 177 cm using the depth of insertion technique described by May and colleagues.[8] For the retrograde route, the mean duration of examination was 89 ± 35 minutes with a mean depth of insertion of 182 ± 165 cm. These data were representative of the first 20 to 30 cases performed at each participating institution. The time involved for SBE seems to be similar; in the study by Kawamura and colleagues,[62] 83 minutes were required for the anterograde approach and 90 minutes for the anal route without description of distance traversed. Similarly the study by Tsujikawa and colleagues[61] reported a mean of 63 ± 20 minutes for the oral route with a mean of 270 cm traversed, and 70 ± 19 min for the retrograde approach with a mean of 199 cm. Examination time for spiral enteroscopy seems to be accelerated compared with balloon-assisted enteroscopy. In the initial study published by Ackerman and colleagues, the Discovery small bowel overtube was used with either the Fujinon EN–450T5 or the Olympus SIF–Q180 enteroscopes. Mean examination times for the anterograde approach ranged from 26 to 29 (±10) cm with estimated depth of insertion of 243 to 256 (±80) cm.

LONG-TERM OUTCOMES

Data regarding long-term outcomes post-DBE have been limited. In a prospective study by Gerson and Semrad, 274 patients who had undergone DBE between August 2004 and September 2006 were invited to participate.[63] One hundred and one (37%)

patients completed the initial follow-up period, which occurred a mean of 10.5 ± 5 (range 2–26) months post-DBE. The most common findings on DBE examination were AVMs found in 50 (43%) patients using the anterograde approach. At 12 months of follow-up, 43% of the patients did not report further bleeding or anemia. 24% reported new or ongoing overt bleeding (with or without transfusions), and 35% reported ongoing iron therapy or transfusions. In the 32 patients with subsequent procedures post-DBE, AVMs were found in eight (25%), a submucosal GIST tumor in one patient, and a subsequent patient underwent repair of a paraesophageal hernia. 85 (31%) patients were subsequently contacted for the second follow-up assessment 30+7 (range 18-47) months post-DBE. Seven patients died of causes not related to bleeding. At 30 months of follow-up, 59 (59%) of patients reported no further bleeding, 20 (24%) new or recurrent overt bleeding with or without transfusions and/or iron therapy, and 15 (28%) ongoing need for iron and/or transfusions. Patients with initial normal DBE examinations or AVMs were most likely to experience recurrent bleeding. Patients with normal initial DBE examinations or AVMs were most likely to experience recurrent bleeding. Most patients did not undergo total enteroscopy, so that a normal examination implied visualization of normal mucosa to the extent of the examination. Because most patients were referred for DBE from outside centers, they were not required to return for an examination from the opposite approach if the initial examination did not reveal any pathologic findings. Limitations of the current study included the low rate of total enteroscopy, lack of data regarding usage of aspirin, non-steroidal anti-inflammatory agents and/or plavix, and lack of laboratory values post-DBE examinations.

COMPLICATIONS

Complications related to standard sedated endoscopic procedures have included sedation-related complications, aspiration pneumonia, and respiratory infections. DBE has been associated with intestinal cramping in 2% to 20% of patients.[9,51] The use of CO_2 has been associated with decreased reporting of postprocedure abdominal cramping.[64] Complications that seem to be associated with DBE have included perforations and pancreatitis.

Perforations Associated with Deep Enteroscopy

Perforations occurred in 5 (0.2%) of 2591 DBE examinations reported in **Table 3**. The perforations were described in association with DBE and the following clinical scenarios: (1) a patient with lymphoma undergoing chemotherapy who sustained a perforation in areas of necrosis;[10] (2) peristomal perforation in a patient with fresh ileostomy;[9] (3) a patient with an actively bleeding AVM postcautery who presented 2 days later with peritonitis and was found to have a perforation at the site of cautery;[52] (4) duodenal perforation, details not listed;[54] (5) jejunal perforation attributed to a balloon rupture that occurred after tattooing the distal extent of examination.[65]

A large retrospective study by Mensink and colleagues[66] demonstrated that in 2367 DBE examinations, the perforation rate was 0.3%. Participating centers had performed at least 200 DBE cases per year. A complication registration system was used in 8/10 (80%) of the centers. Overall there were 40 complications (rate of 1.7%) occurring in 13/1728 (0.8%) diagnostic cases and 27/412 (4.3%) therapeutic cases. Perforations occurred in five (0.8%) subjects including three (0.2%) patients post-APC for AVMs, and two (3%) patients poststricture dilation.

Recently, a large retrospective study was conducted in the United States to examine DBE complications. Of 2478 DBE examinations recorded, complications occurred in 20 (0.9%) patients. The DBE examinations included 1691 (68%) anterograde examinations, 722 (29%) retrograde, five per stoma, and 65 (3%) by endoscopic retrograde cholangiopancreatography (ERCP).[67] Perforations occurred in 11 (0.4%) examinations including three (0.2%) anterograde examinations and eight (1.2%) retrograde DBEs. Patients with inflammatory bowel disease or altered surgical anatomy were more likely to experience complications. Of the 3% of patients with surgically altered anatomy, perforations occurred in 1/59 (0.6%) anterograde examinations, 5/60 (8%) retrograde DBEs, and 1/5 (20%) peristomal examinations. Eight (73%) of the perforations occurred during diagnostic DBE examinations. Four of eight (50%) rectal DBE perforations occurred in patients with prior ileal anal anastomoses. Based on these available data, deep enteroscopy should be performed with caution in patients with altered surgical anatomy.

In a series of 178 therapeutic DBEs performed in 139 patients, serious complications were reported in six (3.4%) of the procedures.[68] Three perforations were reported in patients after polyectomy of large (>3 cm) polyps; two patients postpolypectomy of large polyps experienced GI bleeding.

Data regarding perforations associated with SBE and spiral enteroscopy are limited. In a series of 78 patients undergoing SBE, a mucosal tear was observed in one patient with Crohn disease when the tip of the enteroscope pressed against a longitudinal ulcer scar during insertion of the overtube.[61] The tear was treated with endoclips, and no perforation was observed on subsequent CT scan. In another series of 37 SBE procedures, a perforation occurred in a case of ulcerative colitis postoperatively and was believed to be due to the sliding tube being caught in the mucosa of the ileal pouch when the sliding tube was inserted along the enteroscope.[62] Another case report of SBE reported perforation associated with jejunal ulcerations from metastatic adenocarcinoma of unknown primary; the perforation occurred during insertion of the enteroscope before detection of the lesions that were subsequently found on laparotomy.[69]

Based on the experience described earlier, perforation associated with deep enteroscopy is increased compared with standard endoscopic procedures. Traction and distension in association with deep enteroscopy of a weakened intestinal wall may occur in patients with altered surgical anatomy, ulcerative, or neoplastic disorders.

Pancreatitis

The incidence of pancreatitis is increased in association with deep enteroscopy for unclear reasons. Pancreatitis occurred in seven (0.3%) patients in the Mensink study; six occurred in diagnostic DBE cases.[66] The seventh case occurred in a patient who underwent DBE-assisted ERCP postpapillotomy. Six of the seven cases presented with abdominal pain less than 24 hours post-DBE. The location of pancreatitis occurred in the body or tail in four patients, the head of the pancreas in one patient, and the entire pancreas in two patients. The incidence of pancreatitis did not seem to increase with the use of the therapeutic DBE enteroscope. Pancreatitis was reported in 6 (0.2%) cases in the multicenter United States study; one case occurred in a patient undergoing retrograde DBE examination.[67] None of the procedures involved therapeutic interventions in the area of the ampulla.

The mechanism for post-DBE pancreatitis remains unclear. Potential explanations might include pancreatic duct obstruction by direct compression of the papilla with the inflated balloon, an increase in duodenal intraluminal pressure caused by the overtube and gastrointestinal shortening technique, reflux of duodenal contents into the pancreatic duct due to intraluminal hypertension caused by the inflated balloon, or injury or ischemia due to stretching and shortening of the proximal small bowel.

Gastrointestinal Hemorrhage Post-Double-Balloon Enteroscopy

Gastrointestinal hemorrhage does not seem to be increased post-DBE compared with standard endoscopic procedures. Post-DBE bleeding was reported in four (0.2%) of patients post-DBE in the United States multicenter study in association with the following clinical scenarios:[67] (1) a patient post-APC therapy for a red papule in the ileum; the patient presented with hematochezia postprocedure; there was spontaneous cessation of bleeding while the patient was observed overnight in the hospital; (2) a patient postlaparotomy 3 years before DBE for metastatic melanoma who presented with abdominal pain post-DBE; intraperitoneal bleeding was demonstrated on CT scan; the patient was admitted to the hospital for supportive care and recovered uneventfully; (3) overt bleeding following polypectomy of a hemangioma in the ileum treated with epinephrine injection and hemoclip application; the patient was observed overnight and the bleeding stopped; (4) a patient with Peutz Jeghers syndrome post-polypectomy of a 4-cm polyp that was intussuscepting and causing pain; the morning after the procedure the patient had melena which was self-limiting and did not require endoscopic or other interventions; the patient was hospitalized for 1 day.

Polypectomy seems to be a risk factor for post-DBE hemorrhage. In the Mensink study, the incidence of bleeding post-DBE was 0.8% overall but occurred in 18 (3%) therapeutic cases, all postpolypectomy. Similarly, the prevalence of GI bleeding postpolypectomy of large lesions was 2/178 (1%) in another study performed by May and colleagues.[68]

COST-EFFECTIVENESS OF DEEP ENTEROSCOPY

Given the time and expense involved in deep enteroscopy, it is important to determine whether this endoscopic technique is cost-effective compared with current technology. Two cost models have been published to date. Gerson and Kamal published a cost-effectiveness model examining outcomes 1 year post-DBE.[34] The base-case patient was a 50-year-old man with obscure overt bleeding after a normal upper and lower endoscopy. Management strategies included no therapy with transfusions, push enteroscopy, intraoperative enteroscopy, angiography, initial anterograde DBE followed by retrograde DBE if the patient had ongoing bleeding, and initial capsule endoscopy followed by CE-guided DBE. Patients were not allowed to undergo subsequent testing with a different modality if the original examination was normal or if the patient experienced recurrent hemorrhage (for example a push enteroscopy was not followed by CE or DBE if the patient had ongoing or recurrent hemorrhage). Total costs and quality-adjusted life years were examined. A 1-year time horizon was chosen as the natural history of bleeding from AVMs remains poorly understood. Quality of life estimates (QALYs) were derived from the existing medical literature for patients with GI bleeding or hospitalization. Costs were estimated from the perspective of a third-party payer. The cost for an anterograde DBE approach was estimated using the Current Procedural Terminology (CPT) codes of 44376 for diagnostic procedures and 44378 for therapeutic procedures.

The results of the 1-year model demonstrated that the no-therapy arm was the least expensive and associated with the lowest fraction of QALYs. The initial DBE arm was the most effective strategy; it was more expensive compared with no therapy or push enteroscopy but less costly compared with angiography, capsule-directed DBE, or IOE. The incremental cost-effectiveness ratio was $20,833 per

QALY gained. Important model assumptions included the following: 15% of the cohort would have missed lesions on upper or lower endoscopy; 55% of AVMs would continue to bleed without endoscopic therapy; and this rate of bleeding would be reduced to 20% postendoscopic therapy. The results of the 1-year model demonstrated that approximately 86% of the patients would experience cessation of bleeding in the DBE arm compared with 76% in the CE arm and 59% in the no-therapy arm. The effectiveness of the DBE and CE-guided arms were equivalent when the QALY state associated with bleeding exceeded 0.88 or if the miss rate for lesions on upper or lower endoscopy exceeded 23%. However, the initial DBE arm remained less costly and was therefore preferred by extended dominance. However, an initial CE strategy was associated with a decreased DBE workload and potential for endoscopic complications.

In another cost-minimization analysis by Somsouk and colleagues,[70] 5 strategies were compared including initial small bowel radiography, enteroclysis, push enteroscopy, CE, or DBE. Two separate model end-points included one scenario assuming that endoscopic or surgical management was needed, and a second whereby visual diagnosis of a lesion was sufficient to direct medical therapy. The model assumptions differed from those in the model by Gerson and Kamal in that it was assumed that 30% would have no identified lesion, 15% of treated lesions would have recurrent bleeding, and 100% of missed lesions would have recurrent hemorrhage. The model did not include quality of life parameters or a specific time horizon. The sensitivity of CE was assumed to be 75% for all lesions, whereas the sensitivity of CE in the Gerson model varied from 50% to 87% depending on the type of lesion. Patients with ongoing bleeding or lesions identified after small bowel follow through (SBFT) or push enteroscopy could undergo subsequent DBE or IOE for therapy. In the evaluation of subjects with OGIB, the least costly strategy was an initial DBE at a cost of $3824; initial CE cost an incremental $440. In a one-way sensitivity analysis, CE would be preferred when the cost of DBE exceeded $1849 or if the sensitivity of DBE decreased to less than 68%. If DBE was not available, then CE was the preferred strategy. Push enteroscopy was preferred if the cost of CE exceeded $1190, the capsule retention rate exceeded 3%, or if more than 64% of the lesions were located within reach of push enteroscopy. If the goal of the model was simply lesion identification, CE was the least costly strategy at $1826 per subject evaluated. DBE was preferred if the cost of CE exceeded $936, if the cost of DBE was less than $716, if the sensitivity of CE was less than 63%, or if more than 78% of lesions were located in the proximal small bowel.

Modeling in the area of OGIB remains challenging, due to the lack of available data regarding natural history of bleeding and spontaneous cessation from angiodysplastic lesions, and lack of comparative data for the various testing strategies. Therefore, both models did not include specificity of tests for lesions due to the paucity of literature evaluating the false-positive rates of various diagnostic modalities. In addition, there is currently no CPT code for deep enteroscopy so that DBE costs remain estimated. For retrograde procedures, an unlisted code is commonly utilized and reimbursement remains highly variable.

CHANGES TO THE CURRENT ALGORITHM FOR OBSCURE GASTROINTESTINAL BLEEDING

Fig. 1 demonstrates a current algorithm for OGIB. Based on the data presented earlier, some changes could be proposed. First, DBE studies have confirmed a miss rate of 15% to 20% for lesions within reach of a standard endoscope or colonoscope.[12] Lesions most commonly missed include Cameron's erosions, gastric varices, Dieulafoy's lesions, peptic ulcerations, angiodysplastic lesions, and colonic

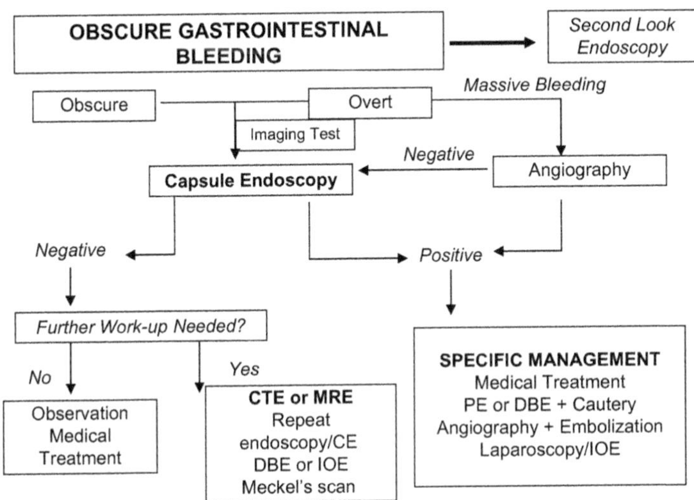

Fig. 1. Management strategy for obscure bleeding. Proposed modifications are in red. CE, capsule endoscopy; CTE, computerized tomographic enterography; DBE, double-balloon enteroscopy; IOE, intraoperative enteroscopy; MRE, magnetic resonance enterography; PE, push enteroscopy. (*Adapted from* Pennazio M, Eisen G, Goldfarb N. ICCE consensus for obscure gastrointestinal bleeding. Endoscopy 2005;37:1046–50; with permission.)

neoplasms. Therefore repeat standard endoscopic examinations may be considered before deep enteroscopy.

The third diagnostic test for obscure bleeding in the algorithm is capsule endoscopy. Many centers recommend an imaging study of the small bowel before CE to avoid capsule retention. The usage of CT enterography has been associated with increased yield in the setting of OGIB,[71] particularly in patients younger than 40 years in whom malignancies or inflammatory bowel disease (IBD) are more likely to be the sources of bleeding.[7] Whereas the incidence of CE retention is approximately 1.4% in obscure bleeding, it can increase to 5% in patients with IBD.[72] If IBD is suspected, small bowel radiography may be useful initially. A recent comparative trial of small bowel series on capsule endoscopy, ileoscopy, and CT enterography demonstrated that the combination of ileoscopy and CT enterography would be preferred over initial CE.[73]

Miss rates of 20% to 30% have been described for CE and DBE.[74] In the setting of a normal CE study and cessation of bleeding, observation can be recommended.[75] However, if the patient continues to experience recurrent bleeding, the choices include repeat CE, proceeding to DBE, or diagnostic imaging with computerized tomographic enterography (CTE) or MRE. The radiographic testing modalities offer the potential for detection of submucosal lesions that may not be visible using other diagnostic modalities. The usage of CTE or MRE was added to **Fig. 1** for patients with ongoing OGIB and negative capsule endoscopy.

SUMMARY

Compared with push enteroscopy, deep enteroscopy is associated with greater potential for detection and therapy for small bowel lesions responsible for OGIB. Whereas initial deep enteroscopy may be a cost-effective approach, initial CE may remain as a preferred initial approach given the time involved with deep enteroscopy, the potential for complications, and limited information regarding the natural history of some vascular or ulcerative small bowel lesions. In addition, bleeding rates from small bowel vascular lesions may be influenced by other concomitant medical therapy such as the use of nonsteroidal antiinflammatory agents, warfarin, clopidogrel, or aspirin. Further studies examining the natural history of small bowel hemorrhage and the impact of endoscopic therapy are warranted.

REFERENCES

1. Szold A, Katz LB, Lewis BS. Surgical approach to occult gastrointestinal bleeding. Am J Surg 1992;163:90–2 [discussion: 92–3].
2. Pennazio M, Arrigoni A, Risio M, et al. Clinical evaluation of push-type enteroscopy. Endoscopy 1995;27:164–70.
3. Foutch PG, Sawyer R, Sanowski RA. Push-enteroscopy for diagnosis of patients with gastrointestinal bleeding of obscure origin. Gastrointest Endosc 1990;36:337–41.
4. Lewis B, Goldfarb N. Review article: the advent of capsule endoscopy – a not-so-futuristic approach to obscure gastrointestinal bleeding. Aliment Pharmacol Ther 2003;17:1085–96.
5. Thomson R, Parkin D, Eccles M, et al. Decision analysis and guidelines for anticoagulant therapy to prevent stroke in patients with atrial fibrillation. Lancet 2000;355:956–62.
6. Junquera F, Feu F, Papo M, et al. A multicenter, randomized, clinical trial of hormonal therapy in the prevention of rebleeding from gastrointestinal angiodysplasia. Gastroenterology 2001;121:1073–9.
7. Raju GS, Gerson L, Das A, et al. American Gastroenterological Association (AGA) Institute technical review on obscure gastrointestinal bleeding. Gastroenterology 2007;133:1697–717.
8. May A, Nachbar L, Schneider M, et al. Push-and-pull enteroscopy using the double-balloon technique: method of assessing depth of insertion and training of the enteroscopy technique using the Erlangen Endo-Trainer. Endoscopy 2005;37:66–70.
9. Mehdizadeh S, Ross A, Gerson L, et al. What is the learning curve associated with double-balloon enteroscopy? Technical details and early experience in 6 U.S. tertiary care centers. Gastrointest Endosc 2006;64:740–50.
10. Yamamoto H, Kita H, Sunada K, et al. Clinical outcomes of double-balloon endoscopy for the diagnosis and treatment of small-intestinal diseases. Clin Gastroenterol Hepatol 2004;2:1010–6.
11. Manabe N, Tanaka S, Fukumoto A, et al. Double-balloon enteroscopy in patients with GI bleeding of obscure origin. Gastrointest Endosc 2006;64:135–40.
12. Fry LC, Bellutti M, Neumann H, et al. Incidence of bleeding lesions within reach of conventional upper and lower endoscopes in patients undergoing double balloon enteroscopy for obscure GI bleeding. Aliment Pharmacol Ther 2008;29:342–9.
13. Benz C, Jakobs R, Riemann JF. Do we need the overtube for push-enteroscopy? Endoscopy 2001;33:658–61.
14. Chong J, Tagle M, Barkin JS, et al. Small bowel push-type fiberoptic enteroscopy for patients with occult gastrointestinal bleeding or suspected small bowel pathology. Am J Gastroenterol 1994;89:2143–6.
15. Davies GR, Benson MJ, Gertner DJ, et al. Diagnostic and therapeutic push type enteroscopy in clinical use. Gut 1995;37:346–52.
16. Schmit A, Gay F, Adler M, et al. Diagnostic efficacy of push-enteroscopy and long-term follow-up of patients with small bowel angiodysplasias. Dig Dis Sci 1996;41:2348–52.

17. Adrain AL, Dabezies MA, Krevsky B. Enteroscopy improves the clinical outcome in patients with obscure gastrointestinal bleeding. J Laparoendosc Adv Surg Tech A 1998;8:279–84.
18. Zaman A, Katon RM. Push enteroscopy for obscure gastrointestinal bleeding yields a high incidence of proximal lesions within reach of a standard endoscope. Gastrointest Endosc 1998;47:372–6.
19. Shackel NA, Bowen DG, Selby WS. Video push enteroscopy in the investigation of small bowel disease: defining clinical indications and outcomes. Aust N Z J Med 1998;28:198–203.
20. Descamps C, Schmit A, Van Gossum A. "Missed" upper gastrointestinal tract lesions may explain "occult" bleeding. Endoscopy 1999;31:452–5.
21. Hayat M, Axon AT, O'Mahony S. Diagnostic yield and effect on clinical outcomes of push enteroscopy in suspected small-bowel bleeding. Endoscopy 2000;32: 369–72.
22. Sharma BC, Bhasin DK, Makharia G, et al. Diagnostic value of push-type enteroscopy: a report from India. Am J Gastroenterol 2000;95:137–40.
23. Landi B, Cellier C, Gaudric M, et al. Long-term outcome of patients with gastrointestinal bleeding of obscure origin explored by push enteroscopy. Endoscopy 2002;34:355–9.
24. Lewis BS, Swain P. Capsule endoscopy in the evaluation of patients with suspected small intestinal bleeding: results of a pilot study. Gastrointest Endosc 2002;56:349–53.
25. Ell C, Remke S, May A, et al. The first prospective controlled trial comparing wireless capsule endoscopy with push enteroscopy in chronic gastrointestinal bleeding. Endoscopy 2002;34:685–9.
26. Mylonaki M, Fritscher-Ravens A, Swain P. Wireless capsule endoscopy: a comparison with push enteroscopy in patients with gastroscopy and colonoscopy negative gastrointestinal bleeding. Gut 2003;52:1122–6.
27. Saurin JC, Delvaux M, Gaudin JL, et al. Diagnostic value of endoscopic capsule in patients with obscure digestive bleeding: blinded comparison with video push-enteroscopy. Endoscopy 2003;35:576–84.
28. Keizman D, Brill S, Umansky M, et al. Diagnostic yield of routine push enteroscopy with a graded-stiffness enteroscope without overtube. Gastrointest Endosc 2003;57:877–81.
29. Romelaer C, Le Rhun M, Beaugerie L, et al. Push enteroscopy for gastrointestinal bleeding: diagnostic yield and long-term follow-up. Gastroenterol Clin Biol 2004; 28:1061–6.
30. Adler DG, Knipschield M, Gostout C. A prospective comparison of capsule endoscopy and push enteroscopy in patients with GI bleeding of obscure origin. Gastrointest Endosc 2004;59:492–8.
31. Mata A, Bordas JM, Feu F, et al. Wireless capsule endoscopy in patients with obscure gastrointestinal bleeding: a comparative study with push enteroscopy. Aliment Pharmacol Ther 2004;20:189–94.
32. Pennazio M, Santucci R, Rondonotti E, et al. Outcome of patients with obscure gastrointestinal bleeding after capsule endoscopy: report of 100 consecutive cases. Gastroenterology 2004;126:643–53.
33. Lara LF, Bloomfeld RS, Pineau BC. The rate of lesions found within reach of esophagogastroduodenoscopy during push enteroscopy depends on the type of obscure gastrointestinal bleeding. Endoscopy 2005;37:745–50.
34. Gerson L, Kamal A. Cost-effectiveness analysis of management strategies for obscure GI bleeding. Gastrointest Endosc 2008;68:920–36.

35. Hartmann D, Schmidt H, Bolz G, et al. A prospective two-center study comparing wireless capsule endoscopy with intraoperative enteroscopy in patients with obscure GI bleeding. Gastrointest Endosc 2005;61:826–32.
36. Desa LA, Ohri SK, Hutton KA, et al. Role of intraoperative enteroscopy in obscure gastrointestinal bleeding of small bowel origin. Br J Surg 1991;78:192–5.
37. Ress AM, Benacci JC, Sarr MG. Efficacy of intraoperative enteroscopy in diagnosis and prevention of recurrent, occult gastrointestinal bleeding. Am J Surg 1992;163:94–8 [discussion: 98–9].
38. Lopez MJ, Cooley JS, Petros JG, et al. Complete intraoperative small-bowel endoscopy in the evaluation of occult gastrointestinal bleeding using the sonde enteroscope. Arch Surg 1996;131:272–7.
39. Zaman A, Sheppard B, Katon RM. Total peroral intraoperative enteroscopy for obscure GI bleeding using a dedicated push enteroscope: diagnostic yield and patient outcome. Gastrointest Endosc 1999;50:506–10.
40. Douard R, Wind P, Panis Y, et al. Intraoperative enteroscopy for diagnosis and management of unexplained gastrointestinal bleeding. Am J Surg 2000;180:181–4.
41. Kendrick ML, Buttar NS, Anderson MA, et al. Contribution of intraoperative enteroscopy in the management of obscure gastrointestinal bleeding. J Gastrointest Surg 2001;5:162–7.
42. Jakobs R, Hartmann D, Benz C, et al. Diagnosis of obscure gastrointestinal bleeding by intra-operative enteroscopy in 81 consecutive patients. World J Gastroenterol 2006;12:313–6.
43. Yamamoto H, Sekine Y, Sato Y, et al. Total enteroscopy with a nonsurgical steerable double-balloon method. Gastrointest Endosc 2001;53:216–20.
44. Hartmann D, Eickhoff A, Tamm R, et al. Balloon-assisted enteroscopy using a single-balloon technique. Endoscopy 2007;39(Suppl 1):E276.
45. Akerman PA, Agrawal D, Cantero D, et al. Spiral enteroscopy with the new DSB overtube: a novel technique for deep peroral small-bowel intubation. Endoscopy 2008;40:974–8.
46. May A, Nachbar L, Ell C. Double-balloon enteroscopy (push-and-pull enteroscopy) of the small bowel: feasibility and diagnostic and therapeutic yield in patients with suspected small bowel disease. Gastrointest Endosc 2005;62:62–70.
47. Ell C, May A, Nachbar L, et al. Push-and-pull enteroscopy in the small bowel using the double-balloon technique: results of a prospective European multicenter study. Endoscopy 2005;37:613–6.
48. Di Caro S, May A, Heine DG, et al. The European experience with double-balloon enteroscopy: indications, methodology, safety, and clinical impact. Gastrointest Endosc 2005;62:545–50.
49. Matsumoto T, Esaki M, Moriyama T, et al. Comparison of capsule endoscopy and enteroscopy with the double-balloon method in patients with obscure bleeding and polyposis. Endoscopy 2005;37:827–32.
50. Hadithi M, Heine GD, Jacobs MA, et al. A prospective study comparing video capsule endoscopy with double-balloon enteroscopy in patients with obscure gastrointestinal bleeding. Am J Gastroenterol 2006;101:52–7.
51. Heine GD, Hadithi M, Groenen MJ, et al. Double-balloon enteroscopy: indications, diagnostic yield, and complications in a series of 275 patients with suspected small-bowel disease. Endoscopy 2006;38:42–8.
52. Kaffes AJ, Koo JH, Meredith C. Double-balloon enteroscopy in the diagnosis and the management of small-bowel diseases: an initial experience in 40 patients. Gastrointest Endosc 2006;63:81–6.

53. Monkemuller K, Weigt J, Treiber G, et al. Diagnostic and therapeutic impact of double-balloon enteroscopy. Endoscopy 2006;38:67–72.
54. Nakamura M, Niwa Y, Ohmiya N, et al. Preliminary comparison of capsule endoscopy and double-balloon enteroscopy in patients with suspected small-bowel bleeding. Endoscopy 2006;38:59–66.
55. Akahoshi K, Kubokawa M, Matsumoto M, et al. Double-balloon endoscopy in the diagnosis and management of GI tract diseases: methodology, indications, safety, and clinical impact. World J Gastroenterol 2006;12:7654–9.
56. Sun B, Rajan E, Cheng S, et al. Diagnostic yield and therapeutic impact of double-balloon enteroscopy in a large cohort of patients with obscure gastrointestinal bleeding. Am J Gastroenterol 2006;101:2011–5.
57. Barreto-Zuniga R, Tellez-Avila FI, Chavez-Tapia NC, et al. Diagnostic yield, therapeutic impact, and complications of double-balloon enteroscopy in patients with small-bowel pathology. Surg Endosc 2008;22:1223–6.
58. Cazzato IA, Cammarota G, Nista EC, et al. Diagnostic and therapeutic impact of double-balloon enteroscopy (DBE) in a series of 100 patients with suspected small bowel diseases. Dig Liver Dis 2007;39:483–7.
59. Zhong J, Ma T, Zhang C, et al. A retrospective study of the application on double-balloon enteroscopy in 378 patients with suspected small-bowel diseases. Endoscopy 2007;39:208–15.
60. Gross SA, Stark ME. Initial experience with double-balloon enteroscopy at a U.S. center. Gastrointest Endosc 2008;67:890–7.
61. Tsujikawa T, Saitoh Y, Andoh A, et al. Novel single-balloon enteroscopy for diagnosis and treatment of the small intestine: preliminary experiences. Endoscopy 2008;40:11–5.
62. Kawamura T, Yasuda K, Tanaka K, et al. Clinical evaluation of a newly developed single-balloon enteroscope. Gastrointest Endosc 2008;68:1112–6.
63. Gerson LB, Batenic M, Newsom S, et al. Long-term outcomes after double balloon enteroscopy for gastrointestinal hemorrhage. Gastrointest Endosc 2009; in press.
64. Domagk D, Bretthauer M, Lenz P, et al. Carbon dioxide insufflation improves intubation depth in double-balloon enteroscopy: a randomized, controlled, double-blind trial. Endoscopy 2007;39:1064–7.
65. Zhi FC, Yue H, Jiang B, et al. Diagnostic value of double balloon enteroscopy for small-intestinal disease: experience from China. Gastrointest Endosc 2007;66:S19–21.
66. Mensink PB, Haringsma J, Kucharzik T, et al. Complications of double balloon enteroscopy: a multicenter survey. Endoscopy 2007;39:613–5.
67. Gerson LB, Chiorean M, Tokar J, et al. Complications associated with double balloon enteroscopy: the U.S. experience. Am J Gastroenterol 2008;103:S95–118.
68. May A, Nachbar L, Pohl J, et al. Endoscopic interventions in the small bowel using double balloon enteroscopy: feasibility and limitations. Am J Gastroenterol 2007;102:527–35.
69. Tominaga K, Iida T, Nakamura Y, et al. Small intestinal perforation of endoscopically unrecognized lesions during peroral single-balloon enteroscopy. Endoscopy 2008;40(Suppl 2):E213–4.
70. Somsouk M, Gralnek IM, Inadomi JM. Management of obscure occult gastrointestinal bleeding: a cost-minimization analysis. Clin Gastroenterol Hepatol 2008;6:661–70.

71. Postgate A, Despott E, Burling D, et al. Significant small-bowel lesions detected by alternative diagnostic modalities after negative capsule endoscopy. Gastrointest Endosc 2008;68:1209–14.
72. Cheifetz AS, Kornbluth AA, Legnani P, et al. The risk of retention of the capsule endoscope in patients with known or suspected Crohn's disease. Am J Gastroenterol 2006;101:2218–22.
73. Solem CA, Loftus EV Jr, Fletcher JG, et al. Small-bowel imaging in Crohn's disease: a prospective, blinded, 4-way comparison trial. Gastrointest Endosc 2008;68:255–66.
74. Ross A, Mehdizadeh S, Tokar J, et al. Double balloon enteroscopy detects small bowel mass lesions missed by capsule endoscopy. Dig Dis Sci 2008;53:2140–3.
75. Lai LH, Wong GL, Chow DK, et al. Long-term follow-up of patients with obscure gastrointestinal bleeding after negative capsule endoscopy. Am J Gastroenterol 2006;101:1224–8.

Endoscopic Retrograde Cholangiopancreatography in the Surgically Modified Gastrointestinal Tract

Andrew S. Ross, MD

KEYWORDS

- ERCP • Gastrointestinal surgery • Bariatric surgery
- Altered anatomy • Endoscopy

Enteroscopy in the surgically altered gastrointestinal tract can present a significant challenge for the endoscopist. There are now eight surgical procedures that may require the use of an enteroscope for postoperative diagnostic or therapeutic endoscopy.[1] To maximize successful interventions, the endoscopist must be aware not only of the type of surgery but also the postoperative anatomy resulting from any given operation.[2]

Although enteroscopy may be performed for a variety of reasons in patients with surgically altered gastrointestinal anatomy, the most common indication by far is the performance of endoscopic retrograde cholangiopancreatography (ERCP). This article focuses on the use of enteroscopy to perform ERCP in patients with surgically altered gastrointestinal anatomy.

SURGERY AND ANATOMY

To date, there are eight surgical procedures described that result in altered gastrointestinal anatomy, and that require nonstandard techniques for the performance of ERCP:[1]

1. Partial gastrectomy with Billroth II gastrojejunostomy
2. Gastrojejunostomy or "bypass" performed for gastric outlet obstruction
3. "Standard" Whipple procedure
4. "Pylorus preserving Whipple" procedure
5. Roux-en-Y gastric bypass performed for obesity
6. Roux-en-Y choledochojejunostomy or hepaticojejunostomy
7. Roux-en-Y biliary diversion, "duodenal switch"
8. Total gastrectomy with Roux-en-Y esophagojejunostomy

Digestive Disease Institute, Virginia Mason Medical Center, 1100 9th Avenue, Mailstop C3-GAS, Seattle, WA 98101, USA
E-mail address: andrew.ross@vmmc.org

Gastrointest Endoscopy Clin N Am 19 (2009) 497–507
doi:10.1016/j.giec.2009.04.009 giendo.theclinics.com
1052-5157/09/$ – see front matter © 2009 Elsevier Inc. All rights reserved.

Several significant challenges to performance of ERCP in a patient with surgically altered gastrointestinal anatomy exist.[1] First, access to the ampulla of Vater or biliary–enteric anastamosis may require the endoscopist to traverse a significant length of small intestine. The length of small intestine that must be traversed to access the major papilla correlates directly with the type of endoscope that must be used. Patients who have undergone a Billroth II gastrojejunostomy typically have the shortest route of access as the afferent limb is anastomosed directly to the gastric remnant. In the case of retrocolic Billroth II anastomosis, the length of bowel that must be traversed can be as short as 30 cm and the major papilla is usually accessible using a standard duodenoscope.[1] Patients who have undergone a gastrojejunostomy or pylorus preserving Whipple procedure have afferent limbs of varying lengths and ERCP can often be performed using a standard duodenoscope, although not uncommonly, a long forward-viewing endoscope or enteroscope is required.[3]

Patients who have Roux-en-Y anastamoses typically require the use of a long forward-viewing endoscope to access the major papilla for the performance of ERCP (**Fig. 1**). The length of the Roux limb typically determines which type of forward-viewing endoscope is required. The longest roux limb is encountered in patients who have undergone a standard Roux-en-Y gastric bypass for bariatric indications or in those individuals in whom bowel resection proximal to the ligament of Treitz has not been performed. The Roux limb in patients who have undergone a Roux-en-Y gastric bypass for weight loss is typically 1 m in length, although limbs of up to 1.5 m are not uncommon.[2] Access to the major papilla using a pediatric colonoscope or enteroscope in patients following Roux-en-Y gastric bypass may fail in a large percentage of cases.[4] Performance of ERCP in these patients may require the use of specialized enteroscopes designed for deep enteral access such as the double-balloon[5] (Fujinon Endoscopy, Wayne, New Jersey), single-balloon[6] (Olympus America, Center Valley, Pennsylvania), or spiral enteroscopy systems[7] (Spirus Medical, Stoughton, Massachusetts). Access to the papilla in patients with long

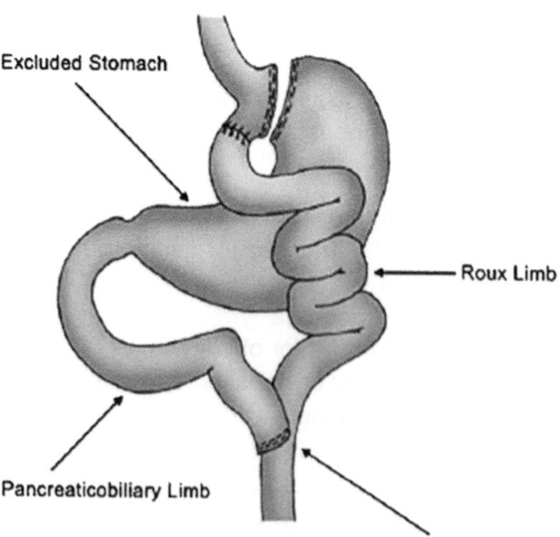

Fig. 1. Postsurgical anatomy observed following a Roux-en-Y gastric bypass. (*Reprinted from* Ross A, Semrad C, Alverdy J, et al. Use of double balloon enteroscopy to perform PEG in the excluded stomach after Roux-en-Y gastric bypass. Gastrointest Endosc 2006;65(5):797–800; with permission from Elsevier.)

Roux limbs has also been successfully reported using a duodenoscope advanced over a wire guide placed initially through a pediatric colonoscope.[4] Other techniques for accessing the major papilla in such patients include surgical access to the excluded stomach through which a standard duodenoscope is passed and the creation of a gastrostomy or jejunostomy, which is then dilated to accommodate the duodenoscope (see later discussion).

There are other significant challenges to performing ERCP in patients with postsurgical anatomy. First, surgical anastomoses were not designed with the endoscope in mind; access to the pancreaticobiliary limb in a patient with Roux-en-Y anatomy often requires an almost 180-degree "U-turn" to access the pancreaticobiliary limb.[1] The use of a forward-viewing endoscope in a retrograde fashion presents its own set of challenges. Due to its location on the medial wall of the duodenum, the papillary orifice is not always visible using a forward-viewing instrument. Because of this; the alignment of the working channel of the endoscope with the papilla for cannulation, especially without the availability of an elevator, can prove difficult. Finally, the use of an enteroscope for the performance of therapeutic ERCP requires the use of enteroscopy-length equipment, the availability of which is limited in many markets.

TECHNICAL ASPECTS OF ERCP IN THE SURGICALLY MODIFIED GASTROINTESTINAL TRACT

Advancement Technique

Before ERCP is attempted in patients with postsurgical anatomy, it is imperative that the endoscopist understands the operation performed and the resultant anatomy. The operative report should be obtained, imaging reviewed and, whenever possible, a discussion with the surgeon who performed the operation should be undertaken.[2] These steps are imperative for preprocedural planning, which includes (at minimum) selection of the proper endoscope, route of sedation, and ensuring the availability of specialized enteroscopy-length ERCP accessories.

For patients with short anastomoses, such as those found in a Billroth II gastrojejunostomy, a duodenoscope may suffice. There are now several published reports describing the technique using a 164-cm long pediatric colonoscope or standard 2.4-m long "standard" enteroscope for the performance of ERCP in patients with postsurgical anatomy.[3,4] The pediatric colonoscope and standard enteroscope are equipped with a 2.8-mm working channel. Successful ERCP has been performed using these instruments with and without the assistance of an overtube. Overtubes may reduce looping in the stomach and duodenum and, in patients who have undergone a gastrectomy or gastric bypass, they are rarely needed. It is preferable to use a variable stiffness colonoscope whenever possible; initial insertion of the endoscope is typically performed on the most flexible setting; the stiffness may be increased once the endoscope is passed into the small intestine to reduce loop formation. Depending on the anatomy, the colonoscope or enteroscope is then advanced to the Roux-en-Y anastomosis or through an afferent limb to the level of the papilla (**Fig. 2**) or pancreaticobiliary anastamosis (**Fig. 3**). In patients with longer intestinal limbs, it may be necessary to use the "hook and pull" technique to advance the endoscope deeper into the small intestine. The use of a colonoscope to place a wire into the pancreaticobiliary limb in patients with Roux-en-Y anatomy followed by advancement of a duodenoscope over the wire has been described.[4]

The double-balloon enteroscopy (DBE) system employs a 2-m endoscope (EN450-T5, Fujinon Endoscopy) with a 145-cm overtube attached (TS-13,140, Fujinon Endoscopy). The working channel is 2.8 mm in diameter. A shorter double-balloon enteroscope has recently become available in some markets. This scope is 152 cm

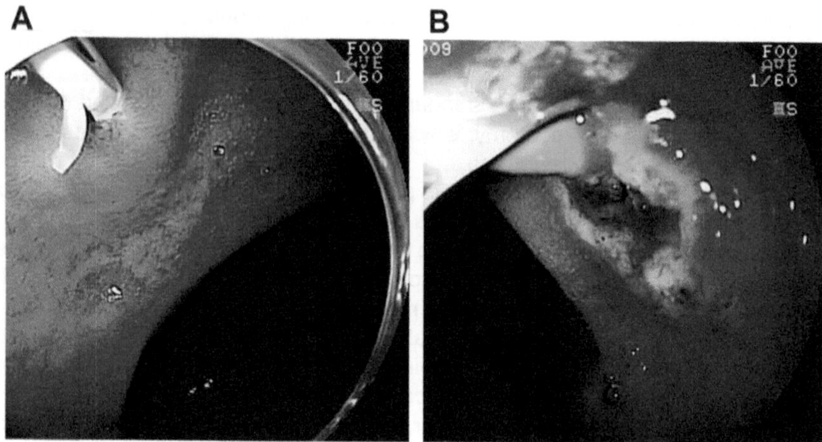

Fig. 2. The major papilla viewed in a retrograde fashion across the duodenum using the double-balloon enteroscope. Needle knife biliary sphincterotomy can be performed following placement of a pancreatic duct (*A*) or bile duct stent (*B*).

in length with a 2.8-mm working channel. The "push and pull" technique for obtaining deep enteral access with the double-balloon system has been well described.[5] This same technique is used when DBE is used to access the major papilla or pancreatico-biliary anastomosis in patients with postsurgical anatomy who require ERCP.[8–13]

The single-balloon enteroscopy (SBE) system uses a 2-m endoscope (SIF-Q180, Olympus America) with a 140-cm overtube attached (ST-SB1, Olympus America). A "push and pull" technique similar to that used for advancement of the double-balloon enteroscope has also been described for SBE. The spiral endoscopy system uses a rotational technique applied to a specially designed overtube combined with a 2-m enteroscope to pleat the small bowel resulting in deep enteral access.[7] To date, the use of the single-balloon or spiral endoscopy systems for the performance of ERCP in postsurgical anatomy has not been described.

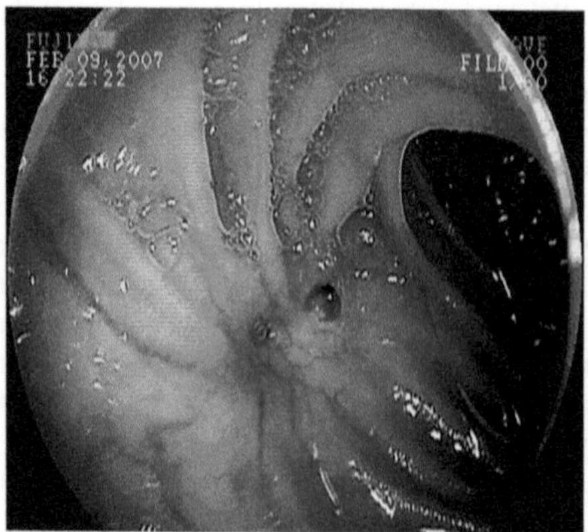

Fig. 3. Endoscopic appearance of a hepaticojejunostomy as visualized using a double-balloon enteroscope.

Regardless of the endoscope used, advancement through a Roux-en-Y anastomosis into the pancreaticobiliary limb can represent a significant challenge. The first issue that arises is the identification of the appropriate limb. On entering the Roux-en-Y anastamosis, the endoscopist will typically visualize two or three potential "openings" into which the endoscope may be passed (**Fig. 4**). One of the openings is not a true passage but represents a "blind end," which is a result of the end-to-side fashion in which the anastamosis is created. The passage visualized directly adjacent to the "blind end" is usually the efferent limb. If the endoscope is inserted into this limb and passed for a distance, fluoroscopy will likely reveal the formation of multiple intestinal loops within the pelvis. Although this limb may contain bile, it will not lead to the papilla. If the efferent limb is inadvertently entered, a tattoo may be placed just past the anastamosis to ensure that passage is not attempted a second time. Navigating the jejuno-jejunal anastomosis can often be disorienting to the endoscopist and it is not uncommon to re-enter an already explored limb.

The pancreaticobiliary limb is usually situated at an almost 180-degree turn once the endoscope is inserted into the Roux-en-Y anastomosis. Entry into the pancreaticobiliary limb is technically challenging. It usually requires the performance of a "U-turn" and, when a variable stiffness colonoscope is used, should be attempted using the most flexible setting. On occasion, changing the patient's position left lateral decubitous or the application of abdominal pressure may prove beneficial. If the DBE system is used, it is useful to perform a reduction maneuver once the jejuno-jejunal anastomosis is reached. Next, the tip of the endoscope is advanced as deep as possible into the pancreaticobiliary limb. The balloon affixed to the endoscope is inflated and the endoscope tip is "hooked" into the limb using a combination of tip deflection and suction while the overtube is advanced through the anastomosis and into the pancreaticobiliary limb.[1] The "push and pull" technique is the used to advance the endoscope to the papilla or biliary anastamosis. In patients who have undergone a pancreaticobiliary diversion for obesity, the Roux-en-Y anastomosis may be accessed more easily using the retrograde approach with a single- or double-balloon enteroscope.[1]

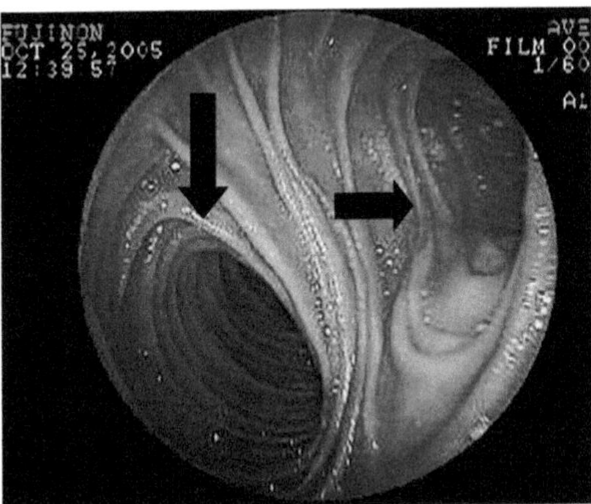

Fig. 4. Typical endoscopic appearance of a Roux-en-Y jejuno-jejunostomy; the vertical arrow demonstrates the entry to the efferent limb; a "blind end" is typically found adjacent to the efferent limb (*horizontal arrow*); this may be incorrectly interpreted as a "third" opening within the anastomosis.

Cannulation

Cannulation of the major papilla using a forward-viewing endoscope presents its own set of challenges. As describe previously, the use of the forward view (as opposed to the side view) afforded by these instruments may prevent complete visualization of the papilla and, in addition, may present difficulties in terms of the angle of approach and vector forces for instrument passage. Additional challenges include the lack of an elevator and inverted orientation of the papilla when retrograde access to the papilla across the duodenum is required.

Standard length ERCP accessories can be used when a colonoscope is used to achieve access to the major papilla. As a pediatric colonoscope is typically used for this purpose, the maximum working channel size is 2.8 mm. As such, a 7 Fr plastic stent is the largest-caliber plastic endoprosthesis that may be used with this instrument. When a 2-m (double- or single-balloon systems) or standard 2.4-m enteroscope is used, specialized equipment must be obtained in advance. An enteroscopy-length sphincterotome, needle knife, extraction balloon and basket are all available through custom order.[1] Because the market for these accessories is limited, delivery of this equipment may take up to 6 weeks, even in major markets. As such, adequate inventories of this specialized equipment should be on hand in high-volume centers. Most other accessories including standard length dilation balloons, stent "pushing" catheters, and wire guides are long enough to be used through the 2-m enteroscope.

Due to the lack of an elevator and typical retrograde access across the duodenum, cannulation of the major papilla is typically performed using a straight single or double lumen catheter (**Fig. 5**). A sphincterotomy is typically performed by placement of a stent into either the pancreatic or bile duct followed by a needle knife sphincterotomy over the stent (see **Fig. 2**). The performance of other therapeutic maneuvers, assuming the appropriate equipment is available, is straightforward. One exception is exchange of accessories when the standard or 2-m enteroscope is used. It is not uncommon for the assistant to "lose" the wire when exchanging accessories due to their increased length relative to the wire guide being used. Wherever possible, the longest wire guide available should be used to help avoid this potential pitfall. In the event that the

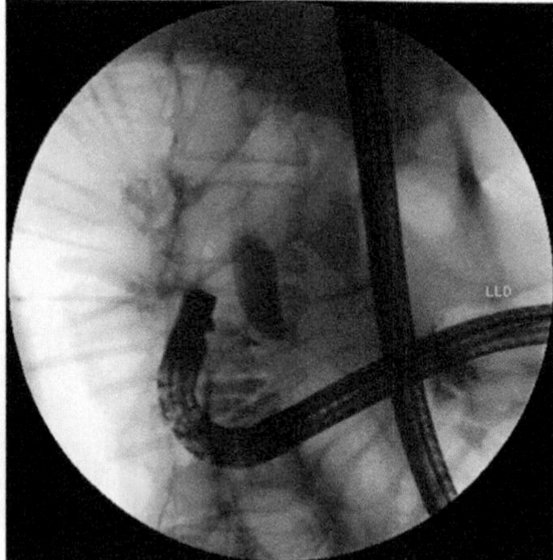

Fig. 5. Fluoroscopic image depicting biliary cannulation in a patient who is post-Roux-en-Y gastric bypass. In this case, a duodenoscope was able to be advanced through the Roux-en-Y anastomosis to the major papilla.

assistant loses the wire, a 60 mL syringe filled with water or saline can be affixed to the accessory being exchanged and counter pressure applied using a static column of water to avoid losing ductal access.

Biliary access in patients with a hepaticojejunostomy (see **Fig. 3**) or choledochojejunostomy is typically easier than in patients with native papillae, however, the anastamosis may be located behind intestinal folds or on a turn in the bowel making visualization difficult.[1] Administration of intravenous sincalide (Kinevac, Bracco Diagnostics, Princeton, New Jersey) at a dose of 0.02 μg/kg can be performed to stimulate the secretion of bile to aid identification of the biliary anastamosis. In patients who have surgical anastamoses of the pancreatic duct (Whipple procedure); the pancreatic anastamosis may prove difficult to identify. Secretin (SecreFlo, Chesapeake Biologic Labs, Baltimore, Maryland) administered intravenously as an 0.2 μg/kg bolus can often be helpful in this regard. For patients with intact papillae and those with surgical pancreaticobiliary reconstruction, a clear plastic cap affixed to the tip of the endoscope improves visualization.

Alternatives to Per Os Endoscopic Access

In many centers, expertise in ERCP in patients with complex postsurgical anatomy may not exist. In addition, endoscopists may not be successful in performing ERCP in all cases. There are several additional options. First, percutaneous transhepatic access by an interventional radiologist can often be achieved, especially in patients with dilated intrahepatic bile ducts. Other alternatives include surgical endoscopic access to the excluded stomach in patients who are post-Roux-en-Y gastric bypass[14,15] or surgical access to the small bowel in patients with other anatomic configurations. ERCP performed through a gastrostomy[16] placed into the excluded stomach or mature jejunostomy[17] has also been reported.

REVIEW OF PUBLISHED DATA

Indications

ERCP is performed for a variety of clinical indications in patients with altered gastrointestinal anatomy. In patients with native papillae, common indications include management of choledocholithiasis and palliation of obstructive jaundice arising from benign or malignant biliary strictures. Many patients who have undergone bariatric surgery have often had a cholecystectomy performed. Papillary stenosis can often be seen in this population, which, on occasion, may require ERCP and sphincterotomy. Finally, indications for using ERCP to perform pancreatic duct therapy in patients with native papillae are identical to those in patients with nonsurgically altered anatomy.

In patients with surgically altered anatomy and biliary or pancreatic anastomosis, the indications for ERCP differ slightly than for patients with native papillae. ERCP is typically performed in this group for anastomotic strictures. Strictures of the pancreatic or biliary anastamosis can be complicated by the formation of stones that require endoscopic removal. Jaundice related to recurrent malignancy can be seen in patients who have undergone a biliary resection and anastomosis for cancer. In this setting, ERCP may be performed to palliate jaundice and for the delivery of photodynamic therapy.

Several groups have now reported their experience performing ERCP in patients with postsurgical anatomy using a duodenoscope, colonoscope, or standard length enteroscope.[3,4] In patients with a Billroth II gastrojejunostomy, complication and technical success rates of ERCP performed in major referral centers are similar to those in patients with normal anatomy.[4] Similarly, ERCP performed with these endoscopes in patients with surgically altered anatomy and anastomoses of the bile or pancreatic duct has also met with high technical success rates.[4] Perhaps the most technically challenging of all cases involves selective cannulation of an intact papilla in patients with long-limb Roux-en-Y anastomoses. In this case, the data are limited to a handful of small case series.

Elton and colleagues[3] first reported the use of a colonoscope or standard length enteroscope to perform ERCP in 18 patients with long-limb gastrojejunostomy performed for a variety of indications. Biliary cannulation was successful in five out of six patients with intact papillae; pancreatic cannulation was achieved in all three patients (with intact papillae) in whom it was attempted.

Wright and colleagues[4] reported on ERCP attempted in 15 patients with native papilla and long-limb Roux-en-Y gastrojejunostomy. As opposed to the report by Elton and colleagues, access to the major papilla was achieved using a duodenoscope advanced over a guidewire placed initially using a colonoscope. In a few cases, the investigators advanced the duodenoscope into the pancreaticobiliary limb over a balloon catheter placed retrograde into the limb. Using this method, the papilla could be reached in 10 of the patients (66.7%) following which therapeutic techniques could be performed in all patients.

Since the introduction of DBE in 2003, several case series have emerged describing experiences using the device for performing ERCP in patients with surgically altered anatomy.[8,12,13,18–30] Sixteen case series have reported the use of the double-balloon enteroscope in 63 patients with a variety of anatomic configurations.[10] In the largest North American series to date,[13] 14 patients with Roux-en-Y anatomy underwent 20 ERCP procedures. The ampulla, biliary, or pancreatic anastamosis could be reached in 85% of cases including all six patients who had undergone a gastric bypass for obesity and therefore had a native papilla. Cannulation was achieved in 80% of patients in whom the ampulla or pancreaticobiliary anastamosis could be reached during procedures that lasted a mean (SD) of 99 (48) minutes. Although 20 procedures were performed, therapeutic interventions were performed in only six cases. The investigators were also able to demonstrate a decreased procedure time with experience, especially in patients with native papillae.

In contrast to North America, most case series from Europe report the use of this device in patients who have undergone Roux-en-Y anastomoses as part of a liver transplant or Whipple procedure, thus limiting the use of this technology, for the most part, to patients with pancreaticobiliary anastamoses. The largest series from Europe[21] reported 18 procedures in 13 patients with the ability to access the pancreaticobiliary anastamosis or native papilla in 17 of 18 cases. Cannulation could be achieved in all but two cases; therapeutic maneuvers were performed in eight. The mean procedure duration was 40 minutes.

A Japanese report has recently detailed the experience performing ERCP using the shorter-length double-balloon enteroscope.[31] In this series, ERCP was performed in 38 patients, 26 of whom had undergone Roux-en-Y total gastrectomy or a Whipple procedure. Pancreaticobiliary anastamoses were reached in 45 of the 48 procedures performed and ERCP was successfully performed in 42 of the 45 cases in which the anastamosis could be reached.

Complications

Although ERCP-related complications such as pancreatitis and bleeding do arise when the procedure is performed on patients with surgically altered intestinal anatomy, the frequency is not increased compared with that observed in patients with normal anatomy who undergo ERCP. By definition, surgically altered intestinal anatomy involve one or more surgical anastomosis of the small bowel or stomach, therefore there is, in theory, a slightly higher risk of bowel perforation in this group.

SUMMARY

The performance of ERCP in patients with postsurgical anatomy is time consuming, technically challenging and often requires a significant level of expertise to optimize chances for success. Despite this, recent advances in techniques for obtaining deep enteral access (double- and single-balloon endoscopy) seem to represent an improvement over previously available technologies and, given time, may result in improved outcomes. In North America, the obesity epidemic will, without a doubt, lead to further increases in bariatric surgery and, thus, increase the patient population with difficult to access pancreaticobiliary anatomy. This group of patients will likely provide a rich source of data to determine whether the use of these new endoscopic techniques for performing ERCP in patients with surgically altered anatomy improves outcomes in a cost-effective, time-efficient manner over other access techniques, namely surgery.

REFERENCES

1. Haber GB. Double balloon endoscopy for pancreatic and biliary access in altered anatomy (with videos). Gastrointest Endosc 2007;66(3 Suppl):S47–50.
2. Stellato TA, Crouse C, Hallowell PT. Bariatric surgery: creating new challenges for the endoscopist. Gastrointest Endosc 2003;57(1):86–94.
3. Elton E, Hanson BL, Qaseem T, et al. Diagnostic and therapeutic ERCP using an enteroscope and a pediatric colonoscope in long-limb surgical bypass patients. Gastrointest Endosc 1998;47(1):62–7.
4. Wright BE, Cass OW, Freeman ML. ERCP in patients with long-limb Roux-en-Y gastrojejunostomy and intact papilla. Gastrointest Endosc 2002;56(2):225–32.
5. Yamamoto H, Sugano K. A new method of enteroscopy – the double-balloon method. Can J Gastroenterol 2003;17(4):273–4.
6. Kawamura T, Yasuda K, Tanaka K, et al. Clinical evaluation of a newly developed single-balloon enteroscope. Gastrointest Endosc 2008;68(6):1112–6.
7. Akerman PA, Agrawal D, Chen W, et al. Spiral enteroscopy: a novel method of enteroscopy by using the Endo-Ease Discovery SB overtube and a pediatric colonoscope. Gastrointest Endosc 2009;69(2):327–32.
8. Monkemuller K, Bellutti M, Neumann H, et al. Therapeutic ERCP with the double-balloon enteroscope in patients with Roux-en-Y anastomosis. Gastrointest Endosc 2008;67(6):992–6.
9. Monkemuller K, Fry LC, Bellutti M, et al. ERCP with the double balloon enteroscope in patients with Roux-en-Y anastomosis. Surg Endosc 2008, in press.
10. Koornstra JJ, Fry L, Monkemuller K. ERCP with the balloon-assisted enteroscopy technique: a systematic review. Dig Dis 2008;26(4):324–9.
11. Bruno M. Double balloon scope for endoscopic retrograde cholangiopancreatography. Neth J Med 2008;66(7):267–8.
12. Chu YC, Yang CC, Yeh YH, et al. Double-balloon enteroscopy application in biliary tract disease – its therapeutic and diagnostic functions. Gastrointest Endosc 2008;68(3):585–91.
13. Emmett DS, Mallat DB. Double-balloon ERCP in patients who have undergone Roux-en-Y surgery: a case series. Gastrointest Endosc 2007;66(5):1038–41.

14. Patel JA, Patel NA, Shinde T, et al. Endoscopic retrograde cholangiopancreatography after laparoscopic Roux-en-Y gastric bypass: a case series and review of the literature. Am Surg 2008;74(8):689–93 [discussion: 93–4].
15. Nakao FS, Mendes CJ, Szego T, et al. Intraoperative transgastric ERCP after a Roux-en-Y gastric bypass. Endoscopy 2007;39(Suppl 1):E219–20.
16. Martinez J, Guerrero L, Byers P, et al. Endoscopic retrograde cholangiopancreatography and gastroduodenoscopy after Roux-en-Y gastric bypass. Surg Endosc 2006;20(10):1548–50.
17. Baron TH, Chahal P, Ferreira LE. ERCP via mature feeding jejunostomy tube tract in a patient with Roux-en-Y anatomy (with video). Gastrointest Endosc 2008;68(1): 189–91.
18. Haruta H, Yamamoto H, Mizuta K, et al. A case of successful enteroscopic balloon dilation for late anastomotic stricture of choledochojejunostomy after living donor liver transplantation. Liver Transpl 2005;11(12):1608–10.
19. Moreels TG, Roth B, Vandervliet EJ, et al. The use of the double-balloon enteroscope for endoscopic retrograde cholangiopancreatography and biliary stent placement after Roux-en-Y hepaticojejunostomy. Endoscopy 2007;39(Suppl 1): E196–7.
20. Chu YC, Su SJ, Yang CC, et al. ERCP plus papillotomy by use of double-balloon enteroscopy after Billroth II gastrectomy. Gastrointest Endosc 2007;66(6): 1234–6.
21. Aabakken L, Bretthauer M, Line PD. Double-balloon enteroscopy for endoscopic retrograde cholangiography in patients with a Roux-en-Y anastomosis. Endoscopy 2007;39(12):1068–71.
22. Koornstra JJ. Double balloon enteroscopy for endoscopic retrograde cholangiopancreaticography after Roux-en-Y reconstruction: case series and review of the literature. Neth J Med 2008;66(7):275–9.
23. Fahndrich M, Sandmann M, Heike M. A facilitated method for endoscopic interventions at the bile duct after Roux-en-Y reconstruction using double balloon enteroscopy. Z Gastroenterol 2008;46(4):335–8.
24. Monkemuller K, Fry LC, Bellutti M, et al. ERCP using single-balloon instead of double-balloon enteroscopy in patients with Roux-en-Y anastomosis. Endoscopy 2008;40(Suppl 2):E19–20.
25. Mehdizadeh S, Ross A, Gerson L, et al. What is the learning curve associated with double-balloon enteroscopy? Technical details and early experience in 6 U.S. tertiary care centers. Gastrointest Endosc 2006;64(5):740–50.
26. Spahn TW, Grosse-Thie W, Spies P, et al. Treatment of choledocholithiasis following Roux-en-Y hepaticojejunostomy using double-balloon endoscopy. Digestion 2007;75(1):20–1.
27. Kawano Y, Mizuta K, Hishikawa S, et al. Rendezvous penetration method using double-balloon endoscopy for complete anastomosis obstruction of hepaticojejunostomy after pediatric living donor liver transplantation. Liver Transpl 2008; 14(3):385–7.
28. Zuber-Jerger I, Klebl F, Schoelmerich J. Endoscopic retrograde cholangiography of a hepaticojejunostomy using double balloon enteroscopy. Dig Surg 2008; 25(3):241–3.
29. Maaser C, Lenze F, Bokemeyer M, et al. Double balloon enteroscopy: a useful tool for diagnostic and therapeutic procedures in the pancreaticobiliary system. Am J Gastroenterol 2008;103(4):894–900.
30. Tsukui D, Yano T, Nakazawa K, et al. Rendezvous technique combining double-balloon endoscopy with percutaneous cholangioscopy is useful for the treatment

of biliary anastomotic obstruction after liver transplantation (with video). Gastrointest Endosc 2008;68(5):1013–5.

31. Matsushita M, Shimatani M, Takaoka M, et al. "Short" double-balloon enteroscope for diagnostic and therapeutic ERCP in patients with altered gastrointestinal anatomy. Am J Gastroenterol 2008;103(12):3218–9.

Novel Applications of Balloon Endoscopy

Michel Delvaux, MD, PhD*, Gérard Gay, MD

KEYWORDS

- Double-balloon endoscopy • Capsule endoscopy
- Abdominal pain • Colonoscopy • Confocal microscopy
- Vasculitides • Intestinal infections

Since double-balloon enteroscopy was introduced by Yamamoto and colleagues in 2001,[1] the technique has developed dramatically and the indications extended, as shown by the previous articles. The use of capsule endoscopy (CE) and double-balloon enteroscopy (DBE) has led to a tremendous increase in knowledge over the last decade about intestinal diseases and the involvement of the small bowel in general conditions such as vasculitides, systemic infections, and autoimmune disorders.

The aim of the present review is to examine the opportunities for DBE, in the light of existing data for indications that have so far not been investigated in large series of patients, but which may help in understanding difficult clinical conditions. The use of DBE in other parts of the alimentary canal is also considered.

EXTENSION OF THE DIAGNOSTIC FIELD OF DOUBLE BALLOON ENTEROSCOPY

Diagnostic Applications of Double Balloon Enteroscopy

At present, almost any suspected intestinal disease might constitute a reason for performing DBE. Some of the most frequent indications, for which the largest amount of data have been gained, have been discussed in the other articles. In most cases, DBE is regarded as an invasive, procedure and requires time and resources, and in western countries at least, the rate of complete examination of the small bowel by a DBE procedure has been reported to be lower than that reported in Japanese series.[2–4] The comparison between these studies is somewhat biased by the heterogeneity of the cases and the variable approaches in the use of DBE. When DBE was initially proposed by Yamamoto and colleagues,[1] CE was not available in Japan and the complete examination of the small bowel was thus considered the primary outcome of these early procedures. In contrast, CE has been in use since 2001/2002 in Europe and the United States for the examination of the small bowel. DBE was introduced

Department of Internal Medicine and Digestive Pathology, Hôpitaux de Brabois, F – 54511 Vandoeuvre les Nancy, France
* Corresponding author.
E-mail address: m.delvaux@chu-nancy.fr (M. Delvaux).

Gastrointest Endoscopy Clin N Am 19 (2009) 509–518
doi:10.1016/j.giec.2009.04.014 giendo.theclinics.com
1052-5157/09/$ – see front matter © 2009 Elsevier Inc. All rights reserved.

later, and was often regarded as a complementary investigation after CE was performed first or as an alternative if CE was contraindicated because of the suspicion of an intestinal stenosis. Several studies have shown that CE can detect lesions that require further assessment by DBE, to obtain biopsies or provide therapy. In a series of 146 patients examined prospectively for occult digestive bleeding, CE was found to accurately predict the route of insertion to be used for subsequent DBE.[5] In this study, CE was found to be possible in most of the patients; intestinal stenosis was suspected in only 4 out of 146 patients and DBE was performed as the first-line examination.

The rationale for performing a diagnostic DBE must be discussed in a global approach based on the combined use of CE, DBE, and radiologic modalities, CT and magnetic resonance imaging (MRI) enteroclysis. Over the last decade, the significant advances in intestinal radiologic and endoscopic examinations have led to examinations of the small bowel in clinical situations that were poorly investigated in the past. Patients with chronic abdominal pain have been included in small proportion in clinical series reporting the outcome of DBE.[3,6,7] The results are not available in the same way in all of these studies. In DiCaro's study,[6] Crohn disease was diagnosed in two of the three patients with abdominal pain. In the other studies,[3,7] the results of DBE were not specified for patients with abdominal pain as most of the patients also presented with chronic anemia. Overall, the diagnostic yield of intestinal examinations in patients with chronic abdominal pain is low. In a retrospective series of patients investigated by barium enteroclysis, a clinically relevant diagnosis was obtained in only 10% of the patients with abdominal pain.[8] In another retrospective study, CT enteroclysis was found to detect more lesions than CE in patients with chronic abdominal pain.[9] CE has also been evaluated in three small series of patients with chronic abdominal pain.[10–12] The diagnostic yield of CE ranged from 6% to 36%, taking into account that the highest diagnostic yield was reported in a study including patients with chronic abdominal pain associated with other clinical signs, such as weight loss, diarrhea, or suspected bleeding.[12] Therefore, it is reasonable to assume that DBE would not have a high diagnostic yield in patients with chronic abdominal pain, in the absence of accompanying signs. DBE should remain a second-line investigation for this indication and CE should be performed first, except for those patients with a suspicion of intestinal stenosis.

Enteric infections and enteric involvement in systemic infections and diseases have also been scarcely investigated. Enteric infections are often observed in immunocompromised conditions, such as cancer,[13] organ transplantation, common variable immunodeficiency,[14] and HIV infection. Cytomegalovirus (CMV) is a common pathogen found in these situations. CMV infection can be recognized from typical endoscopic pictures of bleeding ulcerations of the small intestinal and colonic mucosa with a diffuse inflammatory pattern observed by CE and DBE (**Fig. 1**). However, the diagnosis can be established only by demonstration of CMV inclusions on biopsies. In some cases, lesions may be limited to the small bowel and DBE may be required to obtain these biopsies. However, in critically ill patients, CE should be discussed as the first-line investigation. In a large series of 47 cancer patients, 42 (89.4%) had digestive lesions that contributed to the diagnosis.[13] Gastrointestinal bleeding is a common feature of intestinal CMV infection. In this context, CE and DBE may help to obtain a diagnosis. However, when diffuse intestinal bleeding is observed by CE, DBE should be performed to more precisely examine the lesions at the level of the hemorrhagic segment and obtain biopsies. CMV infection is often associated with graft-versus-host-disease (GVHD), which occurs after bone marrow transplantation. Several studies have shown the usefulness of CE and DBE in the investigation of these patients. In two small series of patients investigated by CE, the typical mucosal

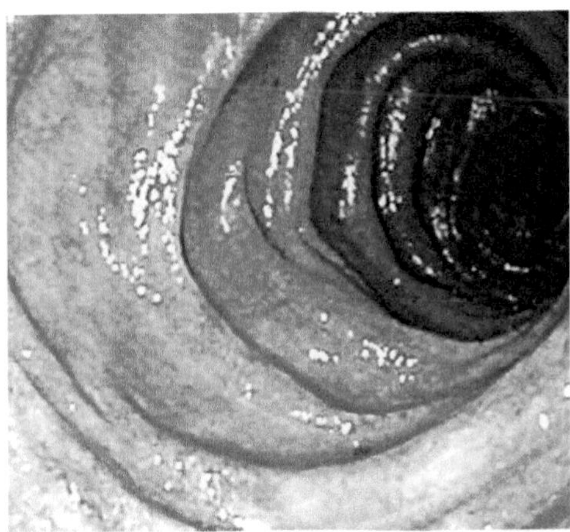

Fig. 1. Diffuse bleeding pattern of the intestinal mucosa in a heart transplant patient with CMV infection.

lesions were detected more frequently than by esophagogastroduodenostomy (EGD).[15,16] The specific role of DBE in this situation has not yet been evaluated in published studies. In patients with lesions seen by CE, DBE and intestinal biopsies may be required to confirm CMV infection, particularly in the case of focal lesions.

The small bowel is frequently involved in systemic diseases such as vasculitides.[17] Lesions have been observed by CE in patients with Behçet disease, Churg and Strauss, Henoch-Schönlein vasculitis, and Wegener granulomatosis.[18–23] These lesions are frequently suggested by an episode of gastrointestinal bleeding.[23,24] On the other hand, the differential diagnosis must be established with any disease causing intestinal ulcers. Some examples of intestinal lesions of vasculitides are shown in **Fig. 2**. In these patients, a combined approach with CE followed by targeted DBE seems to be the most effective.

Additional Diagnostic Procedures During Double Balloon Enteroscopy

Expansion of the diagnostic capabilities of DBE can be achieved using the new devices inserted through the operating channel of the endoscope. Recently, a case report and a short series have been published about the combination of DBE with endoscopic ultrasound (EUS) miniprobes.[25,26] In the case of a tumor seen at DBE as a pseudopedunculated submucosal mass,[25] the complementary examination with a 12-MHz probe inserted through the operating channel of a therapeutic double-balloon enteroscope showed a dumbbell-shaped lesion, extending to the muscularis propria and indicated the need for surgical intervention. In a short series of patients,[26] EUS with a miniprobe introduced through a double-balloon enteroscope could clearly distinguish the different layers of the intestinal wall. It was then tested in seven patients with a protruding lesion (mass or polyp), allowing a clear assessment of the depth of extension of the lesion in four patients.

Recently, a miniprobe has been developed to scan the surface of the digestive mucosa, with the technique of confocal microscopy.[27] The technique has been evaluated initially for the examination of digestive neoplasms. After intravenous injection of fluorescein, the miniprobe is applied to the mucosal surface through the operating channel. Scanning of the mucosa shows the glandular structures and the vessels, allowing a detailed examination of the architecture (**Fig. 3**). A recent short publication

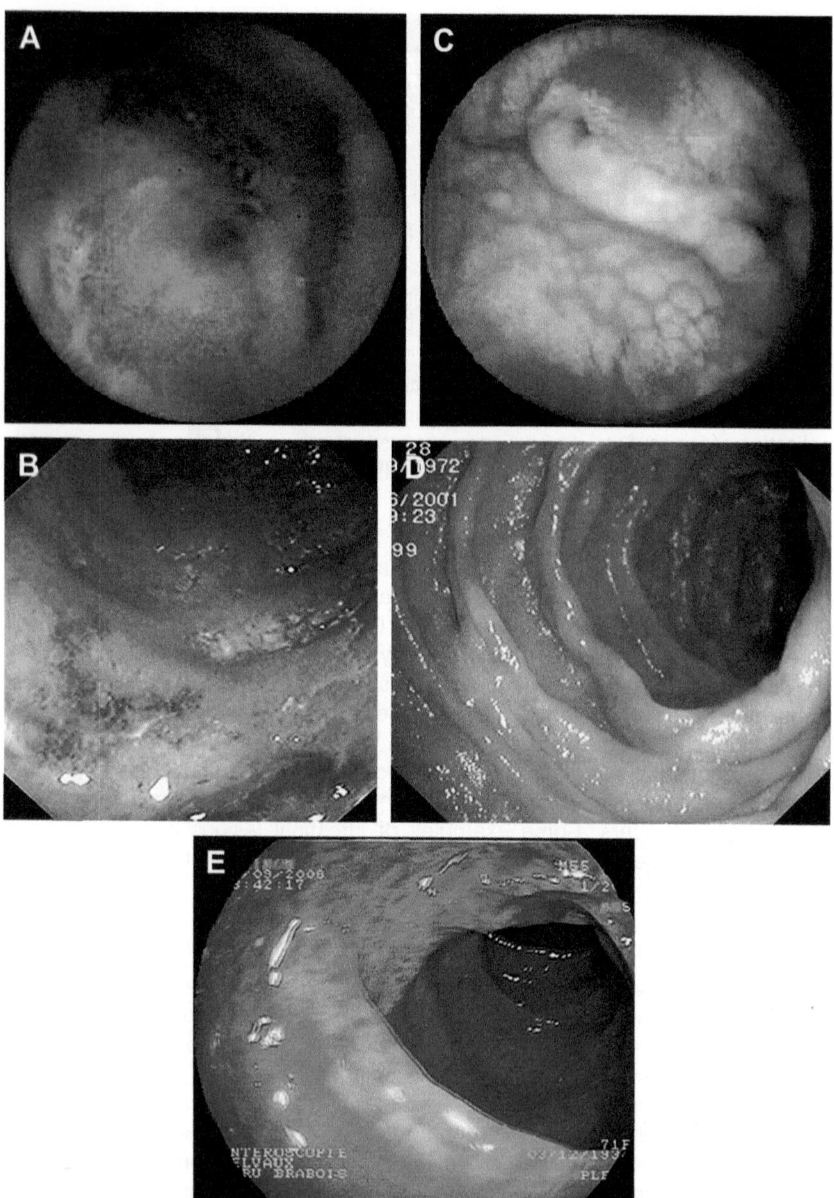

Fig. 2. Examples of vasculitis-related intestinal lesions. (*A*) Churg and Strauss syndrome viewed by CE. (*B*) Rheumatoid purpura (enteroscopy). (*C*) Chronic multifocal ulcerative stenosing enteritis viewed by CE. (*D*) Chronic multifocal ulcerative stenosing enteritis at enteroscopy. (*E*) Antiphospholipid syndrome.

has described the possibility of examining intestinal villi with this technique.[28] Clinical studies will be needed to demonstrate the diagnostic gain over the use of chromoendoscopy, such as Fujinon Intelligent Chromoendoscopy (FICE), with a magnifying endoscope. Potential indications could include the assessment of the intestinal

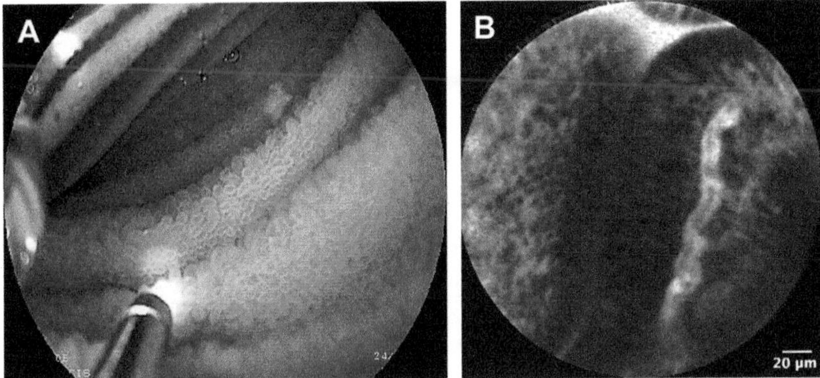

Fig. 3. Confocal microscopy for the examination of the mucosal surface of the jejunum. (*A*) Application of the confocal probe through the operating channel on to the mucosal surface. (*B*) Scanning of an intestinal villus, showing the architecture of the mucosal cells and the submucosa in the center of the villus.

mucosa in patients with refractory celiac disease or other ulcerative disorders of the small bowel.

USE OF DOUBLE BALLOON ENTEROSCOPY IN OTHER AREAS OF THE ALIMENTARY TRACT

Since it has been developed, the technique of DBE has been applied to endoscopic examination of other parts of the digestive tract than the small bowel. Several publications have shown that DBE can be used to investigate patients with surgically modified digestive anatomy, such as the excluded stomach after bariatric surgery, Roux-en-Y anastomosis, and retrograde catheterization of the bile ducts in patients with Billroth II or Roux-en-Y anastomosis. These indications are discussed in a separate article.

Following the experience gained with DBE procedures performed by the retrograde route to examine the ileum, several studies have demonstrated the usefulness of the technique to facilitate cecal intubation in patients with a previously failed colonoscopy.[29–33] In these studies, the success rate of cecal intubation ranged from 88% to 100%. Reasons for previously failed colonoscopy included fixed angles after abdominal surgery, redundant colons with long flexible loops, and in some series, inadequate sedation of the patient. Polypectomies were possible, including resection of large sessile lesions by endoscopic mucosal resection.[29,31]

The authors have applied the same technique using a dedicated double-balloon colonoscope to achieve complete colonoscopy after a previously failed attempt.[34] The double-balloon colonoscope is built on the same principle as the double-balloon enteroscope. The double-balloon colonoscope FC450-B15C (Fujinon Inc. Omiya, Japan) comprises a 182-cm long endoscope and an overtube, both equipped with a latex balloon at their tip (**Fig. 4**A, B). The technical characteristics of the system are reported in **Table 1** and are compared with those of the currently available double-balloon enteroscopes from Fujinon. The colonoscope has an electronic zoom and FICE (**Fig. 4**C). The double-balloon colonoscope is distinguished from the double-balloon enteroscope by its reduced length, which allows for easier insertion of therapeutic devices and a wider variety of accessories, which are often too short to be used through the operating channel of the double-balloon enteroscope (2.40 m in length). The bending part of the tip of the double-balloon colonoscope is

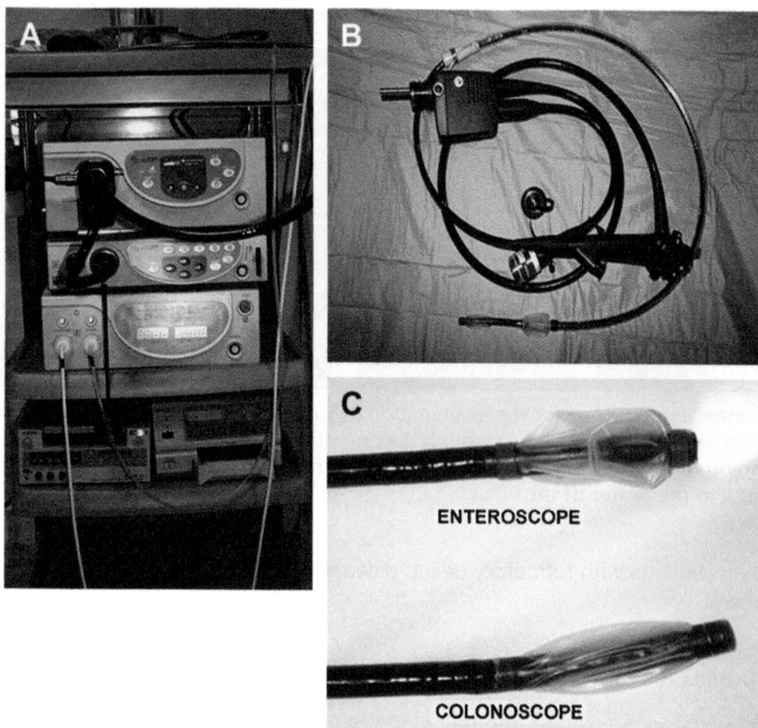

Fig. 4. Double-balloon colonscope. (*A*) Work station with the electronic pump for inflation/deflation of the endoscope and overtube balloons. (*B*) Complete device with the endoscope (Fujinon FC450-B15C) and the dedicated overtube. (*C*) Banding tip of the double-balloon colonoscope, compared with that of the double-balloon enteroscope.

also somewhat longer than that of the current therapeutic double-balloon enteroscopes, making examination of the mucosa behind haustrations and the passage of sharp angles easier.

In the initial report on this technique,[34] the authors had a success rate of 100% for cecal intubation in 29 patients and showed that therapeutic interventions such as electrocoagulation of angiomata and polypectomies were easily performed. The procedure was performed by two operators with the help of fluoroscopy to monitor the progression of the overtube at the beginning of our experience. More than 100 patients with a previously failed colonoscopy attempt because of fixed angles due to postsurgical adhesions or redundant colonic loops at the sigmoid or transverse levels have now been examined (**Fig. 5**). Overall, the authors have succeeded in intubating the cecum in 98% of the patients.[35] The cecum could not be reached in two patients with tortuous and dilated colons, due to adult Hirshprung disease in one case and to acromegaly in the other. The main reason why the double-balloon technique was not helpful in these cases was the widely dilated lumen in the transverse colon that prevented anchorage of the balloons and pleating of the intubated colon on the overtube. No complications were observed in our experience with the double-balloon colonoscope.

Another advantage of the double-balloon technique is that it simplifies the resection of large polyps. The balloon of the overtube helps to stabilize the tip of the endoscope

Table 1
Technical characteristics of available double-balloon endoscopes

	Double-balloon Colonoscope	Double-balloon Enteroscope	
	FC450-B15C	**EN450-P5**	**EN450-T5**
Total length of the shaft (cm)	182	230	230
Working length of the shaft (cm)	152	200	200
External diameter of the shaft (mm)	9.4	8.5	9.4
Working channel (mm)	2.8	2.2	2.8
Deflection angle up-down (degrees)	180	180	180
Deflection angle left-right (degrees)	160	160	160
Depth of the view field (mm)	3–100	5–100	4–100
View angle (degrees)	140	120	140
Length of the overtube (cm)	105	135	135
External diameter of the overtube (mm)	13.2	12.2	13.2

during these often long procedures. Moreover, multiple polyps or piecemeal resections can easily be recovered by leaving the overtube in place and withdrawing and reinserting the scope.[29]

Double-balloon colonoscopy can also be used for colonoscopy performed without sedation, because of better tolerance by the patient, since the progression of the

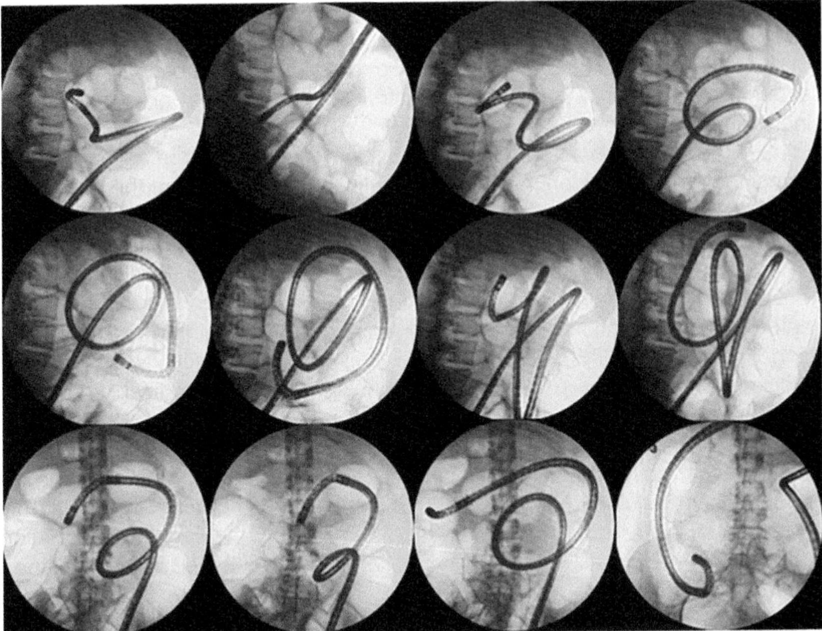

Fig. 5. Radiograph sequence showing the progression of the double-balloon colonoscope with overtube in a patient with fixed angles at the level of the sigmoid and transverse colons.

endoscope occurs while the overtube maintains the colon in a natural shape, avoiding excessive stretching of the mesentery.

SUMMARY

The diagnostic range and the clinical usefulness of DBE is clearly expanding as indications become more numerous, benefiting from the increased interest in small intestinal diseases that has been fostered by the development of several new imaging modalities over the last decade. The combined use of CE and DBE seems to be the most effective approach: CE may direct the route of insertion for targeted DBE procedures;[5] CE can be used as first-line examination in critically ill patients but, on the other hand, DBE is preferred in patients with a suspicion of intestinal stenosis suspected on a CT or MRI scan or after a patency capsule has been retained in the small intestine;[36] DBE has sampling and therapeutic possibilities that complement the diagnostic range of CE. Finally, CE, because it is well tolerated, can easily be repeated during the follow-up of patients with chronic diseases, limiting the number of invasive procedures.

Double-balloon endoscopy seems to be a major advance in the investigation of patients in whom the insertion of conventional endoscopes may be difficult or limited because of surgical modification. Finally, completion of colonoscopy in patients in whom conventional colonoscopy has failed is likely to be a major application for DBE.

REFERENCES

1. Yamamoto H, Sekine Y, Sato Y, et al. Total enteroscopy with a non-surgical steerable double-balloon method. Gastrointest Endosc 2001;53:216–20.
2. Yamamoto H. Clinical outcomes of double-balloon endoscopy for the diagnosis and treatment of small intestinal diseases. Clin Gastroenterol Hepatol 2004;2:1010–6.
3. May A, Nachbar L, Wardak A, et al. Double-balloon enteroscopy: preliminary experience in patients with obscure gastrointestinal bleeding or chronic abdominal pain. Endoscopy 2003;35:985–91.
4. Ell C, May A, Nachbar L, et al. Push-and-pull enteroscopy in the small bowel using the double-balloon technique: results of a prospective European multicenter study. Endoscopy 2005;37:613–6.
5. Gay G, Delvaux M, Fassler I. Outcome of capsule endoscopy in determining indication and route for push-and-pull enteroscopy. Endoscopy 2006;38:49–58.
6. Di Caro S, May A, Heine DG, et al. The European experience with double balloon enteroscopy: indications, methodology, safety and clinical impact. Gastrointest Endosc 2005;62:545–50.
7. Mönkemûller K, Weigt J, Treiber G, et al. Diagnostic and therapeutic impact of double balloon enteroscopy. Endoscopy 2006;38:67–72.
8. Malik A, Lukaszewki K, Caroline D, et al. A retrospective review of enteroclysis in patients with obscure gastrointestinal bleeding and chronic abdominal pain of undetermined etiology. Dig Dis Sci 2005;50:649–55.
9. Rajesh A, Sandrasegaran K, Jennings SG, et al. Comparison of capsule endoscopy with enteroclysis in the investigation of small bowel diseases. Abdom Imaging, in press.
10. Bardan E, Nadler M, Chowers Y, et al. Capsule endoscopy for the evaluation of patients with chronic abdominal pain. Endoscopy 2003;35:688–9.
11. Spada C, Pirozzi GA, Riccioni ME, et al. Capsule endoscopy in patients with chronic abdominal pain. Dig Liver Dis 2006;38:696–8.

12. May A, Manner H, Schneider A, et al. Prospective multicenter trial of capsule endoscopy in patients with chronic abdominal pain, diarrhea and other signs and symptoms. Endoscopy 2007;39:606–12.
13. Torres HA, Kontoyiannis DP, Bodey GP, et al. Gastrointestinal cytomegalovirus disease in patients with cancer: a two decade experience in a tertiary care cancer center. Eur J Cancer 2005;41:2268–79.
14. Stack E, Washington K, Avant GR, et al. Cytomegalovirus enteritis in common variable immunodeficiency. South Med J 2004;97:96–101.
15. Yakoub-Agha I, Maunoury V, Wacrenier A, et al. Impact of small bowel exploration using video-capsule endoscopy in the management of acute gastrointestinal graft-versus-host disease. Transplantation 2004;78:1697–701.
16. Neumann S, Schoppmeyer K, Lange T, et al. Wireless capsule endoscopy for diagnosis of acute intestinal graft-versus-host disease. Gastrointest Endosc 2007;65:403–9.
17. Gay G, Roche JF, Laurent V, et al. Manifestations digestives des maladies systémiques. Médicine Thérapeutique 2007;13:171–85.
18. Hamdulay SS, Cheent K, Ghosh C, et al. Wireless capsule endoscopy in the investigation of intestinal Behçet's syndrome. Rheumatology (Oxford) 2008;47:1231–4.
19. Ersoy O, Harmanci O, Aydinli M, et al. Capability of capsule endoscopy in detecting small bowel ulcers. Dig Dis Sci 2009;54:136–41.
20. Bua J, Lepore L, Martelossi S, et al. Video capsule endoscopy and intestinal involvement in systemic vasculitis. Dig Liver Dis 2008;40:905.
21. Preud'Homme DL, Michail S, Hodges C, et al. Use of wireless capsule endoscopy in the management of severe Henoch-Schonlein purpura. Pediatrics 2006;118:e904–6.
22. Sánchez R, Aparicio JR, Baeza T, et al. Capsule endoscopy diagnosis of intestinal involvement in a patient with Churg-Strauss syndrome. Gastrointest Endosc 2006;63:1082–4.
23. Stancanelli B, Vita A, Vinci M, et al. Bleeding of small bowel in Henoch-Schönlein syndrome: the successful diagnostic role of video capsule endoscopy. Am J Med 2006;119:82–4.
24. Pennazio M. Small-intestinal pathology on capsule endoscopy: spectrum of vascular lesions. Endoscopy 2005;37:864–9.
25. Matsui N, Akahoshi K, Motomura Y, et al. Endosonographic detection of dumbbell-shaped jejunal GIST using double balloon enteroscopy. Endoscopy 2008; 40(Suppl 2):E38–9.
26. Fukumoto A, Manabe N, Tanaka S, et al. Usefulness of EUS with double-balloon enteroscopy for diagnosis of small-bowel diseases. Gastrointest Endosc 2007; 65:412–20.
27. Wang TD, Friedland S, Sahbaie P, et al. Functional imaging of colonic mucosa with a fibered confocal microscope for realtime in vivo pathology. Clin Gastroenterol Hepatol 2007;5:1300–5.
28. Monkemuller K, Neumann H, Fry LC. Endoscopic examination of the small bowel from standard white light to confocal endomicroscopy. Clin Gastroenterol Hepatol 2009;7:e11–2.
29. Kita H, Yamamoto H. New indications of double balloon endoscopy. Gastrointest Endosc 2007;66(3 Suppl):S57–9.
30. Das A. Future perspective of double balloon enteroscopy: newer indications. Gastrointest Endosc 2007;66:S51–3.
31. May A, Nachbar L, Ell C. Push-and-pull enteroscopy using a single-balloon technique for difficult colonoscopy. Endoscopy 2006;38:395–8.

32. Mönkemüller K, Knippig C, Rickes S, et al. Usefulness of the double-balloon enteroscope in colonoscopies performed in patients with previously failed colonoscopy. Scand J Gastroenterol 2007;42:277–8.
33. Pasha SF, Harrison ME, Das A, et al. Utility of double-balloon colonoscopy for completion of colon examination after incomplete colonoscopy with conventional colonoscope. Gastrointest Endosc 2007;65:848–53.
34. Gay G, Delvaux M. Double-balloon colonoscopy after failed conventional colonoscopy: a pilot series with a new instrument. Endoscopy 2007;39:788–92.
35. Gay G, Delvaux M, Frederic M, et al. Double balloon colonoscopy: first experience with a dedicated endoscope-overtube system in patients with previous difficult and incomplete colonoscopy [abstract]. Gastrointest Endosc 2009;69:AB288.
36. Delvaux M, Ben Soussan E, Laurent V, et al. Clinical evaluation of the use of the M2A patency capsule system before a capsule endoscopy procedure, in patients with known or suspected intestinal stenosis. Endoscopy 2005;37:801–7.

Index

Note: Page numbers of article titles are in **boldface** type.

Gastrointest Endoscopy Clin N Am 19 (2009) 519–526
doi:10.1016/S1052-5157(09)00086-5
1052-5157/09/$ – see front matter

© 2009 Elsevier Inc. All rights reserved.
giendo.theclinics.com

D

T

U

V

Moving?

Make sure your subscription moves with you!

To notify us of your new address, find your **Clinics Account Number** (located on your mailing label above your name), and contact customer service at:

Email: journalscustomerservice-usa@elsevier.com

800-654-2452 (subscribers in the U.S. & Canada)
314-447-8871 (subscribers outside of the U.S. & Canada)

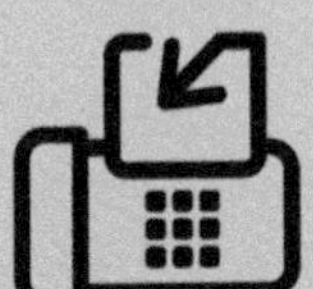

Fax number: 314-447-8029

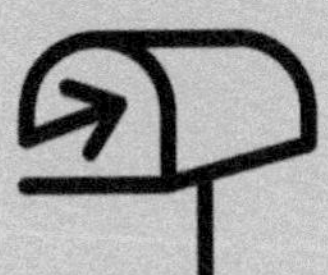

Elsevier Health Sciences Division
Subscription Customer Service
3251 Riverport Lane
Maryland Heights, MO 63043

*To ensure uninterrupted delivery of your subscription, please notify us at least 4 weeks in advance of move.

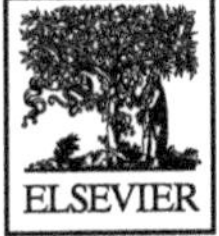

Printed and bound by CPI Group (UK) Ltd, Croydon, CR0 4YY

03/10/2024

01040453-0003